DELIVERING HIGH-QUALITY CANCER CARE

Charting a New Course for a System in Crisis

Committee on Improving the Quality of Cancer Care:
Addressing the Challenges of an Aging Population

Board on Health Care Services

Laura A. Levit, Erin P. Balogh, Sharyl J. Nass, and
Patricia A. Ganz, *Editors*

INSTITUTE OF MEDICINE
OF THE NATIONAL ACADEMIES

THE NATIONAL ACADEMIES PRESS
Washington, D.C.
www.nap.edu

THE NATIONAL ACADEMIES PRESS   500 Fifth Street, NW   Washington, DC 20001

NOTICE: The project that is the subject of this report was approved by the Governing Board of the National Research Council, whose members are drawn from the councils of the National Academy of Sciences, the National Academy of Engineering, and the Institute of Medicine. The members of the committee responsible for the report were chosen for their special competences and with regard for appropriate balance.

This study was supported by Contract Nos. HHSN261200900003C and 200-2011-38807, TO #13 between the National Academy of Sciences and the National Cancer Institute and the Centers for Disease Control and Prevention respectively. This study was also supported by AARP; the American Cancer Society; the American College of Surgeons, Commission on Cancer; the American Society for Radiation Oncology; the American Society of Clinical Oncology; the American Society of Hematology; the California HealthCare Foundation; LIVE**STRONG**; the National Coalition for Cancer Survivorship; the Oncology Nursing Society; and Susan G. Komen for the Cure. Any opinions, findings, conclusions, or recommendations expressed in this publication are those of the author(s) and do not necessarily reflect the view of the organizations or agencies that provided support for this project.

International Standard Book Number-13:   978-0-309-28660-2
International Standard Book Number-10:   0-309-28660-3

Additional copies of this report are available from the National Academies Press, 500 Fifth Street, NW, Keck 360, Washington, DC 20001; (800) 624-6242 or (202) 334-3313; http://www.nap.edu.

For more information about the Institute of Medicine, visit the IOM home page at: **www.iom.edu.**

Printed in the United States of America

The serpent has been a symbol of long life, healing, and knowledge among almost all cultures and religions since the beginning of recorded history. The serpent adopted as a logotype by the Institute of Medicine is a relief carving from ancient Greece, now held by the Staatliche Museen in Berlin.

Cover credit: Original oil painting, "Day 15 Hope," reproduced by permission from Sally Loughridge, *Rad Art: A Journey Through Radiation Treatment* (Atlanta: American Cancer Society, 2012), 31.

Suggested citation: IOM (Institute of Medicine). 2013. *Delivering high-quality cancer care: Charting a new course for a system in crisis.* Washington, DC: The National Academies Press.

"Knowing is not enough; we must apply.
Willing is not enough; we must do."
—Goethe

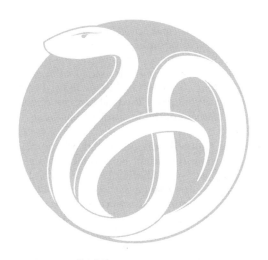

INSTITUTE OF MEDICINE
OF THE NATIONAL ACADEMIES

Advising the Nation. Improving Health.

THE NATIONAL ACADEMIES
Advisers to the Nation on Science, Engineering, and Medicine

The **National Academy of Sciences** is a private, nonprofit, self-perpetuating society of distinguished scholars engaged in scientific and engineering research, dedicated to the furtherance of science and technology and to their use for the general welfare. Upon the authority of the charter granted to it by the Congress in 1863, the Academy has a mandate that requires it to advise the federal government on scientific and technical matters. Dr. Ralph J. Cicerone is president of the National Academy of Sciences.

The **National Academy of Engineering** was established in 1964, under the charter of the National Academy of Sciences, as a parallel organization of outstanding engineers. It is autonomous in its administration and in the selection of its members, sharing with the National Academy of Sciences the responsibility for advising the federal government. The National Academy of Engineering also sponsors engineering programs aimed at meeting national needs, encourages education and research, and recognizes the superior achievements of engineers. Dr. C. D. Mote, Jr., is president of the National Academy of Engineering.

The **Institute of Medicine** was established in 1970 by the National Academy of Sciences to secure the services of eminent members of appropriate professions in the examination of policy matters pertaining to the health of the public. The Institute acts under the responsibility given to the National Academy of Sciences by its congressional charter to be an adviser to the federal government and, upon its own initiative, to identify issues of medical care, research, and education. Dr. Harvey V. Fineberg is president of the Institute of Medicine.

The **National Research Council** was organized by the National Academy of Sciences in 1916 to associate the broad community of science and technology with the Academy's purposes of furthering knowledge and advising the federal government. Functioning in accordance with general policies determined by the Academy, the Council has become the principal operating agency of both the National Academy of Sciences and the National Academy of Engineering in providing services to the government, the public, and the scientific and engineering communities. The Council is administered jointly by both Academies and the Institute of Medicine. Dr. Ralph J. Cicerone and Dr. C. D. Mote, Jr., are chair and vice chair, respectively, of the National Research Council.

www.national-academies.org

YA-CHEN TINA SHIH, Associate Professor, Section of Hospital Medicine, Department of Medicine, Pritzker School of Medicine and Director, the Economics of Cancer Program, The University of Chicago

GEORGE W. SLEDGE, JR., Chief of Oncology and Professor of Medicine, Stanford University School of Medicine

THOMAS J. SMITH, Director of Palliative Medicine and the Harry J. Duffey Family Professor of Palliative Medicine and Professor of Oncology, Johns Hopkins School of Medicine

NEIL S. WENGER, Professor, Division of General Internal Medicine and Health Services Research, University of California, Los Angeles, School of Medicine

Study Staff

LAURA LEVIT, Study Director
ERIN BALOGH, Associate Program Officer
PAMELA LIGHTER, Research Assistant
MICHAEL PARK, Senior Program Assistant
PATRICK BURKE, Financial Associate
SHARYL NASS, Director, National Cancer Policy Forum
ROGER HERDMAN, Director, Board on Health Care Services

Consultants

DANIEL MASYS, Affiliate Professor, Biomedical and Health Informatics, University of Washington

TRACY SPINKS, Project Director, The University of Texas MD Anderson Cancer Center

VICKIE WILLIAMS, Project Coordinator, Young Breast Cancer Survivorship Program, University of California, Los Angeles-LIVE**STRONG** Survivorship Center of Excellence, Jonsson Comprehensive Cancer Center

Reviewers

This report has been reviewed in draft form by individuals chosen for their diverse perspectives and technical expertise, in accordance with procedures approved by the National Research Council's Report Review Committee. The purpose of this independent review is to provide candid and critical comments that will assist the institution in making its published report as sound as possible and to ensure that the report meets institutional standards for objectivity, evidence, and responsiveness to the study charge. The review comments and draft manuscript remain confidential to protect the integrity of the deliberative process. We wish to thank the following individuals for their review of this report:

ROBERT M. ARNOLD, University of Pittsburgh Medical Center

EDWARD J. BENZ, JR., Harvard Medical School and Dana-Farber Cancer Institute

AMY BERMAN, John A. Hartford Foundation

CATHY BRADLEY, Virginia Commonwealth University

DEBORAH BRUNER, Emory University

KAREN S. COOK, Stanford University

DEBRA GORDON, University of Washington School of Medicine

DEBRA J. HOLDEN, RTI International

J. RUSSELL HOVERMAN, The U.S. Oncology Network and Texas Oncology

CARLOS ROBERTO JAÉN, University of Texas Health Science Center at San Antonio

KENNETH W. KIZER, University of California, Davis, Health System
RUTH McCORKLE, Yale University School of Nursing
DIANE E. MEIER, Mount Sinai School of Medicine
LEE N. NEWCOMER, UnitedHealthcare
DAVID B. REUBEN, University of California, Los Angeles
LAWRENCE N. SHULMAN, Dana-Farber Cancer Institute
EDWARD H. WAGNER, Group Health Research Institute

Although the reviewers listed above have provided many constructive comments and suggestions, they were not asked to endorse the conclusions or recommendations nor did they see the final draft of the report before its release. The review of this report was overseen by **HAROLD C. SOX,** Dartmouth Institute for Health Policy and Clinical Practice, and **PATRICIA FLATLEY BRENNAN,** University of Wisconsin–Madison. Appointed by the National Research Council and Institute of Medicine, they were responsible for making certain that an independent examination of this report was carried out in accordance with institutional procedures and that all review comments were carefully considered. Responsibility for the final content of this report rests entirely with the authoring committee and the institution.

Acknowledgments

T he committee and staff are indebted to a number of individuals and organizations for their contributions to this report. The following individuals conducted background research for the committee:

Lindsay Forbes, *Intern, Institute of Medicine (Summer 2011)*
Randy Gale, *Fellow, Institute of Medicine (2010-2011)*
Ana Hincapie, *Mirzayan Science and Technology Fellow, Institute of Medicine (Winter 2012)*
Cher Huang, *Intern, MIT in Washington Program (Summer 2013)*
Adam Schickedanz, *Intern, Institute of Medicine (Summer 2012)*

We extend thanks to Eric Slade and Eric Slade Productions for working with the committee to produce the dissemination video for this report. We also extend special thanks to the following individuals who were essential sources of information, generously giving their time and knowledge to further the committee's efforts.

Peter Bach, *Attending Physician, Memorial Sloan-Kettering Cancer Center*
Dikla Benzeevi, *11-Year Metastatic Breast Cancer Survivor, Breast Cancer Patient Advocate*
Amy Berman, *Senior Program Officer, Hartford Foundation*
Helen Burstin, *Senior Vice President for Performance Measures, National Quality Forum*

Eric Fennel, *Senior Advisor of Policy and Programs, Center for Medicare and Medicaid Innovation*

John Frenzel, *Chief Medical Information Officer, University of Texas MD Anderson Cancer Center*

Kristen McNiff, *Director, Quality and Performance Measurement, American Society of Clinical Oncology*

Mark Miller, *Executive Director, Medicare Payment Advisory Commission*

Stephen Palmer, *Director, Office of e-Health Coordination, Texas Health and Human Services Commission*

Maddie Peterson, *Cancer Survivor*

Willie C. Roberson, *Clergyman/Pastor, Saint's Home Church of God in Christ*

Joesph V. Simone, *President, Simone Consulting*

Ron Walters, *Associate Vice President of Medical Operations and Informatics, The University of Texas MD Anderson Cancer Center*

Peter Yu, *Chair, Health Information Technology Work Group, American Society of Clinical Oncology*

In addition, we thank the individuals who spoke at the October 2012 National Cancer Policy Forum workshop *Delivering Affordable Cancer Care in the 21st Century*. Workshop presentations and discussions informed committee deliberations. Speakers included

Denise R. Aberle, *Professor of Radiology and Bioengineering, David Geffen School of Medicine, University of California, Los Angeles*

Amy P. Abernethy, *Associate Professor, Duke University School of Medicine*

Peter B. Bach, *Attending Physician, Memorial Sloan-Kettering Cancer Center*

Justin E. Bekelman, *Assistant Professor of Radiation Oncology, Member, Abramson Cancer Center*

Otis W. Brawley, *Chief Medical Officer, American Cancer Society*

Renzo Canetta, *Vice President, Oncology Global Clinical Research, Bristol-Myers Squibb Company*

Susan Dentzer, *Editor-in-Chief*, Health Affairs

Craig Earle, *Medical Oncologist, Odette Cancer Centre*

Peter D. Eisenberg, *Medical Director, Marin Specialty Care*

Ezekiel J. Emanuel, *Diane v.S. Levy & Robert M. Levy University Professor, Perelman School of Medicine, University of Pennsylvania*

Robert L. Erwin, *President, Marti Nelson Cancer Foundation*

Harvey V. Fineberg, *President, Institute of Medicine*

James S. Goodwin, *George and Cynthia Mitchell Distinguished Chair in Geriatric Medicine, University of Texas Medical Branch*
Robert J. Green, *Medical Oncologist and Chief Medical Officer, Cancer Clinics of Excellence*
Jessie Gruman, *President, Center for Advancing Health*
Jim C. Hu, *Henry E. Singleton Chair in Urology, University of California, Los Angeles*
Thomas J. Kean, *President and Chief Executive Officer, C-Change*
Barnett S. Kramer, *Director, Division of Cancer Prevention, National Cancer Institute*
Allen S. Lichter, *Chief Executive Officer, American Society of Clinical Oncology*
Mark B. McClellan, *Senior Fellow, The Brookings Institution*
John Mendelsohn, *Co-Director, Khalifa Institute for Personalized Cancer Therapy, The University of Texas MD Anderson Cancer Center*
Therese M. Mulvey, *Physician-in-Chief, Southcoast Centers for Cancer Care*
Lee N. Newcomer, *Senior Vice President, Oncology UnitedHealthcare*
Jeffrey Peppercorn, *Associate Professor of Medicine, Duke University Medical Center*
Scott Ramsey, *Full Member, Cancer Prevention Program, Fred Hutchinson Cancer Research Center*
Lowell E. Schnipper, *Theodore W. & Evelyn G. Berenson Professor, Harvard Medical School*
Joanne Schottinger, *Clinical Lead, Cancer, Kaiser Permanente Care Management Institute*
Deborah Schrag, *Associate Professor of Medicine, Harvard Medical School*
Veena Shankaran, *Assistant Professor of Medical Oncology, University of Washington School of Medicine*
Jennifer Temel, *Associate Professor of Medicine, Harvard Medical School*
Robin Yabroff, *Epidemiologist, National Cancer Institute*

Funding for this study was provided by AARP; the American Cancer Society; the American College of Surgeons, Commission on Cancer; the American Society for Radiation Oncology; the American Society of Clinical Oncology; the American Society of Hematology; the California HealthCare Foundation; Centers for Disease Control and Prevention; LIVE**STRONG**; the National Cancer Institute; the National Coalition for Cancer Survivorship; the Oncology Nursing Society; and Susan G. Komen for the Cure. The committee appreciates the opportunity and support extended by these sponsors for the development of this report.

Finally, many within the Institute of Medicine were helpful to the study staff. We would like to thank Clyde Behney, Marton Cavani, Laura DeStefano, Chelsea Frakes, Jim Jensen, Jillian Laffrey, Tracy Lustig, Abbey Meltzer, Lauren Tobias, and Jennifer Walsh.

Preface

A cancer diagnosis is one of the most feared events. Rarely diagnosed before the late 20th century, cancer now competes with cardiovascular disease as the leading cause of death in North America. With people living longer, the continued use of tobacco products, infectious diseases that transmit cancer-causing viruses and other pathogens, and an obesity epidemic, the cancer burden is projected to increase substantially in the United States over the coming decades. Almost 14 million people, more than 4 percent of the U.S. population, are cancer survivors; by 2012 this will grow to 18 million cancer survivors. Survivors have complex journeys, and even after completing cancer treatment, must engage in medical follow-up care to help manage the long-term and late effects of their treatments, and monitor the possibility of cancer recurrence or development of new secondary cancers.

For the 1.6 million people in the United States who join the ranks of newly diagnosed cancer patients each year, the cancer care system can be overwhelming. The complexity of the cancer care system is driven by the biology of cancer itself, the multiple specialists involved in the delivery of cancer care, as well as a health care system that is fragmented and often ill prepared to meet the individual needs, preferences, and values of patients who are anxious, symptomatic, and uncertain about where to obtain the correct diagnosis, prognosis, and treatment recommendations. Moreover, older individuals comprise the majority of people with cancer. Addressing the unique needs of an aging population of patients diagnosed with cancer, who are already experiencing comorbid conditions and loss of independence, is a critical challenge. We are not prepared to take care of this growing cancer patient population, as few of our standard treatment approaches have been evaluated in this setting. Instead, we extrapolate from trial results and toxicities that emerge from treating younger and healthier patients with the same diagnoses. On top of this, the quality of cancer care varies tremendously.

As someone who has been an oncology practitioner for almost 40 years, I have seen dramatic changes in the treatment of cancer that have benefited my patients—greater precision in diagnosis, surgical treatments that are less radical and disfiguring, diagnoses of earlier stage disease as a result of screening, and more long-term disease-free survivors. However, the human and economic costs of these advances are enormous. Cancer patients often endure protracted periods of primary and adjuvant therapies, multimodal treatments with substantial toxicities and comorbidities, which may take years of physical and psychological recovery, with great financial hardship and social disruption. Palliative care and hospice services are underutilized and usually employed much later in the course of a patient's cancer journey than recommended. Patients and their families often play the role of principal communicator as they visit one cancer treatment specialist after another, conveying the recommendations to subsequent consultants in a serial fashion. Coordination of complex cancer care, using a common electronic health record, with treating specialists who jointly discuss the patient's case and then confer with the patient about their recommendations, is the exception and not the rule. Receipt of psychosocial support at the time of diagnosis and during treatment is also rare, as these "high-touch" services are seldom compensated through health insurance and are usually supported through ad hoc philanthropic funding rather than institutional or clinical practice resources.

We all want the best care for our family members and friends, but our current cancer care delivery system falls short in terms of consistency in the delivery of care that is patient centered, evidence based, and coordinated. We are at an inflection point in terms of repairing the cancer care delivery system. If we ignore the signs of crisis around us, we will be forced to deal with an increasingly chaotic and costly care system, with exacerbation of existing disparities in the quality of cancer care.

How can we change this situation? This report is the result of the thoughtful deliberations of our study committee, as well as the hard work of the Institute of Medicine (IOM) staff who supported our quest for the evidence behind the report's ten recommendations. Those recommendations are based on a unifying conceptual framework for improving the quality of cancer care. This report also rests on the foundation of the transformative 1999 IOM report *Ensuring Quality Cancer Care*, which called for improvements in the technical quality of cancer care, the use of evidence-based guidelines to direct care, the use of electronic data capture and quality monitoring, as well as the assurance of access to cancer care for all, including high-quality end-of-life care. While that report generated much attention in the oncology community, and drove some concerted action among oncology professional organizations and the federal government, a critical review of progress since the report's recommendations were issued identified many continuing gaps and new challenges that could not have been anticipated. Sadly, the key recommendations regarding implementation of evidence-based care and quality monitoring have had limited uptake, and are needed even more today due to the expansion in cancer diagnostics, imaging, and therapeutics in the past decade, as well as the expected growth in the number of new cancer patients. The cost of cancer care is rising much faster than for other diseases, and there are few systematic efforts or incentives to eliminate waste and the use of ineffective therapies.

Facing this crisis, the committee's vision for tackling these challenges and creating a high-quality cancer care delivery system is based on the IOM's extensive work defining the quality of health care, with its patient-centered focus and emphasis on the needs, values, and preferences of patients, including advance care planning. Patient-centered care is at the core of a high-quality cancer care delivery system, as depicted by the study committee's conceptual framework, and is something that is feasible in every clinical care setting, and can be supported by existing information technology if necessary (e.g., guidelines, evidence syntheses, pathways). Patient-clinician communication that focuses on information sharing about the diagnosis, prognosis, and treatment options, and that elicits the patient's preferences for treatment is central to high-quality cancer care. Surrounding the patient and their family caregivers are members of a well-prepared cancer care delivery team that is able to ensure coordinated and comprehensive patient-centered care and close collaboration with other health care professionals not directly involved in cancer care delivery, such as geriatric specialists and primary care clinicians. Because evidence-based care is also at the heart of a high-quality cancer care delivery system, research must fill important gaps in our knowledge, especially pertaining to how best to treat older cancer patients and others who have multiple comorbid conditions in addition to cancer. Further, clinical trials and comparative effectiveness research must include data collection that reflects patient-reported outcomes, as well as information about other relevant patient characteristics and behaviors, to provide accurate information that will inform future patients about what they can expect to experience from recommended cancer treatments.

A high-quality and efficient information technology infrastructure is critical to collecting these outcome data from ongoing clinical practice at the point of care, along with specific information about the cancer, its treatment, and the clinical outcomes of treatments received over time. That data collection system, as depicted in the conceptual framework, will be at the center of a rapid learning health care system which will, in turn, rely on regular assessments of the quality of care delivered in relationship to the costs of the associated care. Understanding how well we are doing with individual cancer patients, as well as groups of similar patients, could allow us to develop strategies for performance improvement and identify gaps in care that need our attention. Finally, in the high-quality cancer care delivery system of the future, payment models and financial incentives must focus on improving the affordability and quality of care for patients and payers. Eliminating disparities in access to high-quality cancer care for all members of our society remains a challenge; however, without relevant patient-centered information and quality measurement, we will not be able to create a more equitable system.

Although the committee's conceptual framework may seem far removed from much current oncology practice, the committee believes that most elements of the framework are in place or are being developed. In many ways, oncology care is an extreme example of the best and worst in the health care system today—highly innovative targeted diagnostics and therapeutics alongside escalating costs that do not consistently relate to the clinical value of treatments, tremendous waste and inefficiencies due to poor coordination of care, and lack of adherence to evidence-based guidelines with frequent use of ineffective or inappropriate treatments.

In the setting of this crisis, there are many opportunities. If we can use this framework to successfully address the challenges to delivering high-quality oncology care, the same principles will be transferrable to other complex and chronic conditions that place continued demands on the health care system. In my closing years as an oncology professional, I dream of a cancer care delivery system that will ensure access to high-quality, patient-centered, evidence-based care, and that patients with cancer will have care teams supported by a system that enables them to provide compassionate and timely care.

It has been my privilege to serve as the chair of this study committee and to learn so much from the other committee members who worked extremely hard and collaboratively to refine the recommendations and evidence that we present in this report. As someone who was a reviewer of the 1999 IOM report, I feel that I have come full circle in helping to lead the efforts of this committee. I am sure that a decade from now, someone else will be reviewing these recommendations and they will either be commenting about how foolish we were or complimenting us on our vision and prescience. I hope the latter is the case and that this report will chart a new course for the cancer care delivery system that ensures high-quality, evidence-based care for all.

Patricia A. Ganz, *Chair*
Committee on Improving the Quality of Cancer Care:
Addressing the Challenges of an Aging Population

Contents

APPENDIXES

Boxes, Figures, and Tables

BOXES

FIGURES

Acronyms

AACN	American Association of Colleges of Nursing
AAMC	Association of American Medical Colleges
ABIM	American Board of Internal Medicine
ACA	Patient Protection and Affordable Care Act
ACO	accountable care organization
ACoS	American College of Surgeons
ACOVE	Assessing Care of Vulnerable Elders
ACS	American Cancer Society
ADLs	activities of daily living
AHRQ	Agency for Healthcare Research and Quality
ALK	anaplastic lymphoma kinase
AML	acute myeloid leukemia
APRN	advanced practice registered nurse
ASCO	American Society for Clinical Oncology
ASP	average sales price
ASTRO	American Society for Radiation Oncology
AWP	average wholesale price
BPCA	Best Pharmaceuticals for Children Act
CBO	Congressional Budget Office
CDC	Centers for Disease Control and Prevention
CDRP	Cancer Disparities Research Partnership
CED	coverage with evidence development
CER	comparative effectiveness research

CMOH   Consultants in Medical Oncology and Hematology
CMS   Centers for Medicare & Medicaid Services
CoC   Commission on Cancer
COI   conflict of interest
COME HOME   Community Oncology Medical Homes
CPG   clinical practice guideline
CPR   cardiopulmonary resuscitation
CRCHD   Center to Reduce Cancer Health Disparities
CT   computed tomography
CTCAE   Common Terminology Criteria for Adverse Events

DCPC   Division of Cancer Prevention and Control
DNP   doctorate of nursing practice

ECHO   Extension for Community Healthcare Outcomes
EGFR   epidermal growth factor receptor
EHB   essential health benefit
EHR   electronic health record
ER   estrogen receptor

FDA   Food and Drug Administration
FMAP   Federal Medical Assistance Percentages
FPL   federal poverty level

GAO   Government Accountability Office
GDG   guideline development group
GDP   gross domestic product
GME   graduate medical education

HER   human epidermal growth factor receptor-2
HHS   U.S. Department of Health and Human Services
HIPAA   Health Insurance Portability and Accountability Act
HITECH   Health Information Technology for Economic and
              Clinical Health
HRSA   Health Resources and Services Administration

IADLs   instrumental activities of daily living
IMRT   intensity-modulated radiotherapy
IOM   Institute of Medicine
IRB   institutional review board
IT   information technology

MAP	Measures Applications Partnership
MB-CCOP	Minority-Based Community Clinical Oncology Programs
MedPAC	Medicare Payment Advisory Commission
MMA	Medicare Prescription Drug, Improvement, and Modernization Act
NCCN	National Comprehensive Cancer Network
NCCS	National Coalition for Cancer Survivorship
NCDB	National Cancer Data Base
NCI	National Cancer Institute
NCPF	National Cancer Policy Forum
NCTN	National Clinical Trials Network
NIA	National Institute on Aging
NIH	National Institutes of Health
NPP	National Priorities Partnership
NQF	National Quality Forum
NQMC	National Quality Measures Clearinghouse
NSQIP	National Surgical Quality Performance Improvement Program
ONC	Office of the National Coordinator for Health Information Technology
PA	physician assistant
PACT	Planning Actively for Cancer Treatment [Act of 2013]
PCMH	patient-centered medical home
PCORI	Patient-Centered Outcomes Research Institute
PCPI	Physician Consortium for Performance Improvement
PET	positron emission tomography
PPS	prospective payment system
PREA	Pediatric Research Equity Act
PRO	patient-reported outcome
PROMIS	Patient-Reported Outcome Measurement Information System
QOPI	Quality Oncology Practice Initiative
RCT	randomized controlled trial
RN	registered nurse

SEER	Surveillance, Epidemiology, and End Results
SES	socioeconomic status
SR	systematic review
USPSTF	U.S. Preventive Services Task Force
VA	U.S. Department of Veterans Affairs
VBID	value-based insurance design
VBP	value-based purchasing

Summary[1]

In the United States, approximately 14 million people are cancer survivors and more than 1.6 million people are newly diagnosed with cancer each year. By 2022, it is projected that there will be 18 million cancer survivors and, by 2030, 2.3 million people are expected to be newly diagnosed with cancer each year. However, more than a decade after the Institute of Medicine (IOM) first addressed the quality of cancer care in the United States, the barriers to achieving excellent care for all cancer patients remain daunting. The growing demand for cancer care, combined with the complexity of the disease and its treatment, a shrinking workforce, and rising costs, constitute a crisis in cancer care delivery (see Box S-1).

The complexity of cancer impedes the ability of clinicians, patients, and their families to formulate plans of care with the necessary speed, precision, and quality. As a result, decisions about cancer care are often not evidence-based. Many patients also do not receive adequate explanation of their treatment goals, and when a phase of treatment concludes, they frequently do not know what treatments they have received or the consequences of their treatments for their future health. In addition, many patients do not receive palliative care to manage their symptoms and side effects from treatment. Most often this occurs because the clinician lacks knowledge of how to provide this care (or how to make referrals to pal-

---

[1] This summary does not include references. Citations for the findings presented in the summary appear in the subsequent chapters.

BOX S-1
The Crisis in Cancer Care Delivery

Studies indicate that cancer care is often not as patient-centered, accessible, coordinated, or evidence-based as it could be, detrimentally impacting patients. The following trends amplify the problem:

- The number of older adults is expected to double between 2010 and 2030, contributing to a 30 percent increase in the number of cancer survivors from 2012 to 2022 and a 45 percent increase in cancer incidence by 2030.
- Workforce shortages among many of the professionals involved in providing care to cancer patients are growing, and training programs lack the ability to rapidly expand. The care that is provided is often fragmented and poorly coordinated. In addition, family caregivers and direct care workers are administering a substantial amount of care with limited training and support.
- The cost of cancer care is rising faster than are other sectors of medicine, having increased from $72 billion in 2004 to $125 billion in 2010; costs are expected to increase another 39 percent to $173 billion by 2020.
- Advances in understanding the biology of cancer have increased the amount of information a clinician must master to treat cancer appropriately.
- The few tools currently available for improving the quality of cancer care— quality metrics, clinical practice guidelines, and information technology—are not widely used and all have serious limitations.

---

liative care consultants) or does not identify palliative care management as an important component of high-quality cancer care.

Complicating the situation further are the changing demographics in the United States that will place new demands on the cancer care delivery system, with the number of adults older than 65 rapidly increasing. The population of those 65 years and older comprises the majority of patients who are diagnosed with cancer and who die from cancer, as well as the majority of cancer survivors. The oncology workforce may soon be too small to care for the growing population of individuals diagnosed with cancer. Meanwhile, the Centers for Medicare & Medicaid Services (CMS), the single largest insurer for this population, is struggling financially. In addition, the costs of cancer treatments are escalating unsustainably, making cancer care less affordable for patients and their families and creating disparities in patients' access to high-quality cancer care.

To address the increasing challenges clinicians face in trying to deliver high-quality cancer care, this report charts a new course for cancer care. There is great need for high-quality, evidence-based strategies to guide cancer care and ensure efficient and effective use of scarce resources. Responding to these new and continuing challenges, this IOM report updates the 1999 report and revisits the need to improve the quality of cancer care.

The IOM appointed an independent committee of experts with a broad range of expertise, including patient care and cancer research, patient advocacy, health economics, ethics, and health law. The committee was charged with examining challenges to and opportunities for the delivery of high-quality cancer care and formulating recommendations for improvement. The committee's recommendations aim to ensure the delivery of high-quality cancer care across the care continuum, from diagnosis through end of life. Prevention, risk reduction, and screening were not addressed by the committee. Another way to conceptualize the period of the cancer care continuum that this report addresses is through the three overlapping phases of cancer care: (1) the acute phase, (2) the chronic phase, and (3) the end-of-life phase (see Figure S-1).

Cancer care for older adults, as noted throughout this report, is especially complex. Age is one of the strongest risk factors for cancer, and there are many important considerations to understanding the prognoses of older adults with cancer and formulating their care plans, such as altered physiology, functional and cognitive impairment, multiple coexisting morbidities, increased side effects of treatment, distinct goals of care, and the increased need for social support. The current health care delivery system is poorly prepared to address these concerns comprehensively. Thus, meeting the needs of the aging population will be an integral part of improving the quality of cancer care.

CONCEPTUAL FRAMEWORK

The committee's conceptual framework for improving the quality of cancer care takes into account the heterogeneity of clinical settings where cancer care is delivered as well as the existing models of high-quality care. The central goal of its conceptual framework is delivering comprehensive, patient-centered, evidence-based, high-quality cancer care that is accessible and affordable to the entire U.S. population, regardless of the setting where cancer care is provided. The committee identified six components of a high-quality cancer care delivery system that will be integral to this transformation:

1. Engaged patients: A system that supports all patients in making informed medical decisions consistent with their needs, values, and preferences in consultation with their clinicians who have

4

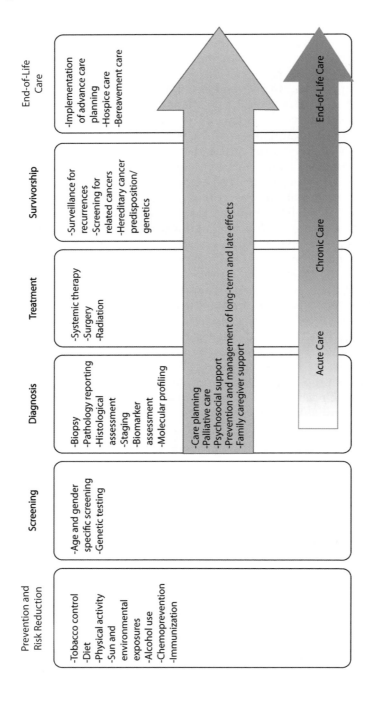

FIGURE S-1 Domains of the cancer care continuum with examples of activities in each domain. The blue arrow identifies components of high-quality cancer care that should span the cancer care continuum from diagnosis through end-of-life care. The green arrow identifies three overlapping phases of cancer care, which is a way of conceptualizing the period of the cancer care continuum that is the focus of this report.

expertise in patient-centered communication and shared decision making (see Chapter 3).

2. An adequately staffed, trained, and coordinated workforce: A system that provides competent, trusted, interprofessional cancer care teams that are aligned with patients' needs, values, and preferences, as well as coordinated with the patients' noncancer care teams and their caregivers (see Chapter 4).

3. Evidence-based cancer care: A system that uses scientific research, such as clinical trials and comparative effectiveness research (CER), to inform medical decisions (see Chapter 5).

4. A learning health care information technology (IT) system for cancer: A system that uses advances in IT to enhance the quality and delivery of cancer care, patient outcomes, innovative research, quality measurement, and performance improvement (see Chapter 6).

5. Translation of evidence into clinical practice, quality measurement, and performance improvement: A system that rapidly and efficiently incorporates new medical knowledge into clinical practice guidelines; measures and assesses progress in improving the delivery of cancer care and publicly reports performance information; and develops innovative strategies for further improvement (see Chapter 7).

6. Accessible, affordable cancer care: A system that is accessible to all patients and uses new payment models to align reimbursement to reward care teams for providing patient-centered, high-quality care and eliminating wasteful interventions (see Chapter 8).

Figure S-2 illustrates the interconnectivity of the committee's six components for a high-quality cancer delivery system.

Prioritization

The committee recognizes that improving the quality of the cancer care delivery system will take substantial time and effort to achieve and that implementation will require efforts by all stakeholders in the cancer care community. The committee numbered its six components for high-quality cancer care in order of priority for implementation, taking into account both the need and the feasibility of achieving each component of the framework. Thus, achieving a system that supports patient decision making is the top priority, followed by an adequately staffed, trained, and coordinated workforce, evidence-based cancer care, a learning health care IT system, the translation of evidence into practice, measurement of outcomes and performance improvement, and, finally, accessible and af-

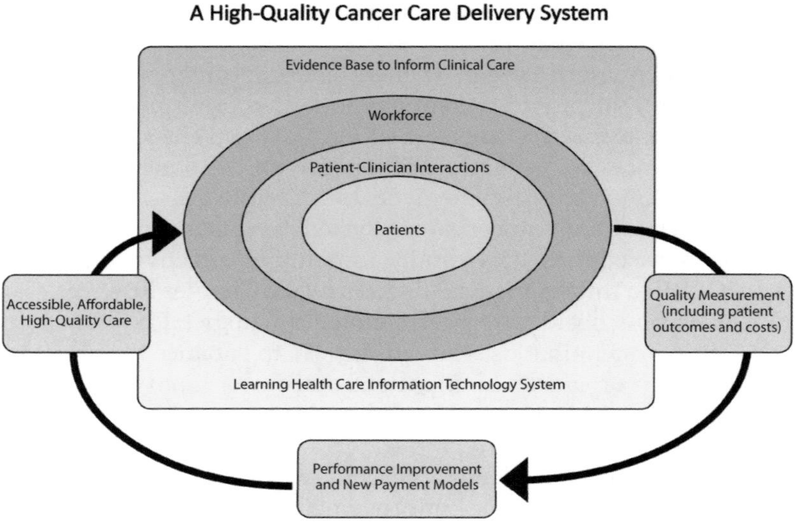

A High-Quality Cancer Care Delivery System

FIGURE S-2 An illustration of the committee's conceptual framework for improving the quality of cancer care.

fordable cancer care. The top priorities for implementation are depicted within the rectangle in Figure S-2, with the most important component in the center (i.e., patients). The committee recognizes the importance of access and affordability in a high-quality cancer care delivery system but expects the Patient Protection and Affordable Care Act (ACA) to make substantial changes in these areas of health care. Because much of the law has not yet been implemented, these issues will need to be revisited once the law's full impact is known.

Approach to Implementation

The committee utilizes a variety of approaches in its recommendations to improve the quality of cancer care. In many circumstances, the recommendations provide specific direction to individual stakeholders. However, fully achieving the goals of the committee's framework will also necessitate collaboration among relevant stakeholders to define the best path to implementation. Although there are numerous challenges to such collaboration, examples of ongoing collaborations among diverse stakeholders in the cancer community already exist and there may be greater incentives for such coordinated efforts in the current environment. For example, the ACA is focusing national attention and resources on improving the coordination and quality of the U.S. health care system. Many stakeholders are already making changes in response to health care reform and the committee's framework provides guidance on this process. In addition, the current financial situation in the United States is placing pressure on the health care delivery system to develop actionable solutions for eliminating waste in care while maintaining or improving quality. Again, the committee's conceptual framework charts a new course for achieving this task.

RECOMMENDATIONS

The committee structured its recommendations for action around the six components outlined in its conceptual framework. Each component is discussed briefly below and elaborated on in more detail in the respective chapters. Box S-2 provides an overview of the committee's recommendations.

BOX S-2
Goals of the Recommendations

1. Provide patients and their families with understandable information about cancer prognosis, treatment benefits and harms, palliative care, psychosocial support, and costs.
2. Provide patients with end-of-life care that meets their needs, values, and preferences.
3. Ensure coordinated and comprehensive patient-centered care.
4. Ensure that all individuals caring for cancer patients have appropriate core competencies.
5. Expand the breadth of data collected in cancer research for older adults and patients with multiple comorbid conditions.
6. Expand the depth of data collected in cancer research through a common set of data elements that capture patient-reported outcomes, relevant patient characteristics, and health behaviors.
7. Develop a learning health care information technology system for cancer that enables real-time analysis of data from cancer patients in a variety of care settings.
8. Develop a national quality reporting program for cancer care as part of a learning health care system.
9. Implement a national strategy to reduce disparities in access to cancer care for underserved populations by leveraging community interventions.
10. Improve the affordability of cancer care by leveraging existing efforts to reform payment and eliminate waste.

Patient-Centered Communication and Shared Decision Making

Patients are at the center of the committee's conceptual framework (see Figure S-2), which conveys the most important goal of a high-quality cancer care delivery system: meeting the needs of patients with cancer and their families. Such a system should support all patients in making informed medical decisions that are consistent with their needs, values, and preferences. In the current system, information to help patients understand their cancer prognoses, treatment benefits and harms, palliative care, psychosocial support, and costs of care is often unavailable or not regularly communicated. Additionally, patient-clinician communication and shared decision making is often less than optimal, impeding the delivery of patient-centered, high-quality cancer care. For example, several recent studies found that approximately 65 to 80 percent of cancer patients with poor prognoses incorrectly believed their treatments could result in a cure.

Recommendation 1: Engaged Patients

Goal: The cancer care team should provide patients and their families with understandable information on cancer prognosis, treatment benefits and harms, palliative care, psychosocial support, and estimates of the total and out-of-pocket costs of cancer care.

To accomplish this:

- The National Cancer Institute, the Centers for Medicare & Medicaid Services, the Patient-Centered Outcomes Research Institute, as well as patient advocacy organizations, professional organizations, and other public and private stakeholders should improve the development of this information and decision aids and make them available through print, electronic, and social media.
- Professional educational programs for members of the cancer care team should provide comprehensive and formal training in communication.
- The cancer care team should communicate and personalize this information for their patients at key decision points along the continuum of cancer care, using decision aids when available.
- The cancer care team should collaborate with their patients to develop a care plan that reflects their patients' needs, values, and preferences, and considers palliative care needs and psychosocial support across the cancer care continuum.

- The Centers for Medicare & Medicaid Services and other payers should design, implement, and evaluate innovative payment models that incentivize the cancer care team to discuss this information with their patients and document their discussions in each patient's care plan.

Patients with advanced cancer[2] face specific communication and decision-making needs. Clinicians should discuss these patients' options, such as implementing advance care plans, emphasizing palliative care and psychosocial support, and maximizing quality of life by timely use of hospice care. These difficult conversations do not occur as frequently or as timely as they should, resulting in care that may not be aligned with patient preferences.

Recommendation 2: Engaged Patients

Goal: In the setting of advanced cancer, the cancer care team should provide patients with end-of-life care consistent with their needs, values, and preferences.

To accomplish this:

- Professional educational programs for members of the cancer care team should provide comprehensive and formal training in end-of-life communication.
- The cancer care team should revisit and implement their patients' advance care plans.
- The cancer care team should place a primary emphasis on providing cancer patients with palliative care, psychosocial support, and timely referral to hospice care for end-of-life care.
- The Centers for Medicare & Medicaid Services and other payers should design, implement, and evaluate innovative payment models that incentivize the cancer care team to counsel their patients about advance care planning and timely referral to hospice care for end-of-life care.

The Workforce Caring for Patients with Cancer

A diverse team of professionals provides cancer care, reflecting the complexity of the disease, its treatments, and survivorship care. These

---

[2] Cancer that has spread to other places in the body and usually cannot be cured or controlled with treatment.

teams include professionals with specialized training in oncology, such as medical, surgical, and radiation oncologists and oncology nurses, as well as other specialists and primary care clinicians. In addition, family caregivers (e.g., relatives, friends, and neighbors) and direct care workers (e.g., nurse aides, home health aides, and personal and home care aides) provide a great deal of care to cancer patients. Patients, at the center of the committee's conceptual framework, are encircled by the workforce (see Figure S-2), depicting the idea that high-quality cancer care depends on the workforce providing competent, trusted interprofessional care that is aligned with patients' needs, values, and preferences. To achieve this standard, the workforce must include adequate numbers of health care clinicians with training in oncology. New models of interprofessional, team-based care are an effective mechanism of responding to the existing workforce shortages and demographic changes, as well as in promoting coordinated and patient-centered care.

Recommendation 3: An Adequately Staffed, Trained, and Coordinated Workforce

Goal: Members of the cancer care team should coordinate with each other and with primary/geriatrics and specialist care teams to implement patients' care plans and deliver comprehensive, efficient, and patient-centered care.

To accomplish this:

- **Federal and state legislative and regulatory bodies should eliminate reimbursement and scope-of-practice barriers to team-based care.**
- **Academic institutions and professional societies should develop interprofessional education programs to train the workforce in team-based cancer care and promote coordination with primary/geriatrics and specialist care teams.**
- **Congress should fund the National Workforce Commission, which should take into account the aging population, the increasing incidence of cancer, and the complexity of cancer care, when planning for national workforce needs.**

The workforce must also have the distinct set of skills necessary to implement the committee's conceptual framework for a high-quality cancer care delivery system. The recent IOM report *Retooling for an Aging America: Building the Health Care Workforce* recommended enhancing the geriatric competency of the general health care workforce. The committee endorses this recommendation as it is especially important to cancer care, where the majority of patients are older adults. Currently, many clinicians also lack essential cancer core competencies.[3]

Recommendation 4: An Adequately Staffed, Trained, and Coordinated Workforce

Goal: All individuals caring for cancer patients should have appropriate core competencies.

To accomplish this:

- Professional organizations that represent clinicians who care for patients with cancer should define cancer core competencies for their memberships.
- Cancer care delivery organizations should require that the members of the cancer care team have the necessary competencies to deliver high-quality cancer care, as demonstrated through training, certification, or credentials.
- Organizations responsible for accreditation, certification, and training of nononcology clinicians should promote the development of relevant core competencies across the cancer care continuum.
- The U.S. Department of Health and Human Services and other funders should fund demonstration projects to train family caregivers and direct care workers in relevant core competencies related to caring for cancer patients.

The Evidence Base for High-Quality Cancer Care

Because a high-quality cancer care delivery system uses results from scientific research, such as clinical trials and CER, to inform medical decisions, the committee's conceptual framework (see Figure S-2) depicts the evidence base as supporting patient-clinician interactions. The committee envisions clinical research that gathers evidence of the benefits and harms of various treatment options, so that patients, in consultation with their clinicians, can make treatment decisions that are consistent with their needs, values, and preferences.

Currently, many medical decisions are not supported by sufficient evidence. Additionally, research participants are often not representative of the population with the disease, which makes it difficult to generalize

---

[3] The tasks or functions that providers of health care should be able to do or perform.

the research results to a specific patient. Another limitation of the current evidence base is that it frequently does not capture information about the impact of a treatment regimen on quality of life, functional and cognitive status, symptoms, and overall patient experience with the disease. Given that the majority of cancer patients are over 65 years and have comorbid conditions complicated by other health (e.g., physical and cognitive deficits) and social (e.g., limited or absent social support, low health literacy) risks, the committee is particularly concerned about the lack of clinical research focused on older adults and individuals with multiple chronic diseases.

Recommendation 5: Evidence-Based Cancer Care

Goal: Expand the breadth of data collected on cancer interventions for older adults and individuals with multiple comorbid conditions.

To accomplish this:

- **The National Cancer Institute, the Agency for Healthcare Research and Quality, the Patient-Centered Outcomes Research Institute, and other comparative effectiveness research funders should require researchers evaluating the role of standard and novel interventions and technologies used in cancer care to include a plan to study a population that mirrors the age distribution and health risk profile of patients with the disease.**
- **Congress should amend patent law to provide patent extensions of up to 6 months for companies that conduct clinical trials of new cancer treatments in older adults or patients with multiple comorbidities.**

Recommendation 6: Evidence-Based Cancer Care

Goal: Expand the depth of data available for assessing interventions.

To accomplish this:

- **The National Cancer Institute should build on ongoing efforts and work with other federal agencies, the Patient-Centered Outcomes Research Institute, clinical and health services researchers, clinicians, and patients to develop a common set of data elements that captures patient-reported outcomes, relevant patient characteristics, and health behaviors that researchers** should collect from randomized clinical trials and observational studies.

A Learning Health Care Information Technology System for Cancer

The committee's conceptual framework for a high-quality cancer care delivery system calls for implementation of a learning health care IT system: a system that "learns" by collecting data on care outcomes and cost in a systematic manner, analyzing the captured data both retrospectively and through prospective studies, implementing the knowledge gained from these analyses into clinical practice, evaluating the outcomes of the changes in care, and generating new hypotheses to test and implement into clinical care.

A learning health care IT system is a key requirement for implementing the components of the committee's conceptual framework for high-quality cancer care. In the committee's conceptual framework (see Figure S-2), a learning health care IT system supports patient-clinician interactions by providing patients and clinicians with the information and tools necessary to make well-informed medical decisions. It plays an integral role in developing the evidence base from research (e.g., clinical trials and CER) and by capturing data from real-world care settings that researchers can then analyze to generate new knowledge. Further, it is used to collect and report quality metrics data, implement performance improvement initiatives, and allow payers to identify and reward high-quality care.

Many of the elements needed to create a learning health care system are already in place for cancer, including electronic health records, cancer registries, a robust infrastructure for cancer clinical trials, and biorepositories that are linked with clinical data. Unfortunately, they are incompletely implemented, have functional deficiencies, and are not integrated in a way that creates a true learning health care system. In addition, relevant regulations that govern clinical care and research could pose a challenge to a learning health care system. The learning system will either need to comply with the relevant regulations or, alternatively, the regulations may need to be updated to accommodate such a system.

Recommendation 7: A Learning Health Care Information Technology System for Cancer

Goal: Develop an ethically sound learning health care information technology system for cancer that enables real-time analysis of data from cancer patients in a variety of care settings.

To accomplish this:

- Professional organizations should design and implement the digital infrastructure and analytics necessary to enable continuous learning in cancer care.
- The U.S. Department of Health and Human Services should support the development and integration of a learning health care information technology system for cancer.
- The Centers for Medicare & Medicaid Services and other payers should create incentives for clinicians to participate in this learning health care system for cancer, as it develops.

Translating Evidence into Practice, Measuring Quality, and Improving Performance

A high-quality cancer care delivery system should translate evidence into clinical practice, measure quality, and improve the performance of clinicians. This involves developing clinical practice guidelines (CPGs) to assist clinicians in quickly incorporating new medical knowledge into routine care. Also critical are measuring and assessing a system's progress in improving the delivery of cancer care, publicly reporting the information gathered, and developing innovative strategies to further performance improvement. In the figure illustrating the committee's conceptual framework (see Figure S-2), knowledge translation and performance improvement are part of a cyclical process that measures the outcomes of patient-clinician interactions and implements innovative strategies to improve the accessibility, affordability, and quality of care.

CPGs translate evidence into practice by synthesizing research findings into actionable steps clinicians can take when providing care. The development of CPGs is not straightforward or consistent because the evidence base supporting clinical decisions is often incomplete and includes studies and systematic reviews of variable quality. In addition, organizations that develop CPGs often use fragmented processes that lack transparency, and they are plagued by conflicts of interest. The committee endorses the standards in the IOM report *Clinical Practice Guidelines We Can Trust* to address these problems and produce trustworthy CPGs.

Performance improvement initiatives can also be used to translate evidence into practice. These tools have been described as systematic, data-guided activities designed to bring about immediate, positive change in the delivery of health care in a particular setting, as well as across settings. They can improve the efficiency, patient satisfaction, health outcomes, and costs of cancer care. These efforts are typically implemented in a single organization or health system; as a result, they often lack the pace, magnitude, coordination, and sustainability to transform health care delivery nationwide.

Cancer care quality measures provide a standardized and objective means for assessing the quality of cancer care delivered. Measuring performance has the potential to drive improvements in care, inform patients, and influence clinician behavior and reimbursement. There are currently serious deficiencies in cancer care quality measurement in the United States, including pervasive gaps in existing measures, challenges in the measure development process, lack of consumer engagement in measure development and reporting, and the need for data to support meaningful, timely, and actionable performance measurement. A number of groups representing clinicians who provide cancer care, including the American Society of Clinical Oncology and the American College of Surgeons' Commission on Cancer, have instituted voluntary reporting programs, through which program participants have demonstrated improvements. U.S. Department of Health and Human Services (HHS) has also attempted to influence quality measurement for cancer care through various mandatory reporting programs.

Recommendation 8: Quality Measurement

Goal: Develop a national quality reporting program for cancer care as part of a learning health care system.

To accomplish this, the U.S. Department of Health and Human Services should work with professional societies to:

- **Create and implement a formal long-term strategy for publicly reporting quality measures for cancer care that leverages existing efforts.**
- **Prioritize, fund, and direct the development of meaningful quality measures for cancer care with a focus on outcome measures and with performance targets for use in publicly reporting the performance of institutions, practices, and individual clinicians.**
- **Implement a coordinated, transparent reporting infrastructure that meets the needs of all stakeholders, including patients, and is integrated into a learning health care system.**

Accessible and Affordable Cancer Care

The committee's conceptual framework for a cancer care delivery system is one in which all people with cancer have access to high-quality, affordable cancer care. Several IOM reports have called on the U.S. government to ensure that all people have health insurance coverage. Expanding health insurance coverage is a primary goal of the ACA, which is expected to result in 25 million individuals gaining insurance coverage. However, much of the ACA has not yet been implemented and its full impact on access to cancer care is unknown. Many individuals will likely remain uninsured or underinsured. There are also major disparities in cancer outcomes among individuals who are of lower socioeconomic status, are racial or ethnic minorities, or lack insurance coverage. Many of these disparities are exacerbated by these individuals' lack of access to cancer care.

Recommendation 9: Accessible, Affordable Cancer Care

Goal: Reduce disparities in access to cancer care for vulnerable and underserved populations.

To accomplish this, the U.S. Department of Health and Human Services should:

- **Develop a national strategy that leverages existing efforts by public and private organizations.**
- **Support the development of innovative programs.**
- **Identify and disseminate effective community interventions.**
- **Provide ongoing support to successful existing community interventions.**

The affordability of cancer care is equally as important as accessibility in a high-quality cancer delivery care system. The committee's conceptual framework (see Figure S-2) illustrates the concept of using quality measurement and new payment models to reward the cancer care team for providing patient-centered, high-quality care and eliminating wasteful interventions. The current fee-for-service reimbursement system encourages a high volume of care, but it fails to reward the provision of high-quality care. This system is leading to higher cancer care costs, which are negatively impacting patients and their families. One survey found that more than one-third of personal bankruptcies in the United States are due to medical problems and that three out of four families studied had insurance at the onset of illness. From a system perspective, health care costs, including the costs of cancer care, are on an unsustainable trajectory and could pose serious fiscal consequences for the United States.

Payers are experimenting with numerous models that could be employed to reward clinicians for providing high-quality cancer care, such as rewarding care that is concordant with CPGs, coordinated, based on meaningful patient-clinician communication and shared decision making, and includes palliative care and psychosocial support throughout treatment, advance care planning, and timely referral to hospice care (e.g., bundled payments, accountable care organizations, oncology patient-centered medical homes, care pathways, coverage with evidence development, and value-based purchasing and competitive bidding programs). Clinicians are also undertaking efforts to discourage wasteful interventions, such as the Choosing Wisely Campaign.

Recommendation 10: Accessible, Affordable Cancer Care

Goal: Improve the affordability of cancer care by leveraging existing efforts to reform payment and eliminate waste.

To accomplish this:

- **Professional societies should identify and publicly disseminate evidence-based information about cancer care practices that are unnecessary or where the harm may outweigh the benefits.**
- **The Centers for Medicare & Medicaid Services and other payers should develop payment policies that reflect the evidence-based findings of the professional societies.**
- **The Centers for Medicare & Medicaid Services and other payers should design and evaluate new payment models that incentivize the cancer care team to provide care that is based on the best available evidence and aligns with their patients' needs, values, and preferences.**
- **If evaluations of specific payment models demonstrate increased quality and affordability, the Centers for Medicare & Medicaid Services and other payers should rapidly transition from traditional fee-for-service reimbursements to new payment models.**

CONCLUSIONS

This report outlines a conceptual framework to improve the quality of cancer care for patients. Changes across the board are urgently needed. All participants and stakeholders, including clinicians, patients and their families, researchers, quality metrics developers, and payers, as well as

HHS, other federal agencies, and industry, must reevaluate their current roles and responsibilities in cancer care and work together to develop a high-quality cancer care delivery system, starting with improving patient-clinician interactions. By working toward this shared goal, the cancer care community can improve the quality of life and outcomes for people facing a cancer a diagnosis.

1

Introduction

In the United States, approximately 14 million people are cancer survivors and more than 1.6 million people are newly diagnosed with cancer each year (ACS, 2013). By 2022, it is projected that there will be 18 million cancer survivors and, by 2030, 2.3 million people are expected to be newly diagnosed with cancer each year (ACS, 2013; Smith et al., 2009). However, more than a decade after the Institute of Medicine (IOM) first addressed the quality of cancer care in the United States (IOM and NRC, 1999), the barriers to achieving excellent care for all cancer patients remain daunting. The growing demand for cancer care, combined with the complexity of the disease and its treatment, a shrinking workforce, and rising costs, constitute a crisis in cancer care delivery (see Box 1-1).

The complexity of cancer impedes the ability of clinicians, patients, and their families to formulate plans of care with the necessary speed, precision, and quality. As a result, decisions about cancer care are often not evidence-based (IOM, 2008b, 2012). Many patients also do not receive adequate explanation of their treatment goals, and when a treatment phase concludes, they frequently do not know what treatments they have received or the consequences of their treatments for their future health (IOM, 2011b). In addition, many patients do not receive palliative care to manage their cancer symptoms and the side effects from treatment. Most often this occurs because the clinician lacks knowledge of how to provide this care (or how to make referrals to palliative care consultants) or does not identify palliative care management as an important component of high-quality cancer care.

Complicating the situation further are the changing demographics in

---

BOX 1-1
The Crisis in Cancer Care Delivery

Studies indicate that cancer care is often not as patient-centered, accessible, coordinated, or evidence-based as it could be, detrimentally impacting patients. The following trends amplify the problem:

- The number of older adults is expected to double between 2010 and 2030, contributing to a 31 percent increase in the number of cancer survivors from 2012 to 2022 and a 45 percent increase in cancer incidence by 2030.
- Workforce shortages among many of the professionals involved in providing care to cancer patients are growing and training programs lack the ability to rapidly expand. The care that is provided is often fragmented and poorly coordinated. In addition, family caregivers and direct care workers are administering a substantial amount of care with limited training and support.
- The cost of cancer care is rising faster than are other sectors of medicine, having increased from $72 billion in 2004 to $125 billion in 2010; costs are expected to increase another 39 percent to $173 billion by 2020.
- Advances in understanding the biology of cancer have increased the amount of information a clinician must master to treat cancer appropriately.
- The few tools currently available for improving the quality of cancer care— quality metrics, clinical practice guidelines, and information technology— are not as widely used as they could be and all have serious limitations.

SOURCES: de Moor et al., 2013; He et al., 2005; IOM, 2008c, 2009b, 2011a; Mariotto et al., 2011; NCI, 2007; NRC, 2009; Reinhard and Levine, 2012; Smith et al., 2009; Spinks et al., 2012.

---

the United States that will place new demands on the cancer care delivery system, with the number of adults older than 65 rapidly increasing (He et al., 2005; Smith et al., 2009). The population of those 65 years and older comprises the majority of patients who are diagnosed with cancer and die from cancer, as well as the majority of cancer survivors (NCI, 2012, 2013; NVSS, 2012). In addition, there is a major structural crisis looming in cancer care delivery: the oncology workforce may soon be too small to care for the growing population of individuals diagnosed with cancer (IOM, 2009b). Meanwhile, the Centers for Medicare & Medicaid Services (CMS), the single largest insurer for this older population, is struggling with financial solvency (Goldberg, 2013; Medicare Trustees, 2013). In addition, the costs of cancer treatments are escalating unsustainably, making cancer care less affordable for patients and their families, and creating disparities in patients' access to high-quality cancer care

(IOM, 2013; Kantarjian and experts in chronic myeloid leukemia, 2013; Stump et al., 2013; Sullivan et al., 2011).

To address the increasing challenges clinicians face in trying to deliver high-quality cancer care, this report charts a new course for cancer care. There is great need for high-quality, evidence-based strategies to guide cancer care and ensure efficient and effective use of scarce resources.

CHANGES IN CANCER CARE SINCE 1999

The IOM's National Cancer Policy Board first examined the quality of cancer care in the United States in 1999. The resulting report, *Ensuring Quality Cancer Care,* concluded that "for many Americans with cancer, there is a wide gulf between what could be construed as the ideal and the reality of their experience with cancer care" (IOM and NRC, 1999, p. 2). The report recommended steps to improve cancer care and the evidence base for cancer care, and to overcome barriers of access to high-quality cancer care.

These recommendations led to a number of efforts targeted at improving the delivery of cancer care. The Secretary of the U.S. Department of Health and Human Services (HHS) established the Quality of Cancer Care Committee to work on issues identified in the report. A number of organizations used the report to develop core indicators of quality of cancer care and recommendations for improving the quality of cancer care, including the Agency for Healthcare Research and Quality (AHRQ), the National Quality Forum (NQF), and the National Dialogue on Cancer (a collaboration organized by former President George H.W. Bush and Senator Dianne Feinstein, now known as C-Change). In response to the report, the American Society of Clinical Oncology (ASCO) undertook a national study of the quality of care delivered by oncologists, called the National Initiative on Quality Cancer Care (ASCO, 2013). In addition, the Cancer Quality Alliance, a diverse group of stakeholders committed to advocating for improvements in the quality of cancer care, used the 1999 IOM report and several other reports to develop five cancer case studies depicting a vision for high-quality cancer care and a blueprint for action (Rose et al., 2008). The report also provided major input for the quality of cancer care legislation drafted by the Senate Health, Education, Labor, and Pension Committee.[1]

Box 1-2 provides examples of the progress to date in implementing the IOM's 1999 recommendations and examples of the recommendations that are still relevant. However, cancer care has changed substantially since this report was released.

---

[1] Quality of Care for Individuals with Cancer Act. S. 2965. 107th Cong. (2d Sess. 2002).

BOX 1-2
Examples of Progress to Date in Implementing the
Institute of Medicine's 1999 Recommendations

Recommendation 1: Ensure patients undergoing procedures that are technically difficult to perform and have been associated with higher mortality in lower volume settings receive care at facilities with extensive experience.

Progress to date
- Mortality rates for select complex cancer operations declined after certain patients were redirected to high-volume cancer centers.
- Low-volume clinicians are participating in programs designed to improve the quality of their care.

Current gaps
- The capacity at high-volume centers is insufficient to provide care for all complex cancer cases.

Recommendation 2: Use systematically developed guidelines based on the best available evidence for prevention, diagnosis, treatment, and palliative care.

Progress to date
- The National Comprehensive Cancer Care Network, the American Society of Clinical Oncology, and the American Society of Radiation Oncology have worked with clinical experts to develop guidelines for more than 135 cancers or processes of care.

Current gaps
- Clinicians' adoption and reporting of adherence to these guidelines is voluntary and not widespread.
- Existing guidelines are not comprehensive and were often developed using consensus processes, not always meeting current standards.

Recommendation 3: Measure and monitor the quality of care using a core set of quality measures.

Progress to date
- A select number of cancer care measures have been developed and endorsed for use in quality reporting.
- These measures are largely process oriented.

Current gaps
- There is no nationally mandated program to which clinicians report data for core measures related to cancer.
- There are pervasive gaps in existing cancer measures.

Recommendation 4: Ensure the following elements of quality care for each individual with cancer:
- *Experienced professionals who make recommendations about initial cancer management, which are critical to determining long-term outcome*

- *An agreed-upon care plan that outlines goals of care*
- *Access to the full complement of resources necessary to implement the care plan*
- *Access to high-quality clinical trials*
- *Policies to ensure full disclosure of information about appropriate treatment options*
- *A mechanism to coordinate care*
- *Psychosocial support services and compassionate care*

Progress to date
- Many clinicians use multidisciplinary care planning to provide coordinated care to cancer patients.
- Medicare, several states, and new insurance plans included in Health Insurance Marketplaces created by the Patient Protection and Affordable Care Act (ACA) cover standard or routine costs of clinical trials.
- Patient-focused educational materials are available to clinicians when discussing appropriate treatment options with patients.

Current gaps
- Continuing geographic, financial, and social barriers prevent patients from seeking and receiving multidisciplinary care planning and comprehensive cancer care.
- Many cancer patients are not informed about their treatment options and their preferences are not elicited.
- Palliative care is not integrated with cancer care across the continuum from diagnosis to end of life.
- Many cancer patients receive inadequate psychosocial support.

Recommendation 5: Ensure quality of care at the end of life, particularly the management of cancer-related pain and timely referral to palliative and hospice care.

Progress to date
- Screening tools are available to monitor the frequency and severity of patients' symptoms and to guide patients to supportive and palliative care services.
- Most cancer centers in the United States have inpatient palliative care consult teams.

Current gaps
- Patients with advanced cancer frequently receive palliative care late in their disease course, which compromises quality of life and quality of care for them and their families.
- Patients with advanced cancer nearing the end of life are frequently referred to hospice only days to weeks before death, if at all, compromising quality of life and quality of care for them and their families.

continued

BOX 1-2 Continued

Recommendation 6: Federal and private research sponsors, such as the National Cancer Institute, the Agency for Health Care Policy and Research (now called the Agency for Healthcare Research and Quality), and various health plans, should invest in clinical trials to address questions about cancer care management.

Progress to date
  • This recommendation has not been implemented because of the current nature of clinical trials.
Current gaps
  • Cancer care management is addressed in Recommendation 8.

Recommendation 7: A cancer data system that can provide quality benchmarks for use by systems of care (e.g., hospitals, provider groups, and managed care systems) is needed.

Progress to date
  • Some large health care systems have implemented electronic health records (EHRs) that capture data fields relevant to cancer care.
Current gaps
  • There is no standardized system for all cancer care providers to report on quality benchmarks.
  • Current EHRs were not designed to collect and report quality metrics but rather as records of individual patient information.

Recommendation 8: Public and private sponsors of cancer care research should support national studies of recently diagnosed individuals with cancer, using information sources with sufficient detail to assess patterns of cancer care and factors associated with the receipt of good care; research sponsors should also support training for cancer care providers interested in health services research.

Progress to date
  • The American Recovery and Reinvestment Act, which directed $1.1 billion to comparative effectiveness research (CER), has accelerated CER activity.

Cancer care has always been highly complex, due to diagnostic challenges (imaging, pathology); multimodal, multispecialty treatment strategies (surgery, radiation, chemotherapy); a narrow therapeutic/toxic ratio for many treatments; and long-term and late effects of disease and treatment that contribute to morbidity and mortality (Zapka et al., 2012). Recent results from The Cancer Genome Atlas project (NCI, 2013a), which

- The Patient-Centered Outcomes Research Institute (PCORI) was created by the ACA.

Current gaps
  - CER for cancer is just beginning.
  - There are shortages of funding for and investigators trained in health services research.

Recommendation 9: Services for the un- and underinsured should be enhanced to ensure entry to, and equitable treatment within, the cancer care system.

Progress to date
  - State and federal programs are directing funds to screening for and early detection of cancer in underserved populations.
  - The ACA introduced new programs to improve access for many uninsured individuals.

Current gaps
  - The uninsured population continues to grow despite ongoing implementation of the ACA, and was exacerbated by the Great Recession.
  - Uninsurance is associated with poorer outcomes and lower survival rates.
  - Underinsurance is a growing problem with the increased cost of cancer treatments, including tiered copayments for expensive cancer therapies.

Recommendation 10: Studies are needed to examine why specific segments of the population (e.g., members of certain racial or ethnic groups, older patients) do not receive appropriate cancer care.

Progress to date
  - Programs have been introduced to increase the involvement of cancer centers designated by the National Cancer Institute in developing research, education, and outreach programs to reduce cancer health disparities.

Current gaps
  - There are ongoing disparities, including later stage diagnoses and poorer outcomes for racial and ethnic minorities with cancer.

SOURCE: Adapted from Spinks et al., 2012. Reprinted with permission from John Wiley and Sons.

has characterized hundreds of individual tumors originating from common cancer sites (e.g., breast, lung, prostate, ovary), using state-of-the-art genomic, molecular, and proteomic technologies, have provided startling information about the extreme heterogeneity of cancers that were once thought to have a more uniform biology (Hayano et al., 2013; Joung et al., 2013; Liang et al., 2012; Wang et al., 2013). Cancer treatments have evolved to reflect this new information on the nature of the disease, with more treatments targeting specific molecular aberrations.

Large randomized clinical trials of muli-agent chemotherapy, the standard at the time of the 1999 report on quality cancer care, have given way to smaller trials of targeted agents, in which companion diagnostic tests are often needed to assess whether the patient's tumor is likely to be susceptible to the planned treatment. Today, many patients need to be screened in order to identify patients whose tumors have the relevant mutations for trials that study new targeted treatments or combinations of treatments.

In addition, as noted above, there has been a major expansion in the number of individuals receiving treatment, and the population is older and more diverse than it was in 1999. Moreover, a number of recent federal laws, including the Patient Protection and Affordable Care Act of 2010 (ACA),[2] have changed the context in which cancer care is practiced. Thus, the factors creating an imperative for change in the cancer care system today are not the same as during the drafting of the 1999 report (see Chapter 2 for a detailed discussion of these trends).

COMMITTEE CHARGE

The charge to the committee was to revisit the quality of cancer care more than a decade after publication of the first IOM report, *Ensuring Quality Cancer Care* (1999). The committee examined what has changed, what challenges remain, whether new problems have arisen, and how health care reform might affect quality care, with a specific focus on the aging U.S. population (see Box 1-3). Although the committee was not asked to undertake an examination of the barriers to adoption of the previous 1999 recommendations, the committee invited Joe Simone, President, Simone Consulting, and chair of the 1999 study, to discuss the challenges associated with implementation of the earlier recommendations.

The IOM appointed an independent committee with a broad range of expertise, including patient care and cancer research, patient advocacy, health economics, ethics, and health law. Brief biographies of the 17 members of the Committee on Improving the Quality of Cancer Care: Addressing the Challenges of an Aging Population are presented in Appendix B. This report, which updates the 1999 report in response to the new and continuing challenges described above, presents the committee's findings and recommendations.

---

[2] Patient Protection and Affordable Care Act, Public Law 111-148, 111th Congress (March 23, 2010).

BOX 1-3
Charge to the Committee on Improving the
Quality of Cancer Care:
Addressing the Challenges of an Aging Population

An Institute of Medicine (IOM) committee will examine issues related to the quality of cancer care with a specific focus on the demographic changes that will rapidly accelerate the number of new cancer diagnoses at a time when workforce shortages are predicted. The study will consider quality of care from the perspectives of key stakeholders, including patients, health care providers, and payers. Using other foundational IOM reports as a starting point, the committee will examine opportunities for and challenges to the delivery of high-quality cancer care to an aging population and formulate recommendations for improvement. The committee will

- Review various aspects of quality cancer care, including the coordination and organization of care, outcomes reporting, quality metrics, and disparities in care;
- Consider the growing need for survivorship care, palliative care, and informal caregiving;
- Consider the increasing complexity and cost of cancer care, for example through incorporation of biomarkers to predict response to therapy;
- Consider potential opportunities to improve the quality of care by aligning incentives to promote more effective models of care delivery or through specific payment reforms; and
- Consider how patients can identify, find, and access high-quality cancer care.

SCOPE OF THE REPORT

This report presents a conceptual framework for improving the quality of cancer care. Two concepts important for understanding the scope of the report include (1) the continuum of cancer care and (2) the importance of addressing the unique needs of older adults with cancer.

The Continuum of Cancer Care

The committee's recommendations aim to ensure the delivery of high-quality cancer care across the care continuum from diagnosis and treatment to maintaining the health of survivors and providing end-of-life care consistent with patients' needs, values, and preferences. The provision of patient-centered care planning, palliative care, and psychosocial care; the prevention and management of long-term and late effects of cancer treatment; and family caregiver support should span the cancer care continuum from diagnosis through end-of-life care. The full cancer care continuum also includes the domains of prevention and risk reduction and screening; however, these domains are outside the scope of this report (see Figure 1-1). An opportunity to improve the quality of cancer care exists in each of the steps of care delivery, as well as in the transitions between the types of care (Zapka et al., 2003). Although the diagram is linear, a patient might enter the cancer care continuum at any of the stages and might not necessarily progress through each of the stages in sequence.

Another way to conceptualize the period of the cancer care continuum that is the focus of this report is through the three overlapping phases of cancer care: (1) the acute phase, (2) the chronic phase, and (3) the end-of-life phase. These phases correspond to the three phases commonly used in the NCI's studies on the cost of cancer care (i.e., the initial, continuing, and last year of life phases) (Brown et al., 2002; Yabroff et al., 2011). The relationship of the three phases to the overall cancer care continuum is depicted by the green arrow in Figure 1-1.

The acute phase of cancer care occurs immediately after a person is diagnosed with cancer, and generally includes surgical interventions and initial chemotherapy and radiation therapies, as well as palliative and psychosocial care as needed by the patient. Although acute care is often associated with hospitalization for complex conditions, newly diagnosed cancer patients will generally have minimal contact with the inpatient hospital setting. Even many surgical treatments for cancer require only short hospital stays. A large proportion of cancer care is delivered by individual medical oncology practices, where chemotherapy is administered and other treatments are coordinated with surgeons and radiation oncologists.

Cancer treatment and management follow the acute period of care. This period can be conceptualized as the chronic phase, similar to what might be applied to the management of diabetes or congestive heart failure. The goal of care is to provide patients with long-term surveillance for cancer recurrence and, in some patients, prolonged adjuvant or maintenance therapies (e.g., adjuvant endocrine therapy for breast cancer, daily oral tyrosine kinase treatment for chronic myelogenous leukemia). Patients can also receive palliative and psychosocial care during this phase to manage residual effects of the cancer and its treatment. This period can continue for months to years after the initial diagnosis. It includes both patients who are disease-free, as well as the growing number of cancer patients whose disease is controlled but not cured (as in chronic myelogenous leukemia). This phase usually includes multiple clinicians who may or may not be working in the same system of care. Coordination of care with primary care clinicians during this time is variable.

A substantial number of cancer patients will eventually experience

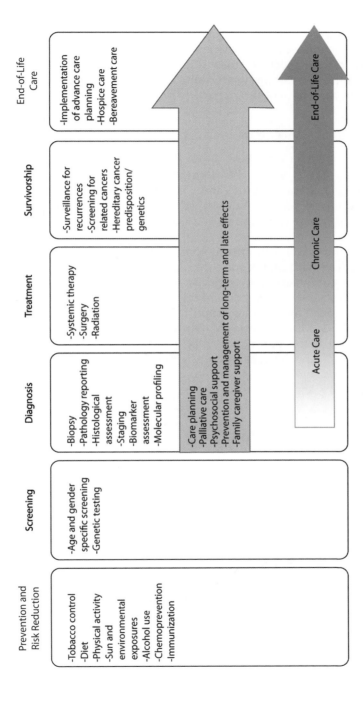

FIGURE 1-1 Domains of the cancer care continuum with examples of activities in each domain. The blue arrow identifies components of high-quality cancer care that should span the cancer care continuum from diagnosis through end-of-life care. The green arrow identifies three overlapping phases of cancer care, which are a way of conceptualizing the period of the cancer care continuum that is the focus of this report.

SOURCE: Adapted from National Cancer Institute figure on the "Cancer Control Continuum" (NCI, 2013b).

a cancer recurrence or progression of their disease. In addition, a minority of patients will have advanced, incurable disease from the time of diagnosis. When cancer-directed therapies are no longer beneficial for the patient, the primary focus of their care should be on palliative care, psychosocial support, and timely referral to hospice care. These patients are in the end-of-life phase of their care.

Cancer Care in Older Adults

Cancer care for older adults, as noted throughout this report, is especially complex. Age is one of the strongest risk factors for cancer. As mentioned above, the majority of cancer diagnoses and cancer deaths occur in individuals 65 years and older, and the majority of cancer survivors are in this age range (see Figures 1-2, 1-3, and 1-4) (NCI, 2012, 2013c; NVSS, 2012).

There are many important considerations to understanding the prognoses of older adults with cancer and formulating their care plans, such as altered physiology, functional and cognitive impairment, multiple coexisting morbidities, increased side effects of treatment, distinct goals of care, and the increased need for of social support. Their ability to participate in clinical trials has been limited, and thus the evidence base for informing treatment decisions in this population is lacking (Scher and Hurria, 2012). The current health care delivery system is poorly prepared to address

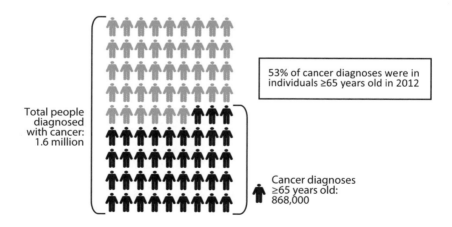

FIGURE 1-2 The majority of cancer diagnoses are in older adults.
SOURCE: NCI, 2012.

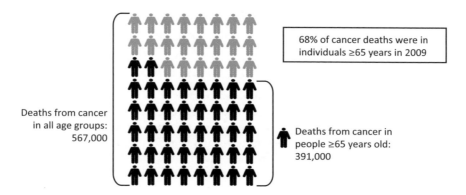

FIGURE 1-3 The majority of cancer deaths are in older adults.
SOURCE: NVSS, 2012.

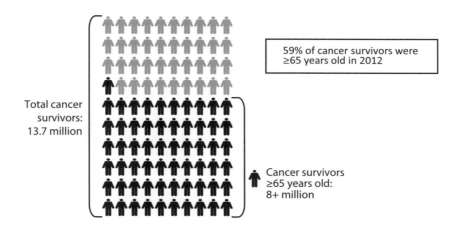

FIGURE 1-4 The majority of cancer survivors are older adults.
NOTE: The committee adopted the National Coalition for Cancer Survivorship's definition of a cancer survivor, which states that a survivor is any person who has been diagnosed with cancer, from the time of diagnosis through the balance of life (IOM and NRC, 2005).
SOURCE: NCI, 2013c.

these concerns comprehensively. Thus, meeting the needs of the aging population will be an integral part of improving the quality of cancer care.

DEFINING HIGH-QUALITY CARE

The various stakeholders involved in cancer care bring different perspectives on quality. Patients, for example, tend to evaluate care based on whether they receive the most effective and timely treatment for their particular ailment so that they may return to normal life as soon as possible. Health care clinicians, on the other hand, may focus on technical competence and how well care is executed. A health plan might evaluate quality based on efficiency and appropriate use of resources (IOM and NRC, 1999).

The IOM has a long history of analyzing the quality of care and recommending improvements to the health care delivery system. Since the 1999 report was released, the IOM has produced a number of foundational consensus studies addressing particular aspects of high-quality cancer care (e.g., *Interpreting the Volume-Outcome Relationship in the Context of Cancer Care* [IOM, 2001]; *From Cancer Patient to Cancer Survivor: Lost in Transition* [IOM and NRC, 2005]; *Cancer Care of the Whole Patient: Meeting Psychosocial Health Needs* [IOM, 2008a]) and health care generally (e.g., *Crossing the Quality Chasm: A New Health System for the 21st Century; Best Care at Lower Cost: The Path to Continuously Learning Health Care in America* [IOM, 2001, 2012]) as well as the impact of changing demographics on the health care workforce (*Retooling for an Aging America: Building the Health Care Workforce* [IOM, 2008c]). In addition, past workshops hosted by the IOM's National Cancer Policy Forum (NCPF) have addressed a number of issues relevant to improving the quality of cancer care, including the oncology workforce, survivorship care, informal caregiving, assessing value in cancer care, molecularly targeted therapies, treatment planning, a learning health care system for cancer, and the affordability of cancer care (IOM, 2007, 2009a,b, 2010a,b, 2011b, 2013). IOM forums convene workshops in which stakeholders examine policy issues, but they are not formulated to generate consensus recommendations.

The IOM has defined quality of care as "the degree to which health services for individuals and populations increase the likelihood of desired health outcomes and are consistent with current professional knowledge" (IOM, 1990, p. 21). In its 1999 report on ensuring the quality of cancer care, the IOM elaborated on this definition and defined poor quality as "overuse (e.g., unnecessary tests, medication, and procedures, with associated risks and side effects); underuse (e.g., not receiving lifesaving surgical procedures); or misuse (e.g., medicines that should not be given together, poor surgical technique)" (IOM and NRC, 1999, p. 79). The IOM defined good quality care as "providing patients with appropriate services in a technically competent manner, with good communication, shared decision making, and cultural sensitivity" (IOM and NRC, 1999, p. 79).

The 1999 report adopted Avedis Donabedian's approach to evaluating quality based on structure, process, and outcomes (Donabedian, 1980). Structural quality refers to the ability of a health care system to meet the needs of patients or communities; process quality refers to the technical skills of health care clinicians and their interactions with patients; and outcomes quality refers to changes in patients' health status (e.g., morbidity and mortality) (IOM and NRC, 1999).

The IOM's report *Crossing the Quality Chasm* furthered the conceptualization of high-quality care by identifying six aims for the 21st-century health care system. It stated that health care should be (1) safe—avoiding injuries to patients from the care that is intended to help them; (2) effective—providing services based on scientific knowledge to all who could benefit and refraining from providing services to those not likely to benefit; (3) patient-centered—providing care that is respectful of and responsive to individual preferences, needs, and values, and ensuring that patient values guide all clinical decisions; (4) timely—reducing waits and sometimes harmful delays for both those who receive and those who give care; (5) efficient—avoiding waste, including waste of equipment, supplies, ideas, and human resources; and (6) equitable—providing care that does not vary in quality because of personal characteristics, such as gender, ethnicity, geography, and socioeconomic status (IOM, 2001a).

More recently, a number of other groups have identified additional components of high-quality health care. For example, in commissioning a new facility for Walter Reed National Military Center, Congress mandated that an independent committee oversee the development of the design plans. This committee initiated its task by developing a definition of a world-class medical facility. It determined that these facilities should (1) be designed using evidence-based design principles that facilitate care processes; (2) employ a well-trained, competent, and compassionate workforce; (3) provide coordinated, evidence-based care; (4) meet all relevant quality metric benchmarks and reporting requirements; and (5) appoint pragmatic and visionary leaders (Kizer, 2010; NCR BRAC HSAS, 2009).

AHRQ's conceptualization of medical neighborhoods—which are oriented around patient-centered medical homes (PCMHs) and include all other clinicians involved in caring for patients, the community, and social services—also include key features of high-quality care. According to AHRQ, high-functioning medical neighborhoods (1) delineate the roles of the clinicians and institutions in the system; (2) share clinical information;

(3) develop individualized care plans for patients; (4) coordinate patients' transition between care settings; (5) focus on patient preferences; and (6) link clinical and nonclinical services (e.g., personal care services, home-delivered meals, or school-based health care). For patients with cancer, a medical neighborhood could be centered on the cancer care team rather than a primary care PCMH (Taylor et al., 2011). Both of these efforts represent high-level examinations of structural and operational aspects of high-quality health care delivery.

In recent years there have also been several efforts to define high-quality of care for specific aspects of cancer care delivery. The IOM's report *Cancer Care for the Whole Patient* concluded that "attending to psychosocial needs should be an integral part of quality cancer care" (IOM, 2008a, p. 8). Recently, Parry and colleagues (2013) developed a conceptual model for cancer survivorship care. Similar to the cancer care framework presented in this report, care planning and meeting the needs of patients and their families are at the center of their survivorship care framework. Their framework aims to use survivorship care plans to produce the short-term goals of improving patients' adherence to follow-up care; clinicians' management of long-term and late effects of treatment and comorbid conditions; and health care resources use, and the long-term goals of better health outcomes and lower costs.

Similarly, McCorkle and colleagues (2011) adapted the Chronic Care Model to cancer care because cancer patients increasingly need long-term surveillance and treatment. The primary features of this model are productive interactions between patients and their clinicians; enabled and empowered patients; proactive and prepared practice teams; a practice home for patients with cancer (i.e., a single clinical team that takes responsibility for meeting a patient's care needs across the continuum of care); and collaborative care plans.

CONCEPTUAL FRAMEWORK

The committee's conceptual framework for improving the quality of cancer care takes into account the heterogeneity of clinical settings where cancer care is delivered as well as the existing models of high-quality care summarized above. The central goal of its conceptual framework is to deliver patient-centered, evidence-based, high-quality cancer care that is accessible and affordable to the entire U.S. population regardless of the setting where cancer care is provided. The committee identified six components of a high-quality cancer care delivery system that will be integral to this transformation:

1. Engaged patients: A system that supports all patients in making informed medical decisions consistent with their needs, values, and preferences in consultation with clinicians who have expertise in patient-centered communication and shared decision making (see Chapter 3).

2. An adequately staffed, trained, and coordinated workforce: A system that provides competent, trusted, interprofessional cancer care teams that are aligned with patients' needs, values, and preferences, as well as coordinated with the patients' noncancer care teams and their caregivers (see Chapter 4).

3. Evidence-based cancer care: A system that uses scientific research, such as clinical trials and comparative effectiveness research (CER), to inform medical decisions (see Chapter 5).

4. A learning health care information technology (IT) system for cancer: A system that uses advances in IT to enhance the quality and delivery of cancer care, patient outcomes, innovative research, quality measurement, and performance improvement (see Chapter 6).

5. Translation of evidence into clinical practice, quality measurement, and performance improvement: A system that rapidly and efficiently incorporates new medical knowledge into clinical practice guidelines; measures and assesses progress in improving the delivery of cancer care and publicly reports performance information; and develops innovative strategies for further improvement (see Chapter 7).

6. Accessible, affordable cancer care: A system that is accessible to all patients and uses new payment models to align reimbursement to reward care teams for providing patient-centered, high-quality care and eliminating wasteful interventions (see Chapter 8).

Figure 1-5 illustrates the interconnectivity of the committee's six components for a high-quality cancer care delivery system. Patients are at the center of the committee's conceptual framework, recognizing that the system's most important goal is to meet the care needs of patients with cancer and their families, through patient-centered communication and shared decision making. The workforce encircles the patients, depicting the idea that high-quality cancer care depends on the workforce to provide competent, trusted, interprofessional care aligned with patients' needs, values, and preferences. The evidence base and a rapid learning IT system support patient-clinician interactions and provide patients and clinicians with the information and decision support necessary to make well-informed medical decisions. The arrows in the figure depict the cy-

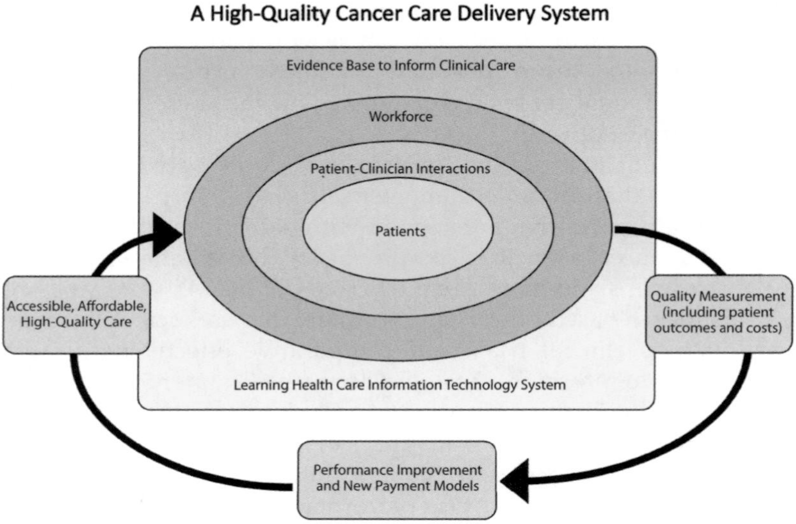

A High-Quality Cancer Care Delivery System

FIGURE 1-5 An illustration of the committee's conceptual framework for a high-quality cancer care delivery system.

clical process of measuring the outcomes of patient-clinician interactions and implementing innovative strategies and new payment models to improve the accessibility, affordability, and quality of care.

Prioritizing the Components of the Framework

The committee recognizes that improving the quality of cancer care will take substantial time and effort to achieve and implementation will require efforts by all stakeholders in the cancer care community. The committee numbered its six components for high-quality cancer care in order of priority for implementation, taking into account both the need and the feasibility of achieving each component of the framework. Thus, achieving a system that supports patient decision making is the top priority, followed by an adequately staffed, trained, and coordinated workforce, evidence-based cancer care, a learning health care IT system, the translation of evidence into practice, measurement of outcomes, and performance improvement, and, finally, accessible and affordable cancer care. The top priorities for implementation are depicted within the rectangle in Figure 1-5, with the most important component in the center (i.e., patients). The committee recognizes the importance of access and affordability in a high-quality cancer care delivery system but expects the

ACA to make substantial changes in these areas of health care. Because much of the law has not yet been implemented, these issues will need to be revisited once the law's full impact is known.

Approach to Implementing the Framework

The committee utilizes a variety of approaches in its recommendations to improve the quality of cancer care. In many circumstances, the recommendations provide specific direction to individual stakeholders. It directs recommendations to patients; members of the cancer care team (including both academic and community oncology clinicians, primary care clinicians, and other specialists); and health care delivery organizations that are directly involved in the provision of cancer care. It also targets the federal government, where appropriate, because the government is in a position to develop national strategies and to influence the policies that affect the behavior of those involved in the provision of cancer care. In addition, as the dominant health insurance provider for cancer patients and survivors, the federal government has a responsibility to assure that its payments for services meet quality standards and are not harmful to patients.

In many cases, change may start with individual organizations that undertake localized efforts or pilot projects to implement improvements in the cancer care delivery system. There are already many ongoing activities related to the committee's recommendations that would fall in this category. In some cases, fully achieving the goals of the committee's framework may also necessitate collaboration among relevant stakeholders to define the best path to implementation. Although there are numerous challenges to such collaboration, examples of ongoing collaborations among diverse stakeholders in the cancer community already exist, and there may be greater incentives for such coordinated efforts in the current environment. For example, the ACA is focusing national attention and resources on improving the coordination and quality of the U.S. health care system, such as promoting accountable care organizations and other innovative payment models that reward clinicians for working as a team and providing high-quality care. Many stakeholders are already making changes in response to health care reform, and the committee's framework provides guidance on this process. In addition, the current financial situation in the United States is placing pressure on the health care delivery system to develop actionable solutions for eliminating waste in care while also maintaining or improving quality. Again, the committee's conceptual framework charts a new course for achieving this task.

METHODS OF THE STUDY

The committee deliberated during four in-person meetings and numerous conference calls between May 2012 and April 2013. During its second meeting, the committee met in conjunction with the NCPF's workshop on *Delivering Affordable Cancer Care in the 21st Century*. The goals of the workshop included (1) summarizing current evidence on the overuse, underuse, and misuse of medical technology throughout the continuum of cancer care; (2) identifying modifiable problems in the cancer care delivery system and suggesting changes to address them; and (3) discussing policy issues related to the value, cost containment, and reimbursement of cancer care, as well as the economic incentives for innovation and technology diffusion in cancer care. As part of this study, the committee reviewed published literature, including the prior NCPF workshops and IOM consensus studies, and sought input from stakeholders in cancer care. The committee used the IOM's *Ensuring Quality Cancer Care* report (1999) as a foundation for examining challenges to and opportunities for the delivery of high-quality cancer care and formulating recommendations for improvement.

ORGANIZATION OF THE REPORT

The committee structured its report around the six components of its conceptual framework. This introductory chapter has described the background, charge to the committee, conceptual framework, and methods for the report. Chapter 2 provides additional background information on the current landscape and trends in cancer care. Chapters 3 through 8 elaborate on the committee's six components for a high-quality cancer care system and present the committee's recommendations for action.

Chapter 2: The Current Cancer Care Landscape: An Imperative for Change, focuses on demographic changes in the United States; trends in cancer diagnoses, cancer survivorship, cancer treatment, and cancer care costs; the unique needs of older adults with cancer; and policy initiatives that may impact cancer care. It also provides a summary of the key stakeholders involved in the cancer care delivery system.

Chapter 3: Patient-Centered Communication and Shared Decision Making, focuses on strategies and tools for improving patient-centered communication and shared decision making, as well as the unique communication and decision-making needs of patients with advanced cancers.

Chapter 4: The Workforce Caring for Patients with Cancer, focuses on ensuring that there is an adequate supply of clinicians to meet the rising demand for cancer care and that the workforce has the training and skills necessary to provide high-quality cancer care.

Chapter 5: The Evidence Base for High-Quality Cancer Care, focuses on improving the evidence base that supports cancer care decisions by improving the breadth and depth of data that are collected in clinical research and improving the use of IT to collect, organize, and assess data from various sources.

Chapter 6: A Learning Health Care Information Technology System for Cancer, focuses on using technological advancements to improve cancer care delivery, patient health, cancer research, quality measurement, performance improvement, and reimbursement for high-quality cancer care.

Chapter 7: Translating Evidence into Practice, Measuring Quality, and Improving Performance, focuses on translating evidence into practice through quality metrics, clinical practice guidelines, and performance improvement initiatives.

Chapter 8: Accessible and Affordable Cancer Care, focuses on access to cancer care and on the role of payers, clinicians, and patients in improving affordability and quality of cancer care.

REFERENCES

ACS (American Cancer Society). 2013. *Cancer facts and figures 2013.* http://www.cancer.org/acs/groups/content/@epidemiologysurveilance/documents/document/acspc-036845.pdf (accessed April 19, 2013).

ASCO (American Society of Clinical Oncology). 2013. *National Initiative on Cancer Care Quality (NICCQ).* http://www.asco.org/institute-quality/national-initiative-cancer-care-quality-niccq (accessed July 30, 2013).

Brown, M. L., G. F. Riley, N. Schussler, and R. Etzioni. 2002. Estimating health care costs related to cancer treatment from SEER-Medicare data. *Medical Care* 40(8 Suppl):IV-104-117.

de Moor, J. S., A. B. Mariotto, C. Parry, C. M. Alfano, L. Padgett, E. E. Kent, L. Forsythe, S. Scoppa, M. Hachey, and J. H. Rowland. 2013. Cancer survivors in the United States: Prevalence across the survivorship trajectory and implications for care. *Cancer Epidemiliogy, Biomarkers, & Prevention* 22(4):561-570.

Donabedian, A. 1980. Explorations in Quality Assessment and Monitoring. In *The definition of quality and approaches to its assessment.* Vol. 1. Ann Arbor, MI: Health Administration Press.

Goldberg, L. 2013. *The Medicare trustees report in perspective.* http://healthaffairs.org/blog/2013/06/07/the-medicare-trustees-report-in-perspective (accessed June 13, 2013).

Hayano, T., M. Garg, D. Yin, M. Sudo, N. Kawamata, S. Shi, W. Chien, L. W. Ding, G. Leong, S. Mori, D. Xie, P. Tan, and H. P. Koeffler. 2013. Sox7 is down-regulated in lung cancer. *Journal of Experimental Clinical Cancer Research* 32:17.

He, W., M. Sengupta, V. A. Velkoff, and K. A. DeBarros. 2005. *65+ in the United States: 2005.* http://www.census.gov/prod/2006pubs/p23-209.pdf (accessed May 3, 2012).

IOM (Institute of Medicine). 1990. *Medicare: A strategy for quality assurance.* 2 vols. Washington, DC: National Academy Press.

———. 2001a. *Crossing the quality chasm: A new health system for the 21st century.* Washington, DC: National Academy Press.

————. 2001b. *Interpreting the volume-outcome relationship in the context of cancer care.* Washington, DC: National Academy Press.

————. 2007. *Implementing cancer survivorship care planning.* Washington, DC: The National Academies Press.

————. 2008a. *Cancer care for the whole patient: Meeting psychosocial health needs.* Washington, DC: The National Academies Press.

————. 2008b. *Knowing what works in health care: A roadmap for the nation.* Washington, DC: The National Academies Press.

————. 2008c. *Retooling for an aging America: Building the health care workforce.* Washington, DC: The National Academies Press.

————. 2009a. *Assessing and improving value in cancer care: Workshop summary.* Washington, DC: The National Academies Press.

————. 2009b. *Ensuring quality cancer care through the oncology workforce: Sustaining care in the 21st century: Workshop summary.* Washington, DC: The National Academies Press.

————. 2010a. *A foundation for evidence-driven practice: A rapid learning system for cancer care: Workshop summary.* Washington, DC: The National Academies Press.

————. 2010b. *Policy issues in the development of personalized medicine in oncology: Workshop summary.* Washington, DC: The National Academies Press.

————. 2011a. *Clinical practice guidelines we can trust.* Washington, DC: The National Academies Press.

————. 2011b. *Patient-centered cancer treatment planning: Improving the quality of oncology care: Workshop summary.* Washington, DC: The National Academies Press.

————. 2012. *Best care at lower cost: The path to continuously learning health care in America.* Washington, DC: The National Academies Press.

————. 2013. *Delivering affordable cancer care in the 21st century: Workshop summary.* Washington, DC: The National Academies Press.

IOM and NRC (National Research Council). 1999. *Ensuring quality cancer care.* Washington, DC: National Academy Press.

————. 2005. *From cancer patient to cancer survivor: Lost in transition.* Washington, DC: The National Academies Press.

Joung, J. G., D. Kim, K. H. Kim, and J. H. Kim. 2013. Extracting coordinated patterns of DNA methylation and gene expression in ovarian cancer. *Journal of the American Medical Informatics Association* 20(4):637-642.

Kantarjian, H., and experts in chronic myeloid leukemia. 2013. The price of drugs for chronic myeloid leukemia (CML); A reflection of the unsustainable prices of cancer drugs: From the perspective of a large group of CML experts. *Blood* epub ahead of print:doi:10.1182/blood-2013-1103-490003.

Kizer, K. W. 2010. What is a world-class medical facility? *American Journal of Medical Quality* 25(2):154-156.

Liang, H., L. W. Cheung, J. Li, Z. Ju, S. Yu, K. Stemke-Hale, T. Dogruluk, Y. Lu, X. Liu, C. Gu, W. Guo, S. E. Scherer, H. Carter, S. N. Westin, M. D. Dyer, R. G. Verhaak, F. Zhang, R. Karchin, C. G. Liu, K. H. Lu, R. R. Broaddus, K. L. Scott, B. T. Hennessy, and G. B. Mills. 2012. Whole-exome sequencing combined with functional genomics reveals novel candidate driver cancer genes in endometrial cancer. *Genome Research* 22(11):2120-2129.

Mariotto, A. B., K. R. Yabroff, Y. Shao, E. J. Feuer, and M. L. Brown. 2011. Projections of the cost of cancer care in the United States: 2010-2020. *Journal of the National Cancer Society* 103(2):117-128.

McCorkle, R., E. Ercolano, M. Lazenby, D. Schulman-Green, L. S. Schilling, K. Lorig, and E. H. Wagner. 2011. Self-management: Enabling and empowering patients living with cancer as a chronic illness. *CA: A Cancer Journal for Clinicians* 61(1):50-62.

Medicare Trustees (The Boards of Trustees, Federal Hospital Insurance and Federal Supplementary Medical Insurance Trust Funds). 2013. *Annual Report.* Washington, DC: The Centers for Medicare & Medicaid Services.

NCI (National Cancer Institute). 2007. *Cancer trends progress report— 2007 update: Costs of cancer care.* http://progressreport.cancer.gov/2007/doc_detail.asp?pid=1&did=2007& chid=75&coid=726&mid= (accessed May 13, 2013).

———. 2012. *SEER Stat Fact Sheets: All Sites.* http://seer.cancer.gov/statfacts/html/all.html (accessed April 19, 2013).

———. 2013a. *The Cancer Genome Atlas.* http://cancergenome.nih.gov/ (accessed July 30, 2013).

———. 2013b. *Cancer control continuum.* http://cancercontrol.cancer.gov/OD/continuum. html (accessed June 13, 2013).

———. 2013c. *Estimated U.S. Cancer Prevalence Counts: Method.* http://dccps.nci.nih.gov/ ocs/prevalence/prevalence.html (accessed April 19, 2013).

NCR BRAC HSAS (National Capital Region Base Realignment and Closure Commission Health Systems Advisory Submcommittee of the Defense Health Board). 2009. *Achieving world class: An independent review of the design plans for the Walter Reed National Military Medical Center and the Fort Belvoir Community Hospital.* Washington, DC: Department of Defense.

NRC (National Research Council). 2009. *Computational technology for effective health care: Immediate steps and strategic direction.* Washington, DC: The National Academies Press.

NVSS (National Vital Statistics System). 2012. *Deaths: Leading Causes for 2009.* http://www. cdc.gov/nchs/data/nvsr/nvsr61/nvsr61_07.pdf (accessed April 19, 2013).

Parry, C., E. E. Kent, L. P. Forsythe, C. M. Alfano, and J. H. Rowland. 2013. Can't see the forest for the care plan: A call to revisit the context of care planning. *Journal of Clinical Oncology* 31:1-3.

Reinhard, S. C., and C. Levine. 2012. *Home alone: Family caregivers providing complex chronic care.* http://www.aarp.org/home-family/caregiving/info-10-2012/home-alone-family-caregivers-providing-complex-chronic-care.html (accessed March 29, 2013).

Rose, C., E. Stovall, P. A. Ganz, C. Desch, and M. Hewitt. 2008. Cancer Quality Alliance: Blueprint for a better cancer care system. *CA: A Cancer Journal for Clinicians* 58(5):266-292.

Scher, K. S., and A. Hurria. 2012. Under-representation of older adults in cancer registration trials: Known problem, little progress. *Journal of Clinical Oncology* 30(17):2036-2038.

Smith, B. D., G. L. Smith, A. Hurria, G. N. Hortobagyi, and T. A. Buchholz. 2009. Future of cancer incidence in the United States: Burdens upon an aging, changing nation. *Journal of Clinical Oncology* 27(17):2758-2765.

Spinks, T., H. W. Albright, T. W. Feeley, R. Walters, T. W. Burke, T. Aloia, E. Bruera, A. Buzdar, L. Foxhall, D. Hui, B. Summers, A. Rodriguez, R. Dubois, and K. I. Shine. 2012. Ensuring quality cancer care: A follow-up review of the Institute of Medicine's 10 recommendations for improving the quality of cancer care in America. *Cancer* 118(10):2571-2582.

Stump, T. K., N. Eghan, B. L. Egleston, O. Hamilton, M. Pirollo, J. S. Schwartz, K. Armstrong J. R. Beck, N. J. Meropol, and Y. Wong. 2013. Cost concerns of patients with cancer. *Journal of Oncology Practice* doi:10.1200/JOP.2013.00092.

Sullivan, R., J. Peppercorn, K. Sikora, J. Zalcberg, N. J. Meropol, E. Amir, D. Khayat, P. Boyle, P. Autier, I. F. Tannock, T. Fojo, J. Siderov, S. Williamson, S. Camporesi, J. G. McVie, A. D. Purushotham, P. Naredi, A. Eggermont, M. F. Brennan, M. L. Steinberg, M. De Ridder, S. A. McCloskey, D. Verellen, T. Roberts, G. Storme, R. J. Hicks, P. J. Ell, B. R. Hirsch, D. P. Carbone, K. A. Schulman, P. Catchpole, D. Taylor, J. Geissler, N. G. Brinker, D. Meltzer, D. Kerr, and M. Aapro. 2011. Delivering affordable cancer care in high-income countries. *Lancet Oncology* 12(10):933-980.

Taylor, E. F., T. Lake, J. Nysenbaum, G. Peterson, and D. Meyers. 2011. *Coordinating care in the medical neighborhood: Critical components and available Mechanisms. White paper*. Rockville, MD: Agency for Healthcare Research and Quality.

Wang, C., T. Pecot, D. L. Zynger, R. Machiraju, C. L. Shapiro, and K. Huang. 2013. Identifying survival associated morphological features of triple negative breast cancer using multiple datasets. *Journal of the American Medical Informatics Association* 20(4):680-687.

Yabroff, K. R., J. Lund, D. Kepka, and A. Mariotto. 2011. Economic burden of cancer in the United States: Estimates, projections, and future research. *Cancer Epidemiology, Biomarkers & Prevention* 20(10):2006-2014.

Zapka, J. G., S. H. Taplin, L. I. Solberg, and M. M. Manos. 2003. A framework for improving the quality of cancer care: The case of breast and cervical cancer screening. *Cancer Epidemiology, Biomarkers & Prevention* 12(1):4-13.

Zapka, J., S. H. Taplin, P. Ganz, E. Grunfeld, and K. Sterba. 2012. Multilevel factors affecting quality: Examples from the cancer care continuum. *Journal of the National Cancer Institute Monographs* 44:11-19.

2

The Current Cancer Care Landscape: An Imperative for Change

This chapter documents the major drivers creating an imperative for change in the cancer care delivery system: (1) the changing demographics in the United States and the increasing number of cancer diagnoses and cancer survivors and (2) the challenges and opportunities in cancer care, including trends in cancer treatment, unique considerations in treating older adults with cancer, unsustainable cancer care costs, and federal efforts to reform health care. The chapter concludes with a section outlining the key stakeholders who will be responsible for transforming the cancer care delivery system, setting the stage for the report's subsequent chapters, which address the committee's recommendations for overcoming challenges to delivering high-quality cancer care.

CANCER DEMOGRAPHICS

The changing demographics in the United States will exacerbate the most pressing challenges to delivering high-quality cancer care. From 2010 to 2050, the United States is expected to grow from more than 300 million to 439 million people, an increase of 42 percent (Vincent and Velkoff, 2010). Although the overall growth rate of the population is slowing, the older adult population, defined in this report as individuals over the age of 65, continues to experience remarkable growth (Mather, 2012; Smith et al., 2009). The diversity of the population is also increasing (Smith et al., 2009). This section explores these trends in detail as well as trends in cancer diagnosis and survivorship.

The Aging Population

Between 1980 and 2000, the older adult population grew from 25 million to 35 million and it is expected to comprise an even larger proportion of the population in the future (Smith et al., 2009). Projections show that by 2030, nearly one in five U.S. residents will be age 65 and older. By 2050, the older adult population is expected to reach 88.5 million, more than double that in 2010 (Vincent and Velkoff, 2010). The baby boomer generation, the first of whom turned 65 in 2011, is largely responsible for the projected population increase. As the baby boomer generation ages, the older adult population over 85 years will rapidly increase: in 2010, around 14 percent of older adults were 85 years of age and older; by 2050, that proportion is expected to grow to more than 21 percent (see Figure 2-1) (Vincent and Velkoff, 2010). Thus, not only is the U.S. population getting older, the older adult population is getting older.

Increasing Diversity of the Population

Growing racial and ethnic diversity in the United States are important demographic trends influencing the delivery of high-quality cancer care. The two major factors contributing to this increasing diversity include (1) immigration and (2) differences in fertility and mortality rates (Shrestha and Heisler, 2011). From 1980 to 2000, racial and ethnic minorities (i.e., non-White) grew from 46 million to 83 million and are expected to expand

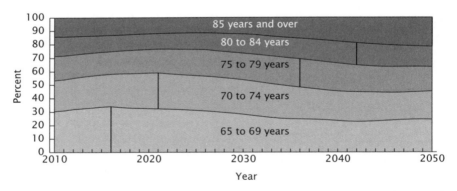

FIGURE 2-1 Distribution of the projected older population by age in the United States, 2010 to 2050.
NOTE: Vertical line indicates the year that each age group is the largest proportion of the older population. Data are from the U.S. Census Bureau's 2008 National Population Projections.
SOURCE: Vincent and Velkoff, 2010.

to 157 million by 2030 (see Table 2-1 and Figure 2-2) (Smith et al., 2009).[1] The Hispanic population, for example, is one of the fastest-growing segments of the U.S. population; if current demographic trends continue, the proportion of Hispanic individuals will rise from 12.6 percent of the population in 2000 to 30.2 percent in 2050 (Shrestha and Heisler, 2011).

Racial and ethnic minorities are much younger than the overall U.S. population. As a result, the older adult population in the United States is not as racially and ethnically diverse as the U.S. population as a whole. As the minority population ages over the next four decades, the older adult population is expected to become more diverse. Minorities are projected to comprise 42 percent of the older adult population by 2050, a 20 percent increase from 2010 (Vincent and Velkoff, 2010). The Hispanic population age 65 and older is projected to increase by more than sixfold from 2010 to 2050, compared to the non-Hispanic population, which is expected to double during this same time period (Vincent and Velkoff, 2010).

The male-to-female ratio in the older adult population is also expected to shift in the coming decades. The U.S. population has traditionally included more females than males due to women's longer life expectancy. With the life expectancy among males quickly rising, the percentage of females 65 years and older will decrease from 57 percent of the older population in 2010 to 55 percent in 2050 (Vincent and Velkoff, 2010).

Trends in Cancer Diagnoses

From 1980 to 2000, the U.S. population grew from 227 million to 279 million (a 23 percent increase). During that same time period, the total yearly cancer incidence increased from 807,000 to 1.34 million (a 66 percent increase) (Smith et al., 2009). Future projections indicate that between 2010 and 2030, the U.S. population will increase from 305 million to 365 million (a 19 percent increase), while the total cancer incidence will rise from 1.6 million to 2.3 million (a 45 percent increase) (Smith et al., 2009). Thus, the incidence of cancer is rapidly increasing (see Figure 2-3).

Men are more likely than women are to be diagnosed with cancer. Current estimates place the overall lifetime risk of developing cancer in men at around one in two and for women around one in three; the incidence rate for all cancers combined is 33 percent higher in men than in women (ACS, 2012b; Eheman et al., 2012). More than 1.6 million individuals will be diagnosed with cancer in 2013 (854,790 in men and 805,500 in women) (NCI, 2013a). The three most common cancers in men

---

[1] Federal standards for collecting information on race and Hispanic origin were established by the Office of Management and Budget in 1997 and revised in 2003. Race and ethnicity are discussed as distinct concepts in this report (OMH, 2010; Shrestha and Heisler, 2011).

TABLE 2-1 Projected U.S. Population, by Race: 2000-2050

Population	2000	2010	2020	2030	2040	2050
Total	282,125 (100.0)	310,233 (100.0)	341,387 (100.0)	373,504 (100.0)	405,655 (100.0)	439,010 (100.0)
White alone	228,548 (81.0)	246,630 (79.5)	266,275 (78.0)	286,109 (76.6)	305,247 (75.2)	324,800 (74.0)
African American alone	35,818 (12.7)	39,909 (12.9)	44,389 (13.0)	48,728 (13.0)	52,868 (13.0)	56,944 (13.0)
Asian alone	10,684 (3.8)	14,415 (4.6)	18,756 (5.5)	23,586 (6.3)	28,836 (7.1)	34,399 (7.8)
All other races	7,075 (2.5)	9,279 (3.0)	11,967 (3.5)	15,081 (4.0)	18,704 (4.6)	22,867 (5.2)

NOTES: In thousands, except as indicated. Resident population. Numbers may not add due to rounding.
SOURCE: Shrestha and Heisler, 2009.

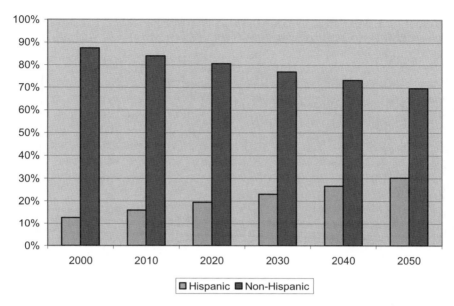

FIGURE 2-2 Hispanics and non-Hispanics as a percentage of the U.S. population, 2000-2050.
NOTE: For the years 2010-2050, data are from the U.S. Census Bureau's 2008 National Population Projections. For 2000, data are from Congressional Research Service extractions from the U.S. Census Bureau's 2004 U.S. Interim National Population Projections.
SOURCE: Shrestha and Heisler, 2011.

are prostate, lung, and colorectal cancer, and the three most common in women are breast, lung, and colorectal cancer (CDC, 2012a,b). The greater incidence of cancer in men is often attributed to higher rates of tobacco use, obesity, physical inactivity, and prostate-specific antigen screening (Andriole et al., 2012; CDC, 2013; KFF, 2013b).

Some minority populations are at an increased risk for cancer (IOM, 1999) (see Table 2-2). African American men consistently have the highest cancer incidence rate of all racial and ethnic groups, with overall rates 15 percent higher than for white men and almost twice that for Asian/Pacific Islander men (Eheman et al., 2012). In addition, the cancer incidence rate is expected to grow faster among racial and ethnic minorities than for Whites (Smith et al., 2009). From 2010 to 2030, the percentage of cancers diagnosed in racial and ethnic minorities is expected to increase from 21 to 28 percent of all cancers (Smith et al., 2009). The causes of these racial and ethnic disparities in risk are complex and overlapping, and they can

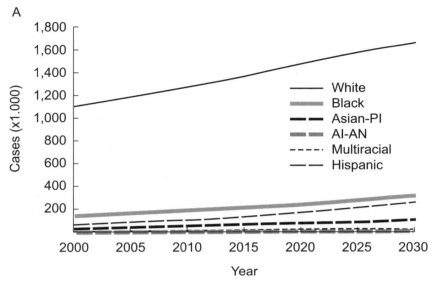

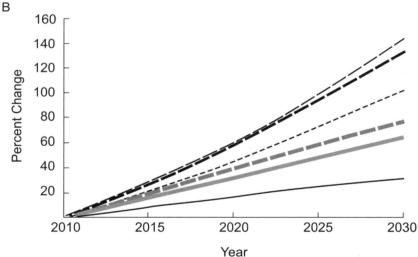

FIGURE 2-3 Projected cases (A) and percent change (B) of all invasive cancers in the United States by race and ethnicity.

NOTE: AI = American Indian; AN = Alaska Native; PI = Pacific Islander.

SOURCE: Smith, B. et al: *J Clin Oncol* 27(17), 2009: 2758-2765. Reprinted with permission. © 2009 American Society of Clinical Oncology. All rights reserved.

TABLE 2-2 Cancer Incidence Rates by Race, 2006-2010, from 18 SEER Geographic Areas

Cancer Incidence Rates by Race and Ethnicity

Race/Ethnicity	Male	Female
All Races	535.9 per 100,000 men	411.2 per 100,000 women
White	539.1 per 100,000 men	424.4 per 100,000 women
African American	610.4 per 100,000 men	397.5 per 100,000 women
Asian/Pacific Islander	335.06 per 100,000 men	291.5 per 100,000 women
American Indian/ Alaska Native	351.3 per 100,000 men	306.5 per 100,000 women
Hispanic	409.7 per 100,000 men	323.2 per 100,000 women

NOTE: SEER = Surveillance, Epidemiology, and End Results program.
SOURCE: NCI, 2013a.

include socioeconomic status (SES); unequal access to care; differences in behavioral, environmental, and genetic risk factors; and social and cultural biases that influence the quality of care (AACR, 2012; ACS, 2011).

SES is another predictor of cancer incidence and morbidity (Clegg et al., 2009). People with lower SES are disproportionately affected by many cancers, including lung, late-stage prostate, and late-stage female breast cancer (ACSCAN, 2009; Booth et al., 2010; Clegg et al., 2009). These disparities in people with lower SES are often attributed to differences in cancer preventive behaviors, health insurance status, and an inability to access and afford timely screening and appropriate follow-up care (ACSCAN, 2009).

Finally, one of the strongest risk factors for cancer is age (see Figure 2-4) (ACS, 2012b; NCI, 2013a). The median age for a cancer diagnosis is 66 years of age (NCI, 2013a). In general, as age increases, cancer incidence and mortality increase (NCI, 2013a). As more of the population reaches 65 years of age, cancer incidence is expected to increase.

Trends in Cancer Survivorship

The Institute of Medicine previously adopted the National Coalition for Cancer Survivorship's definition of a cancer survivor as a person who has been diagnosed with cancer, from the time of diagnosis through the balance of life (IOM and NRC, 2005). Since the "war on cancer" began in 1971, changes in screening and treatment have contributed to an almost fourfold increase in the number of survivors (NCI, 2012a; Parry et al., 2011). Out of a U.S. population of more than 300 million people, approximately 14 million people are cancer survivors (see Table 2-3) (ACS, 2012c;

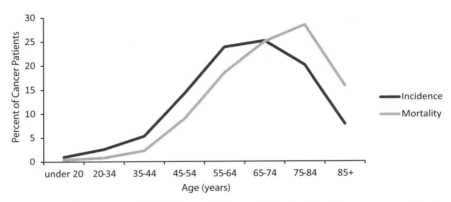

FIGURE 2-4 Age-specific incidence and mortality rates for all cancers combined, 2006-2010.
SOURCE: NCI, 2013a.

U.S. Census Bureau, 2013). Projections estimate that the total number of cancer survivors will reach 18 million (8.8 million males and 9.2 million females) by 2022 (see Figure 2-5) (ACS, 2012c; de Moor et al., 2013).

Average survival time following a cancer diagnosis is growing longer. As a result, there are more adults living with a history of cancer throughout their lifetime (Parry et al., 2011). In the current population of cancer survivors, 64 percent were diagnosed more than 5 years ago and 15 percent were diagnosed more than two decades ago (ACS, 2012c). The majority of these survivors are older adults (ACS, 2012c; Parry et al., 2011). In addition, the number of cancer survivors over the age of 65 years is expected to increase at a faster rate than for any other age group; by 2020, 11 million cancer survivors will be older adults, a 42 percent increase from 2010 (Parry et al., 2011). Box 4-3 in Chapter 4 discusses various workforce strategies that are being utilized to care for this growing population of cancer survivors.

The increases in survival following a cancer diagnosis, however, have not been equitable across all segments of the population (IOM, 1999). Recent policy initiatives, such as the Patient Protection and Affordable Care Act (ACA)[2] provision on understanding health care disparities (see Annex 2-1) and the Healthy People 2020 initiative, are designed to gather data on health care disparities and promote health equity. Current data indicate that there are major disparities in cancer outcomes among people

---

[2] Patient Protection and Affordable Care Act, Public Law 111-148, 111th Congress (March 23, 2010).

TABLE 2-3 Estimated Number of U.S. Cancer Survivors by Sex and Age as of January 1, 2012

	Male		Female	
	Number	Percent	Number	Percent
All ages	6,442,280		7,241,570	
0-14	36,770	1	21,740	<1
15-19	24,860	<1	23,810	<1
20-29	74,790	1	105,110	1
30-39	134,630	2	250,920	3
40-49	350,350	5	647,840	9
50-59	930,140	14	1,365,040	19
60-69	1,705,730	26	1,801,430	25
70-79	1,858,260	29	1,607,630	22
80+	1,326,740	21	1,418,050	20

NOTE: Data are from the Data Modeling Branch, Division of Cancer Control and Population Sciences, National Cancer Institute. Percentages may not sum to 100 percent due to rounding.
SOURCE: American Cancer Society. *Cancer Treatment and Survivorship: Facts and Figures.* Atlanta: American Cancer Society, Inc. ACS, 2012c.

who have lower SES, are racial and ethnic minorities, and people who lack health insurance coverage (ACS, 2011; ACSCAN, 2009; AHRQ, 2011b, 2012b). The committee addresses the importance of ensuring that cancer care is accessible and affordable to all individuals in Chapter 8.

SES is an important factor in cancer survival and cancer death (ACS, 2011; IOM, 1999). For example, the 5-year cancer survival rate is 10 percentage points higher among people who live in affluent areas compared to people who live in poorer areas (Ward et al., 2004). People who have lower SES (measured by years of education) are more likely to die from cancer compared to people who have higher SES, regardless of other demographic factors; this disparity is likely to increase (ACS, 2011). There are several possible explanations for the correlation between low SES and poor cancer survival. Individuals with low SES often lack access to preventive care or cancer treatment due to the high cost of care, lack of health insurance, poor health literacy, or because they live in poor or rural areas that are geographically isolated from clinicians (ACS, 2011). As a result, these individuals may be more likely to be diagnosed with late-stage cancers, which could have been treated more effectively if diagnosed earlier. In addition, an individual's SES can influence the prevalence of

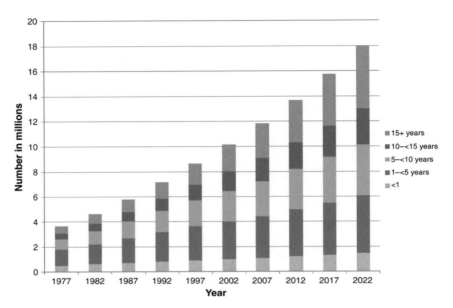

FIGURE 2-5 Estimated and projected number of cancer survivors in the United States from 1977 to 2022 by year since diagnosis.
SOURCE: Reprinted from *Cancer Epidemiology, Biomarkers & Prevention*, 2013, 22(4), 561-570, de Moor, Cancer survivors in the United States: Prevalence across the survivorship trajectory and implications for care, with permission from AACR.

behavioral risk factors for cancer, including tobacco use, poor diet, and physical inactivity, as well as the likelihood of following cancer screening recommendations (ACS, 2011; NCI, 2008). People with less education, for example, are more likely to smoke and those with lower incomes are less likely to exercise than people with higher education and incomes (ACSCAN, 2009).

Some racial and ethnic groups have poorer survival and higher cancer death rates compared to other groups (ACS, 2013b). From 1999 to 2008, overall cancer death rates appreciably declined in every racial and ethnic group except American Indian and Alaska Native populations (Eheman et al., 2012). African Americans have the highest death rate of all racial and ethnic groups; the death rate for all cancers combined is 31 percent higher in African American men compared to White men and 15 percent higher for African American women compared to White women (ACS, 2013a). African Americans also have a lower 5-year overall survival rate from cancer than Whites (60 percent versus 69 percent) (ACS, 2013a).

Asian Americans generally have lower cancer death rates than Whites; however, disparities in survival exist for certain types of cancers, such as stomach and liver cancer (NCI, 2012d; OMH, 2012). Death rates are lower among Hispanics than among non-Hispanic Whites for all cancers combined and for the four most common cancers (prostate, female breast, colorectal, and lung) (ACS, 2012a). Table 2-4 provides overall cancer death rates by race and ethnicity.

As noted previously, the factors contributing to racial and ethnic disparities in cancer outcomes are complex and overlapping, and they can include low SES; unequal access to care; differences in behavioral, environmental, and genetic risk factors; and social and cultural biases that influence the quality of care (AACR, 2012; ACS, 2011). African Americans are often diagnosed at later stages of disease than are Whites, when the severity is greater and the odds of survival are poorer (ACS, 2013a; AHRQ, 2011b, 2012b). Although Hispanics have lower cancer death rates than Whites, they too are often diagnosed at later stages of disease than are Whites (ACS, 2012a). Patient beliefs and choices may contribute to the later stage of diagnosis (Espinosa de los Monteros and Gallo, 2011; Margolis et al., 2003; Stein et al., 2007). Racial and ethnic minorities may be more skeptical about the medical community due to past incidents of mistreatment (IOM, 1999, 2003). In addition, problems in communication and coordination of care may contribute to the disparities in treatment outcomes. According to one study, racial and ethnic minorities and non-English speakers were less likely to report that they had received excellent or very good cancer care than were Whites, and analyses found that a

TABLE 2-4 Death Rates by Race in 2006-2010 from 18 SEER Geographic Areas

Death Rates by Race and Ethnicity		
Race/Ethnicity	Male	Female
All Races	215.3 per 100,000 men	149.7 per 100,000 women
White	213.1 per 100,000 men	149.8 per 100,000 women
African American	276.6 per 100,000 men	171.2 per 100,000 women
Asian/Pacific Islander	132.4 per 100,000 men	92.1 per 100,000 women
American Indian/ Alaska Native	191.0 per 100,000 men	139.0 per 100,000 women
Hispanic	152.1 per 100,000 men	101.2 per 100,000 women

NOTE: SEER = Surveillance, Epidemiology, and End Results program.
SOURCE: NCI, 2013a.

lack of coordination of care was the greatest factor contributing to these differences (Ayanian et al., 2005).

Insurance status is also predictive of an individual's chances of surviving cancer. Uninsured persons and persons enrolled in Medicaid are often diagnosed with cancer at a later stage than are individuals enrolled in other types of insurance (ACS, 2013b; Halpern et al., 2007). Those same individuals are less likely to survive cancer regardless of the stage at diagnosis (ACS, 2008). This difference in cancer outcomes can likely be explained by a number of factors, including these populations' access to care, quality of cancer care, and health literacy. Uninsured and Medicaid enrollees are more likely than are other populations to face barriers in accessing care, such as the inability to find adequate transportation, to take time off from work, to pay out of pocket for the cost of care, or to find physicians who will accept Medicaid insurance or treat them without insurance. Conversely, individuals with private insurance are more likely to receive recommended, appropriate cancer screening and treatment than are individuals who have Medicare and Medicaid insurance, and who are racial and ethnic minorities, or have low SES (ACS, 2008; Harlan et al., 2005).

CHALLENGES AND OPPORTUNITIES IN CANCER CARE

Medical knowledge has expanded in recent years and the pace of advancement is likely to accelerate. There have been breakthroughs in numerous areas of medical research, including genomics, stem cell biology, and molecular biology. This has led to the availability of many more diagnostic tests and treatments for cancer and has moved the practice of oncology toward more molecularly targeted medicine. These advancements, however, have coincided with unsustainable growth in health care spending—spending that is likely to be exacerbated in the future by a cancer care delivery system overwhelmed by many more patients and an increasingly complex patient population with multiple comorbidities. Congress, recognizing that national changes are needed to address these challenges, passed major health care reform legislation as well as a number of other policy initiatives in recent years. Each of these challenges and opportunities is discussed in detail below.

Trends in Cancer Treatment

Once the province of surgeons and local-regional therapies, cancer treatment has evolved rapidly in recent decades. Systemic treatments emerged in the 1950s and 1960s, initially as relatively nonspecific chemotherapies with limited efficacy in some human cancers. Empiricism, rather than an understanding of tumor biology, dominated oncology drug development in this era. In recent years, researchers have developed treatments targeting specific molecular aberrations in cancer cells (e.g., Imatinib for chronic myelogenous leukemia, Trastuzumab for breast cancer). Molecularly targeted treatments have pervaded Food and Drug Administration (FDA) approvals in oncology in the past decade and have improved patient outcomes for many cancers. These agents commonly require a test to assess the drug target in the patient's tumor. As such, companion diagnostic testing (e.g., estrogen receptor [ER] and human epidermal growth factor receptor-2 [HER2] in breast cancer, anaplastic lymphoma kinase [ALK] and epidermal growth factor receptor [EGFR] in non-small-cell lung cancer) has increased in importance. The sheer number of targeted agents has increased the educational burden for cancer care clinicians and the financial burden for the health care system. In the near future, the implementation of genome-based diagnostics will likely alter both the ability to deliver precision medicine and the complexity of cancer treatment (IOM, 2010, 2012b; NRC, 2011).

Unique Considerations in Treating Older Adults with Cancer

There are a number of unique considerations in providing appropriate care to older adults with cancer. Older adults with cancer often have altered physiology, functional impairment (either at the time of diagnosis or as a potential consequence of treatment), multiple and often coexisting morbidities, increased side effects of treatment, and potentially different or additional treatment goals (Yancik, 1997). They may rely more heavily on social support to manage their disease than do younger individuals with cancer (see discussion on caregiving in Chapter 4). In addition, there are limited data from clinical trials to guide treatment decisions in older patients (see discussion in Chapter 5). Older patients—especially frail patients, those with organ dysfunction, or those with poor health status—are often excluded from cancer clinical trials, and the impact of cancer treatment on physical or cognitive function is typically not captured in clinical trials (Hutchins et al., 1999; Talarico et al., 2004; Unger et al., 2006; Yee et al., 2003). Stereotypes held by clinicians about older adults may also deter them from treating patients aggressively (Foster et al., 2010).

Older adults with cancer may have different treatment goals or preferences compared to younger patients with cancer. In a survey of older adults with chronic illness, for example, 74 percent of respondents did not want treatment if it would cause functional impairment, and 88 percent did not want treatment if it would cause cognitive impairment, regardless of the impact on survival (Fried et al., 2002). Clinicians' treatment recommendations are greatly influenced by their patients' age, comorbidity, and health status, and do not always take into account individual preferences (Hurria et al., 2008). Clinicians' communication styles and their own treatment preferences also have an impact on the type of care older adults with cancer receive. In a study of patients 70 years and older with advanced colorectal cancer, patients' preferences for an active or passive role in their chemotherapy decision making did not always match what their physician perceived as their preferred decision-making style (Elkin et al., 2007). Another study found that women who preferred less physician input were less likely to receive chemotherapy, while patients of oncologists who had a strong preference for providing chemotherapy were more likely to receive it (Mandelblatt et al., 2012). Decision aids, discussed in Chapter 3, are one mechanism that can help improve patients' understanding of their prognosis, their treatment options, and the benefits and harms of treatment (Leighl et al., 2011).

A geriatric assessment is a useful tool for assessing the different needs of older adults. A geriatric assessment evaluates an older adult's physiological changes, functional status, comorbid medical conditions, cognition, psychological status, social functioning and support, nutritional status, and polypharmacy. (See Box 2-1 for a description of each domain. Table 2-5 highlights the specific physiological changes that correlate with the aging process. However, it is important to recognize that clinical manifestations may not always be "typical" in an older adult.) Each of these domains is predictive of morbidity and mortality in the geriatric population (Inouye et al., 1998; Landi et al., 2000; Lee et al., 2006; Reuben et al., 1992; Rigler et al., 2002; Seeman et al., 1987; Studenski et al., 2004; Walter et al., 2001). Many of these domains are also predictive of prognosis in younger adults; however, they are particularly important for assessing older adults due to this population's increased risk of social, physical, and mental vulnerability. Clinicians can use geriatric assessments to understand the unique needs of older adults with cancer and the potential benefits and harmsof various care plans (Extermann et al., 2012; Hurria et al., 2011a).

Unsustainable Cancer Care Costs

In the United States, the rising costs of health care is a central fiscal challenge (CBO, 2012b; IOM, 2012a; NRC, 2012; Sullivan et al., 2011). The United States spent $2.7 trillion on health care in 2011, accounting for 17.9 percent of the nation's gross domestic product (GDP) (CMS, 2013a). By 2037, health care costs are anticipated to account for almost 25 percent of the nation's GDP (CBO, 2012a). Estimating future health care spending, however, is challenging, as it depends both on changes within the health care system and the economy as a whole (Fuchs, 2013). From 2015 to 2021,

BOX 2-1
Domains of a Geriatric Assessment

Physiological Changes

It is important for clinicians to recognize the potential for physiological decline in older adults with cancer when devising care plans for this population. The rate of decline and the appearance of resulting physiological consequences due to aging are unique to each individual. Age-related changes, including declines in organ function, can impact an individual's tolerance for cancer therapy and the correct dosing of chemotherapy (Bajetta et al., 2005; Bruno et al., 2001; Crivellari et al., 2000; Extermann et al., 2012; Goldberg et al., 2006; Graham et al., 2000; Haller et al., 2005; Hurria et al., 2005, 2011b; Muss et al., 2007; Toffoli et al., 2001). Table 2-5 summarizes common age-related changes in various organ systems. Periods of stress, such as stress induced by cancer and/or cancer treatment, can further impact an individual's physiological state. For example, older adults often have increased bone marrow fat and decreased bone marrow reserve. In older adults with cancer, this is associated with an increased risk of myelosuppression (i.e., bone marrow suppression) and can lead to complications from chemotherapy, such as anemia and an increased distribution of drugs throughout the body (Dees et al., 2000; Gomez et al., 1998; Repetto et al., 2003).

Functional Status

Functional status is generally measured by assessing an individual's ability to complete activities of daily living (ADLs) (e.g., grooming, dressing, eating, walking) and instrumental activities of daily living (IADLs) (e.g., shopping, housekeeping, accounting, preparing food, using the telephone, traveling). Cancer is associated with an increased need for assistance with these types of activities (Keating et al., 2005; Stafford and Cyr, 1997). It is important that the oncology workforce have tools to assess the functional status of older adults with cancer because this evaluation helps clinicians to determine a patient's risk of treatment toxicity and postoperative complications; ascertain whether a patient receiving chemotherapy is able to seek medical attention if necessary (i.e., use the telephone to call for help, follow instructions, and anticipate and respond to toxicity); and estimate overall survival (Audisio et al., 2005; Extermann et al., 2012; Hurria et al., 2011a; Keating et al., 2005; Stafford and Cyr, 1997). For example, in a clinical trial of older patients with advanced non-small-cell lung cancer, pretreatment IADLs were correlated with survival (Maione et al., 2005). Other studies have shown that declines in physical function persisting over time are associated with poorer overall survival and increased risk of subsequent hospitalization, compared with declines in physical function that are transient (Mor et al., 1994; Sleiman et al., 2009). Measuring functional status at several points along the trajectory of illness may provide valuable prognostic information.

continued

BOX 2-1 Continued

Comorbid Medical Conditions

It is important for the medical team to identify performance status and existing comorbidities in older adults with cancer, because these can impact a patient's prognosis and tolerance for cancer treatment (Birim et al., 2006; Frasci et al., 2000; Steyerberg et al., 2006). The presence of multiple comorbidities is associated with worse survival in adults with cancer (Extermann et al., 2000; Firat et al., 2002; Frasci et al., 2000; Piccirillo et al., 2004; Satariano and Ragland, 1994). Individuals with multiple comorbidities are also likely to experience a decline in functional status over time (Rigler et al., 2002; Studenski et al., 2004). However, further research is needed to understand the longitudinal relationship between comorbidities and subsequent functional status of older adults with cancer (Dacal et al., 2006; Extermann et al., 1998; Hurria et al., 2006; Yancik et al., 2007).

Nutritional Status

Few studies have examined the association between cancer, aging, and nutrition, but existing evidence suggests that nutritional status may have an impact on prognosis and survival. For example, older adults are at an increased risk for mucositis, which impacts an individual's ability to maintain adequate nutrition during cancer therapy. Weight loss in cancer patients is associated with poorer chemotherapy response rates and poorer survival (Dewys et al., 1980). There is also evidence that poor nutritional status is associated with an increased risk of mortality (Landi et al., 2000). In a study of patients with metastatic colorectal cancer, severe malnutrition was associated with greater toxicity and reduced overall survival (Barret et al., 2011).

Cognition

A cognitive assessment in older adults with cancer should be conducted to determine whether a patient has the ability to consent to and adhere to medication regimens in the home. Both aging and cancer therapy have the potential to impact cognitive function. A patient with cognitive impairment will likely need assistance from a family member, friend, or caregiver to maintain safety and remember instructions on taking medications. There is also an association between cognitive function and physical function, so a patient with cognitive impairment may also require assistance with other ADLs/IADLs (Dodge et al., 2005; Sauvaget et al., 2002; Wadley et al., 2008).

Psychological State and Social Support

Many older adults with cancer are at risk for depression, psychological distress, and social isolation. Depression is common in older adults and can be hard to diagnose because the symptoms of cancer and depression often overlap, and the presentation of depression in older adults is often more somatic and less affective or emotional than in younger persons (Weinberger et al., 2009). However, it is important to identify and treat depression in older adults because depressive symptoms are associated with a decline in physical function (Penninx et al., 1998). Similarly, in a recent study, 41 percent of older adults with cancer reported psychological distress, which was correlated with poorer physical function (Hurria et al., 2009). Evidence from both the geriatric and the oncology literature has linked social isolation to a higher risk of death (Kroenke et al., 2006; Reuben et al., 1992; Seeman et al., 1993; Waxler-Morrison et al., 1991). For example, two studies have found that women with breast cancer who get divorced or separated and lack adequate social support are at a higher risk for severe psychological distress (Kornblith et al., 2001, 2003). Social support plays a vital role in the psychological functioning of older adults and can mitigate the psychological impact of stressful life events, such as a cancer diagnosis and cancer treatment (Kornblith et al., 2001). Thus, assessing a patient's psychological state and their social support system can provide important prognostic information.

Polypharmacy

Older adults are likely to have one or more chronic conditions and, as a result, see multiple clinicians and take multiple medications (Gurwitz, 2004; Hajjar et al., 2007; Hanlon et al., 2001; Safran et al., 2005). It is important for clinicians to assess the medications older adults receive in addition to cancer therapy, because the use of multiple medications increases an individual's risk of adverse effects. Drug-drug and drug-disease interactions, for example, can lead to increased or decreased clinical effects, increased drug toxicity, and compromised adherence to therapy (Elmer et al., 2007; Qato et al., 2008; Riechelmann and Del Giglio, 2009). There is also the risk of medication duplication (where medications of the same or similar drug class or therapeutic effect taken concurrently do not provide any additional benefit) and medication underuse (where patients are overwhelmed by the number of medications they have been prescribed and do not take some of them). This assessment should consider dosage and indications of prescription medications, as well as over-the-counter, herbals, and complementary/alternative medications (Qato et al., 2008; Rolita and Freedman, 2008; Yoon and Schaffer, 2006). Evidence suggests that having a pharmacist or interdisciplinary team review a patient's medications can lessen the number of medications a patient must take or identify potential drug-drug interactions (Bregnhoj et al., 2009; Chrischilles et al., 2004; Crotty et al., 2004; Davis et al., 2007; Hanlon et al., 1996; Holmes et al., 2008; Spinewine et al., 2007; Stuijt et al., 2008; Vinks et al., 2009). Clinicians' use of electronic drug databases and indexes on appropriate medication can also help identify unnecessary medications or potential drug-drug interactions (Clauson et al., 2007; Egger et al., 2003; Tulner et al., 2008; Weber et al., 2008). Methods to help clinicians assess the appropriateness of drug prescribing have also been developed, including the Medication Appropriateness Index and the Beers Criteria (Beers, 1997; Beers et al., 1991; Fick et al., 2003; Hanlon et al., 1992; Zhan et al., 2001).

TABLE 2-5 Examples of Age-Related Changes in Each Organ of the Functional System

System or Function	Age-Related Changes
Cardiovascular system	• Decreased maximal heart rate in response to stress • Increased wall stiffness that leads to reduction in early diastolic filling and diastolic dysfunction • Declined ventricular function
Gastrointestinal system	• Decreased secretion of digestive enzymes • Changed peristalsis rate; gastric emptying is prolonged • Decreased basal gastric flow • Changed intestinal motility and absorption • Decreased liver size, volume, and blood flow
Pulmonary system	• Declined lung recoil • Decreased ability to clear secretions • Increased airway resistance
Renal function	• Decreased kidney weight • Decreased renal blood flow • Decreased creatinine clearance • Decreased reabsorption and responsiveness to regulatory hormones
Neurologic system	• Decreased hearing/eyesight • Increased response time • Increased risk of developing delirium • Increased risk of peripheral neuropathy
Hematologic system	• Decreased bone marrow reserve • Increased risk of infection and anemia
Immunologic changes	• Increased susceptibility to infection • Altered T-cell function
Changes in body composition may lead to alterations in drug distribution	• Increased body fat • Decreased lean body mass • Decreased total body water • Increased susceptibility to dehydration

SOURCES: Avorn and Gurwitz, 1997; Baker and Grochow, 1997; Duthie, 2004; Sawhney et al., 2005; Sehl et al., 2005; Vestal, 1997; Yuen, 1990.

the Centers for Medicare & Medicaid Services (CMS) has estimated that health care spending will grow at an average rate of 6.2 percent annually, driven by a number of factors, including the aging of the population and implementation of health care reform (CMS, 2013b). Likewise, although the Congressional Budget Office (CBO) recently revised its 10-year projection of Medicaid and Medicare spending downward by 3.5 percent, it has projected an increase in federal deficits due to the pressures of an aging population, rising health care costs, expansion of federal subsidies for health insurance as part of health care reform, and growing interest payments on federal debt (CBO, 2013a,b,c). The growth in health care spending has slowed in recent years but it is unclear that this trend will continue (Fuchs, 2013; Hartman et al., 2013; Ryu et al., 2013). Regardless, health economist Victor Fuchs (2013) has asserted that national health care spending will continue to pose challenges for the U.S. economy in the future.

Health care costs are a critical challenge to the nation's economic stability. In 2009, health care spending in the United States was 2.5 times greater than the Organisation for Economic Co-operation and Development average (OECD, 2013). Rising health care costs could lead to higher taxes, a decline in the nation's GDP, decreased employment, and a lower standard of living (AHR, 2012; Baicker and Skinner, 2011). They could also threaten the United States' economic competitiveness and perpetuate the stagnation of employee wages seen in the past 30 years (Emanuel and Fuchs, 2008). In addition, increased spending on health care diverts spending from a number of other national priorities, including investments in education, infrastructure, and research (BPC, 2012; Emanuel et al., 2012; Milstein, 2012). Fuchs has said that if the United States solves its health care spending problem, "practically all of our fiscal problems go away. [And if we don't], then almost anything else we do will not solve our fiscal problems" (Kolata, 2012).

Cancer care costs make a substantial contribution to rising health care costs. The costs of direct medical care for cancer are estimated to account for 5 percent of national health care spending (Sullivan et al., 2011); however, one large insurer, UnitedHealthcare, estimated that 11 percent of its costs are for cancer care (IOM, 2013). National expenditures for cancer care accounted for $72 billion in 2004, rose to $125 billion in 2010, and are likely to increase to $158 billion in 2020 due to demographic changes alone (Mariotto et al., 2011; NCI, 2007). Accounting for the rise in cancer care costs, researchers estimated that costs could reach $173 billion in 2020, a 39 percent increase from 2010 (Mariotto et al., 2011). Cancer care costs are growing faster than are costs for other sectors of medicine (Bach, 2009; Elkin and Bach, 2010; Meropol and Schulman, 2007; Yabroff et al., 2011). In fact, Sullivan et al. (2011) suggested that increases in the costs of cancer care could begin to outpace health care inflation as a whole and account for a greater share of total health care spending.

A number of factors influence the cost of cancer care. The overall growth in spending on cancer care is related to both the increased price of cancer care and quantity of cancer care (Bach, 2009; Elkin and Bach, 2010). Cancer care costs are highest in the months following a cancer diagnosis and at the end of life (Yabroff et al., 2011). As more expensive targeted treatments and other new technologies become the standard of care in the near future, the costs of cancer care are projected to escalate rapidly. An editorial from leaders in the cancer community concluded that some of these new treatments are "rightly heralded as substantial advances, but others provide only marginal benefit" (Emanuel et al., 2013). The FDA approved 13 new cancer treatments in 2012; of these, only 1 extended survival by more than a median of 6 months, 2 extended survival for only 4 to 6 weeks, and all cost more than $5,900 per month of treatment (Emanuel et al., 2013).

Drug manufacturers may be facing more pressure to moderate their prices for cancer treatments (Bach et al., 2012; Kantarjian and experts in chronic myeloid leukemia, 2013). For example, Zaltrap (ziv-aflibercept), approved for colorectal cancer treatment, was initially priced at $11,000 per month of treatment, more than twice as much as for the usual dose of a medicine with similar patient outcomes. Pushback from a cancer center prompted Sanofi to provide hospitals and clinicians with a 50 percent discount on the price of Zaltrap (Pollack, 2012). However, patients and payers were still required to cover the full amount of the drug during its initial months on the market. These parties will only benefit from Sanofi's discount once Medicare's average sales price reflects the actual cost of the drug (Conti, 2012). (See Box 8-2 for a more detailed discussion of how Medicare Part B drugs are reimbursed.) Based on a recent estimate, the price of Zaltrap has dropped by almost half since it was marketed but is still more expensive than comparable drugs (Goldberg, 2013).

The FDA approves cancer drugs based on its evaluation of their safety and efficacy, but it does not consider issues of cost or effectiveness in its decisions (The Lewin Group, Inc., 2007). Drug compendia, such as the one produced by the National Comprehensive Cancer Network, often guide the use of off-label prescribing for cancer treatments, though the information in the compendia is of variable quality and often not adequate to support these decisions (Abernethy et al., 2009, 2010). Additional drivers of costs include the current deficiencies in the cancer care delivery system and payment models (see discussion in Chapter 8); diffusion of innovations in clinical practice with variable and often insufficient evidence supporting their use (see Chapter 5); patient and clinician attitudes, beliefs, and practices (see Chapter 3); and legal and regulatory challenges (see Chapter 8).

The consolidation of private oncology practices into hospital-based practices is also driving up cancer care costs (Guidi, 2013; IOM, 2013). Hospitals are able to negotiate with payers to receive higher reimbursement for oncology services than private medical practices because they have more leverage. Hospitals provide many essential services that private medical practices do not offer (such as bed access). Hospitals use this leverage to their advantage when negotiating their charges and link the provision of these essential services with better reimbursement for oncology care (IOM, 2013). In addition, hospital costs are likely to have an increasingly large impact on the total cost of cancer care in the near future, as patients are receiving a greater proportion of their cancer care in hospital outpatient settings (Guidi, 2013).

Health Reform, HITECH, and Other Policy Initiatives

In the past decade, Congress has passed major legislation to improve care for people with cancer: in particular, the Medicare Prescription Drug, Improvement, and Modernization Act, also known as the Medicare Modernization Act (MMA) (2003), the Health Information Technology for Economic and Clinical Health (HITECH) Act (2009), and the ACA (2010) (see discussions on the MMA in Chapter 8 and the HITECH Act in Chapter 6). These laws and other regulatory changes will impact many aspects of cancer care, including access, delivery systems, quality improvement efforts, research infrastructure, and payment and reimbursement.

This section focuses on the impact of the ACA on cancer care and outlines how the changing policy landscape will likely impact cancer patients and survivors. Signed into law in 2010 and upheld in large part by the U.S. Supreme Court in 2012, the ACA is the most substantial piece of health care legislation enacted since Medicare in 1965. Annex 2-1 provides a summary of the ACA provisions most relevant to cancer care.

Expanding Insurance Coverage

One of the ACA's primary goals is to expand insurance coverage to reduce the number of uninsured individuals. Beginning in 2014, nearly all U.S. citizens will be required to have health insurance coverage or pay a penalty. To ensure that individuals are able to obtain the mandated coverage, the ACA provides subsidies for some individuals and creates market reforms to foster increased access to private and public coverage for others.

The ACA offers states the ability to expand public insurance coverage by removing the Medicaid eligibility categories and raising the income threshold. Now, states can choose to allow all non-elderly, non-disabled citizens, and legal U.S. residents with family incomes below 133 percent of the federal poverty level (FPL), or about $30,000 per year for a family of four, to be eligible for Medicaid benefits. Primarily, this extends coverage to low-income, childless adults, providing them with access to preventive care such as colon and breast cancer screenings, among other services. By expanding the reach of public insurance, it is anticipated that more people with cancer can be diagnosed and treated at an earlier stage, thus increasing their chance for survival. However, the Medicaid expansion may not reach as far as initially expected. Following the Supreme Court's decision in June 2012, states have been encouraged, but not required, to expand their Medicaid programs. As of June 2013, 23 states and the District of Columbia plan to expand their Medicaid programs, 6 states are undecided, and 21 are not expanding their Medicaid program at this time (KFF, 2013c). Individuals living in states that do not expand Medicaid will likely turn to the Health Insurance Marketplace for additional coverage or remain uninsured.

The ACA also expands insurance coverage by creating a "one stop shop" for insurance called the Health Insurance Marketplace (formerly, the "Exchange"). States can (1) administer their own, state-based marketplace (17 states); (2) work with the federal government in a partnership (7 states); or (3) default to the federally facilitated Health Insurance Marketplace (21 states) (KFF, 2013d; numbers current as of May 2013). Regardless of the administration, marketplaces will offer multiple tiers of "qualified health plans" for individuals and small businesses to purchase health insurance. To further encourage purchase of an insurance plan, the federal government will provide subsidies for low-income individuals and families (between 100 to 400 percent of the FPL) to help cover premium costs. Until the marketplaces are up and running, temporary high-risk pools offer coverage to those who have been uninsured for at least the previous 6 months due to a preexisting condition, such as cancer; in 2014, these beneficiaries will transition into marketplace-sponsored coverage.

Because young adults are much more likely to be un- or underinsured, the ACA expands their access to coverage by requiring that most private insurers provide young adults with the option to remain on their parents' insurance plans until age 26. Notably, although cancer death rates have declined in all other age groups during the past decade, individuals ages 15 to 29 have not seen decreases in cancer death rates and individuals ages 25 to 29 have seen increases in cancer death rates (Bleyer et al., 2012). In addition, adolescents and young adults have not had comparable gains in 5-year cancer survival compared to younger and older age groups (NCI, 2013b). Although the reasons for this lack of progress are complex and not well understood, they may be due in part to a lack of health insurance and delays in diagnosis (Bleyer et al., 2012; NCI, 2013b). By extending dependent coverage to as many as 3 million young adults and expanding health insurance coverage through Medicaid expansions and the Health Insurance Marketplace, the ACA may improve access to cancer care for the estimated 68,400 adolescents and young adults ages 15 to 39 who are diagnosed with cancer each year (Bleyer et al., 2012; NCI, 2013b; Sommers et al., 2013).

Protecting Consumers and Improving the Quality of Care

In addition to improving health insurance coverage, the ACA protects consumers by mandating changes to the health care system intended to make health insurance more affordable, comprehensive, and widely available, regardless of a person's health status.

The law prohibits common practices used to restrict eligibility, like denying coverage or charging higher premiums for preexisting conditions such as cancer. Historically, such practices have made it difficult, if not impossible, for many cancer survivors to gain meaningful health insurance coverage. Requiring insurers to accept all applicants, regardless of their preexisting condition, is a major improvement for ensuring patients' access to cancer care.

In the past, patients with expensive cancer treatments could quickly reach their annual and lifetime health care coverage limits, placing them at financial risk for covering the cost of potentially lifesaving care. To address this problem, the ACA prohibits many health plans from placing lifetime limits on benefits for specific conditions and restricts the extent to which plans can place annual limits on coverage. Such a change provides important protections for cancer patients and survivors who will no longer have to worry about their coverage being dropped or limits on coverage being applied.

The ACA sets a baseline for necessary services, with the goal of providing meaningful and comprehensive coverage for certain health plans. Qualified health plans will offer coverage in the new marketplaces and will be required to offer a basic level of care, known as the essential health benefits (EHB) package, although the federal government has given states flexibility in determining which health benefits to designate as "essential." The EHB is designed to reflect what "typical employer coverage" provides across 10 broad categories:

1. ambulatory patient services;
2. emergency services;
3. hospitalization;
4. maternity and newborn care;
5. mental health and substance use disorder services (including behavioral health);
6. prescription drugs;
7. rehabilitative and habilitative services and devices;
8. laboratory services;
9. prevention and wellness services and chronic disease management; and
10. pediatric services including oral and vision care.

Also notable for cancer patients are several ACA provisions related to clinical trials. Starting in 2014, many insurers must cover the routine medical costs of patients participating in clinical trials (i.e., costs that would have otherwise been covered if the patient were not involved in the trial). In addition, insurers will no longer be able to deny coverage to individuals participating in cancer clinical trials.

The ACA also increases the health care system's emphasis on prevention. U.S. residents only receive half of recommended preventive care, but it is estimated that more frequent use of these services could save the United States more than 2 million life-years annually (Maciosek et al., 2010). As a result of the ACA, most health plans must cover certain preventive services, like mammography screening, without cost sharing. This includes services recommended by the U.S. Preventive Services Task Force (USPSTF), immunization schedules endorsed by the Centers for Disease Control and Prevention's Advisory Committee on Immunization Practices, and benefits for women and children suggested by the Health Resources and Services Administration.[3] Many, if not all, of the recommended services will also be available to Medicare and Medicaid beneficiaries. States will be eligible for increased Federal Medical Assistance Percentages (also referred to as federal matching funds, or FMAP) if their Medicaid program offers more optional preventive services (those classified as A or B by USPSTF) without cost sharing. A focus on prevention is essential for those at risk for cancer, not only because of increased access to screening and diagnosis but also because emphasis on concepts such as healthy eating, physical activity, and smoking cessation help to reduce risk factors for a wide variety of chronic diseases, including cancer.

Transforming Delivery Systems

In cancer care, a wide variety of treatment options is often available. Individuals' biological characteristics, personal preferences, and clinician recommendations should influence their treatment decisions. The goal of the Patient-Centered Outcomes Research Institute, established by the ACA, is to provide clinicians and patients with evidence-based research to help them make more informed health care decisions (PCORI, 2013).

As a part of the ACA, the U.S. Department of Health and Human Services (HHS) created a National Strategy for Quality Improvement in Health Care ("National Quality Strategy") to support national, state, and local efforts to improve health care quality. The National Quality Strategy

---

[3] *Federal Register.* 2010a. Interim final rules for group health plans and health insurance issuers relating to coverage of preventive services under the Patient Protection and Affordable Care Act. *Federal Register* 75(127):41726-41730.

encourages better care, with a focus on patient-centeredness, reliability, accessibility, and safety while also calling for attention to population health and affordability of care.

Controlling Rising Health Care Costs

The overall aim of the ACA is to make health insurance more available and affordable to Americans. While these efforts ultimately aim to reduce the cost of health care in this country, other provisions of the law focus more directly on cost-saving measures. For example, the ACA created the CMS Innovation Center to allow states and other stakeholders to test new ways to improve the health of their communities, with the ultimate goal of improving patient outcomes while reducing costs. The CMS Innovation Center is evaluating a number of delivery system and payment models, including accountable care organizations, patient-centered medical homes, and bundled payments (see Chapter 8).

KEY STAKEHOLDERS

This section briefly provides an overview of the major stakeholders involved in the cancer care delivery system. Improving the quality of cancer care requires coordination and commitment from all of these parties.

Patients, Families, and Family Caregivers

As mentioned above, there are approximately 14 million people in the United States with a history of cancer, and more than 1.6 million people are newly diagnosed with cancer each year (ACS, 2012c). These individuals, including their family members and caregivers, are the central focus of the cancer care delivery system. There are many nonprofit organizations that work to ensure that patients' cancer needs are met by educating patients, improving quality of care and access to care, promoting beneficial public policy, and providing financial support for research. The importance of patient-centered communication and shared decision making in cancer care is discussed in Chapter 3. The role of family caregivers is discussed in more detail in Chapter 4.

Health Care Clinicians

Many different professionals participate in cancer care, including medical oncologists, radiation oncologists, surgeons, primary care clinicians, geriatricians, nurses, advanced practice registered nurses, physician assistants, psychosocial workers, pharmacists, rehabilitation clinicians, spiritual workers, and other professionals. Ideally, these health care clinicians work together to provide patients with coordinated care across the cancer continuum. Most of these professionals are represented by organizations that work to further the interests of their members, and many of these professional societies conduct ongoing efforts designed to monitor, measure, and improve the quality of cancer care. In addition, these organizations are often involved in developing clinical practice guidelines, which provide members with guidance on the best treatment options and can be used to develop clinician and hospital quality measures. The role of the workforce providing care to patients with cancer in improving the quality of cancer care is discussed in more detail in Chapter 4. The role of professional organizations in developing a learning health care system is discussed in Chapter 6. The role of professional organizations in developing clinical practice guidelines and quality metrics is discussed in more detail in Chapter 7.

Payers

CMS is the federal agency that manages Medicare, the major insurer of U.S. adults over the age of 65. It currently insures more than 49 million Americans. As the second largest payer for cancer care behind private insurers, Medicare has a great deal of influence on the quality of cancer care in the United States (Tangka et al., 2010). This influence will only continue to expand: by 2030, Medicare will cover an estimated 70 percent of Americans who have cancer (reviewed in AHRQ, 2011a). Medicare provides beneficiaries with protection against the cost of many health care services, including inpatient hospital stays, skilled nursing facility stays, home health visits, hospice care, physician visits, outpatient services, and preventive services. It also includes a voluntary prescription drug benefit. Some limitations of the coverage, however, include relatively high deductibles, no limit on out-of-pocket spending, and no coverage for long-term care or dental services. Many beneficiaries have supplemental insurance to cover these gaps in coverage and high cost-sharing requirements (KFF, 2012). However, like Medicare, supplemental coverage can also come with high premiums or cost-sharing requirements, and thus, many low-income Medicare beneficiaries may be unable to acquire additional coverage.

CMS also funds Medicaid jointly with the states. It is the largest health insurance program and the dominant payer of long-term care in the United States. Medicaid currently covers more than 62 million Americans and will undergo massive expansion with the implementation of the ACA in 2014. Medicaid covers primarily low-income individuals and families, as well as individuals living with disabilities and complex health care needs. Medicaid also provides supplemental coverage to many older adults, as some individuals are eligible for both Medicare and Medicaid coverage (KFF, 2013a). Because Medicaid covers such a substantial portion of the U.S. population at disproportionate risk for cancer, it is likely one of the primary payers for cancer care.

The role of payers in improving the accessibility and affordability of cancer care is discussed in more detail in Chapters 3 and 8.

Government Organizations

In the United States, the federal government conducts a number of activities related to improving the quality of cancer care, including programs designed to fund research, conduct public health initiatives, improve patient safety, ensure an adequate health care workforce, and disseminate health information (see Table 2-6). The role of many federal agencies in cancer research is discussed in more detail in Chapter 5. The roles of many other agencies in improving the quality of cancer care are discussed throughout the report (e.g., CMS in the previous section).

Health Information Technology Organizations

Health information technology (health IT), such as electronic health records, plays an important role in advancing cancer care. Multiple organizations, including the Office of the National Coordinator for Health Information Technology, the National Cancer Institute, and CMS, participate in health IT activities that support the effective and meaningful use of such technologies. These organizations are discussed in more detail in Chapter 6.

Organizations Involved in Cancer Care Quality Measurement

A number of organizations track and evaluate the performance of health care clinicians, practices, and hospitals by comparing actual clinical practices to recommended practice. Recommended practices are established based on the best available evidence and existing clinical practice guidelines. In many cases, however, there is little evidence and no relevant clinical practice guidelines to support the recommended practices. This has been a substantial barrier to the development of performance measures (IOM, 2008). These organizations are discussed in more detail in Chapter 7.

TABLE 2-6 Examples of U.S. Governmental Organizations Involved in
Improving Quality of Cancer Care

Organization	Description
AHRQ	The branch of HHS focused on the quality, safety, efficiency, and effectiveness of health care. It funds research that helps people make more informed health care decisions and improves the quality of health care services. Its focus areas are: encouraging the use of evidence to inform health care decisions, fostering patient safety and quality improvement, and encouraging efficiency by increasing access to effective health care and reducing unnecessary costs.
CDC	The branch of HHS focused on promoting health; preventing disease, injury, and disability; and preparing for new and emerging health threats. The mission of the Division of Cancer Prevention and Control (DCPC) is to prevent and control cancer. DCPC works with various groups at the national and state levels to collect data on cancer incidence, mortality, risk factors, and cancer screening; conduct and support research and evaluation; build capacity and partnerships; and educate clinicians, policy makers, and the public. Examples of DCPC programs include the National Breast and Cervical Cancer Early Detection Program, the National Comprehensive Cancer Control Program, the National Program of Cancer Registries, and the Colorectal Cancer Control Program.
CMS	The federal agency that manages Medicare, the major insurer of U.S. adults over the age of 65. It currently insures over 49 million Americans (see discussion in the section on payers). It also funds Medicaid jointly with the states. Medicaid is run by the states to provide health insurance coverage to individuals with lower incomes.
FDA	The regulatory agency that ensures the safety, efficacy, and security of drugs, biological products, and medical devices. The FDA's Office of Hematology and Oncology Products oversees the development, approval, and regulation of drug and biologic treatments for cancer, therapies for cancer prevention, and products for treatment of nonmalignant hematologic conditions. The FDA's Cancer Liaison Program brings the patient advocate's perspective into the evaluation of new cancer drugs and meets with patient advocacy groups to learn their viewpoints and address their concerns regarding cancer drug development.

TABLE 2-6 Continued

Organization	Description
HRSA	The federal agency charged with improving access to health care services for people who are uninsured, vulnerable, or underserved. HRSA offers training and financial support to clinicians caring for these populations. HRSA coordinates the National Center for Health Workforce Analysis, which collects workforce data, develops tools for projecting workforce supply and demand, and evaluates workforce policies and programs. HRSA also administers the National Health Service Corps, which provides scholarships and loan repayment to primary care clinicians practicing in areas with workforce shortages.
NCI	The section of NIH responsible for cancer research and training. The NCI coordinates the National Cancer Program, which conducts research, training, and the dissemination of information on cancer. The NCI supports cancer research conducted at universities, foundations, hospitals, and businesses through grants and cooperative agreements; conducts its own research; provides career awards, training grants, and fellowships for basic and clinical research and treatment programs; supports a national network of cancer centers; and supports cancer research infrastructure through construction grants.
NIA	The section of NIH that supports research on the aging process and diseases and conditions associated with growing older. NIA supports the development of research and clinician scientists in aging and disseminates information about aging to the public, health professionals, and the scientific community.

NOTE: AHRQ = Agency for Healthcare Research and Quality; CDC = Centers for Disease and Control Prevention; CMS = Centers for Medicare & Medicaid Services; FDA = Food and Drug Administration; HHS = U.S. Department of Health and Human Services; HRSA = Health Resources and Services Administration; NCI = National Cancer Institute; NIA = National Institute on Aging; NIH = National Institutes of Health.
SOURCES: AHRQ, 2012a; CDC, 2010, 2011; CMS, 2012; FDA, 2012a,b,c; HRSA, 2012, 2013a,b; NCI, 2012b; NIA, 2012.

REFERENCES

AACR (American Association for Cancer Research). 2012. *AACR cancer progress report 2012: Making research count for patients: A new day.* Philadelphia, PA: American Association for Cancer Resarch.

Abernethy, A. P., G. Raman, E. M. Balk, J. M. Hammond, L. A. Orlando, J. L. Wheeler, J. Lau, and D. C. McCrory. 2009. Systematic review: Reliability of compendia methods for off-label oncology indications. *Annals of Internal Medicine* 150(5):336-343.

Abernethy, A. P., R. R. Coeytaux, K. Carson, D. McCrory, S. Y. Barbour, M. Gradison, R. J. Irvine, and J. L. Wheeler. 2010. *Report on the evidence regarding off-label indications for targeted therapies used in cancer treatment: Technology assessment report.* Rockville, MD: Agency for Healthcare Research and Quality.

ACS (American Cancer Society). 2008. *Cancer facts and figures 2008.* Atlanta, GA: American Cancer Society.

———. 2011. *Cancer facts & figures.* Atlanta, GA: American Cancer Society.

———. 2012a. *Cancer facts & figures for Hispanics/Latinos 2012-2014.* Atlanta, GA: American Cancer Society.

———. 2012b. *Cancer facts & figures 2012.* Atlanta, GA: American Cancer Society.

———. 2012c. *Cancer treatment and survivorship: Facts and figures 2012-2013.* Atlanta, GA: American Cancer Society.

———. 2013a. *Cancer facts & figures for African Americans 2013-2014.* Atlanta, GA: American Cancer Society.

———. 2013b. *Cancer facts & figures 2013.* Atlanta, GA: American Cancer Society.

ACSCAN (American Cancer Society Cancer Action Network). 2009. *Cancer disparities: A chartbook.* Washington, DC: American Cancer Society Cancer Action Network.

AHR (Alliance for Health Reform). 2012. *High and rising costs of health care in the U.S. The challenge: Changing the trajectory.* http://www.allhealth.org/publications/Alliance_for_Health_Reform_121.pdf (accessed March 12, 2013).

AHRQ (Agency for Healthcare Research and Quality). 2011a. *Utilization and cost of anticancer biologic products among Medicare beneficiaries, 2006-2009. Anticancer biologics. Data Points #6.* http://www.ncbi.nlm.nih.gov/books/NBK65148/pdf/dp6.pdf (accessed March 24, 2013).

———. 2011b. *National healthcare disparities report.* Rockville, MD: U.S. Department of Health and Human Services.

———. 2012a. *AHRQ at a glance.* http://www.ahrq.gov/about/mission/glance/index.html (accessed June 26, 2013).

———. 2012b. *National healthcare dispartities report.* Rockville, MD: U.S. Department of Health and Human Services.

Andriole, G. L., E. D. Crawford, R. L. Grubb, 3rd, S. S. Buys, D. Chia, T. R. Church, M. N. Fouad, C. Isaacs, P. A. Kvale, D. J. Reding, J. L. Weissfeld, L. A. Yokochi, B. O'Brien, L. R. Ragard, J. D. Clapp, J. M. Rathmell, T. L. Riley, A. W. Hsing, G. Izmirlian, P. F. Pinsky, B. S. Kramer, A. B. Miller, J. K. Gohagan, and P. C. Prorok. 2012. Prostate cancer screening in the randomized Prostate, Lung, Colorectal, and Ovarian Cancer Screening Trial: Mortality results after 13 years of follow-up. *Journal of the National Cancer Institute* 104(2):125-132.

Audisio, R. A., H. Ramesh, W. E. Longo, A. P. Zbar, and D. Pope. 2005. Preoperative assessment of surgical risk in oncogeriatric patients. *Oncologist* 10(4):262-268.

Avorn, J., and H. H. Gurwitz. 1997. Principles of pharmacology. In *Geriatric Medicine*, 3rd ed., edited by C. K. Cassel, H. J. Cohen, E. B. Larson and D. E. Meier. New York: Springer. Pp. 55-70.

Ayanian, J., A. Zaslavsky, E. Guadagnoli, C. Fuchs, K. Yost, C. Creech, R. Cress, L. O'Connor, D. West, and W. Wright. 2005. Patients' perceptions of quality of care for colorectal cancer by race, ethnicity, and language. *Journal of Clinical Oncology* 23(27):6576-6586.

Bach, P. B. 2009. Limits on Medicare's ability to control rising spending on cancer drugs. *New England Journal of Medicine* 360(6):626-633.

Bach, P. B., L. B. Saltz, and R. E. Wittes. 2012. In cancer care, cost matters. *New York Times*, October 15, 2012, A25.

Baicker, K., and J. S. Skinner. 2011. *Health care spending growth and the future of U.S. tax rates.* http://www.nber.org/papers/w16772 (accessed March 12, 2013).

Bajetta, E., G. Procopio, L. Celio, L. Gattinoni, S. Della Torre, L. Mariani, L. Catena, R. Ricotta, R. Longarini, N. Zilembo, and R. Buzzoni. 2005. Safety and efficacy of two different doses of Capecitabine in the treatment of advanced breast cancer in older women. *Journal of Clinical Oncology* 23(10):2155-2161.

Baker, S. D., and L. B. Grochow. 1997. Pharmacology of cancer chemotherapy in the older person. *Clinics in Geriatric Medicine* 13(1):169-183.

Barret, M., D. Malka, T. Aparicio, C. Dalban, C. Locher, J. M. Sabate, S. Louafi, T. Mansourbakht, F. Bonnetain, A. Attar, and J. Taieb. 2011. Nutritional status affects treatment tolerability and survival in metastatic colorectal cancer patients: Results of an AGEO prospective multicenter study. *Oncology* 81(5-6):395-402.

Beers, M. H. 1997. Explicit criteria for determining potentially inappropriate medication use by the elderly. An update. *Archives of Internal Medicine* 157(14):1531-1536.

Beers, M. H., J. G. Ouslander, I. Rollingher, D. B. Reuben, J. Brooks, and J. C. Beck. 1991. Explicit criteria for determining inappropriate medication use in nursing home residents. UCLA Division of Geriatric Medicine. *Archives of Internal Medicine* 151(9):1825-1832.

Birim, O., A. P. Kappetein, R. J. van Klaveren, and A. J. Bogers. 2006. Prognostic factors in non-small cell lung cancer surgery. *European Journal of Surgical Oncology* 32(1):12-23.

Bleyer, A., C. Ulrich, and S. Martin. 2012. Young adults, cancer, health insurance, socioeconomic status, and the Patient Protection and Affordable Care Act. *Cancer* 118(24): 6018-6021.

Booth, C. M., G. Li, J. Zhang-Salomons, and W. J. Mackillop. 2010. The impact of socioeconomic status on stage of cancer at diagnosis and survival. *Cancer* 116(17):4160-4167.

BPC (Bipartisan Policy Center). 2012. *What is driving U.S. health care spending?* http://bipartisan policy.org/sites/default/files/BPC%20Health%20Care%20Cost%20Drivers%20 Brief%20Sept%202012.pdf (accessed December 16, 2012).

Bregnhoj, L., S. Thirstrup, M. B. Kristensen, L. Bjerrum, and J. Sonne. 2009. Combined intervention programme reduces inappropriate prescribing in elderly patients exposed to polypharmacy in primary care. *European Journal of Clinical Pharmacology* 65(2):199-207.

Bruno, R., N. Vivier, C. Veyrat-Follet, G. Montay, and G. R. Rhodes. 2001. Population pharmacokinetics and pharmacokinetic-pharmacodynamic relationships for docetaxel. *Investigational New Drugs* 19(2):163-169..

CBO (Congressional Budget Office). 2012a. *The 2012 long-term budget outlook.* http:// www.cbo.gov/sites/default/files/cbofiles/attachments/06-05-Long-Term_Budget_ Outlook_2.pdf (accessed December 14, 2012).

———. 2012b. *Health care.* https://cbo.gov/topics/health-care (accessed December 16, 2012).

———. 2013a. *The budget and economic outlook: Fiscal years 2013 to 2023. Publication Number 4649.* https://cbo.gov/sites/default/files/cbofiles/attachments/43907-Budget Outlook.pdf (accessed March 12, 2013).

———. 2013b. How have CBO's projections of spending for Medicare and Medicaid changed since the August 2012 baseline? http://www.cbo.gov/publication/43947 (accessed June 25, 2013).

————. 2013c. The budget and economic outlook: Fiscal years 2013 to 2023. http://www.cbo.gov/publication/43907 (accessed June 25, 2013).

CDC (Centers for Disease Control and Prevention). 2010. *Vision, mission, core values, and pledge.* http://www.cdc.gov/about/organization/mission.htm (accessed June 26, 2013).

————. 2011. *About CDC's Division of Cancer Prevention and Control.* http://www.cdc.gov/cancer/dcpc/about/ (accessed June 27, 2013).

————. 2012a. *Cancer among men.* http://www.cdc.gov/cancer/dcpc/data/men.htm (accessed August 7, 2012).

————. 2012b. *Cancer among women.* http://www.cdc.gov/cancer/dcpc/data/women.htm (accessed August 7, 2012).

————. 2013. *Adult cigarette smoking in the United States: Current estimate.* http://www.cdc.gov/tobacco/data_statistics/fact_sheets/adult_data/cig_smoking (accessed June 7, 2013).

Chrischilles, E. A., B. L. Carter, B. C. Lund, L. M. Rubenstein, S. S. Chen-Hardee, M. D. Voelker, T. R. Park, and A. K. Kuehl. 2004. Evaluation of the Iowa Medicaid Pharmaceutical Case Management Program. *Journal of the American Pharmaceutical Association* 44(3):337-349.

Clauson, K. A., W. A. Marsh, H. H. Polen, M. J. Seamon, and B. I. Ortiz. 2007. Clinical decision support tools: Analysis of online drug information databases. *BMC Medical Informatics and Decision Making* 7:7.

Clegg, L. X., M. E. Reichman, B. A. Miller, B. F. Hankey, G. K. Singh, Y. D. Lin, M. T. Goodman, C. F. Lynch, S. M. Schwartz, V. W. Chen, L. Bernstein, S. L. Gomez, J. J. Graff, C. C. Lin, N. J. Johnson, and B. K. Edwards. 2009. Impact of socioeconomic status on cancer incidence and stage at diagnosis: Selected findings from the surveillance, epidemiology, and end results: National Longitudinal Mortality Study. *Cancer Causes and Control* 20(4):417-435.

CMS (Centers for Medicare & Medicaid Services). 2012. *Centers for Medicare & Medicaid Services (CMS).* http://www.cms.gov (accessed April 26, 2012).

————. 2013a. *National health expenditure data. Historical.* https://www.cms.gov/Research-Statistics-Data-and-Systems/Statistics-Trends-and-Reports/NationalHealthExpendData/NationalHealthAccountsHistorical.html (accessed March 12, 2013).

————. 2013b. *National health expenditure data. Projected.* https://www.cms.gov/Research-Statistics-Data-and-Systems/Statistics-Trends-and-Reports/NationalHealthExpendData/NationalHealthAccountsProjected.html (accessed March 12, 2013).

Conti, R. 2012. Zaltrap economics 101: The pricing and repricing of an expensive drug. *Cancer Letter* 38(43):1-4.

Crivellari, D., M. Bonetti, M. Castiglione-Gertsch, R. D. Gelber, C. M. Rudenstam, B. Thürlimann, K. N. Price, A. S. Coates, C. Hürny, J. Bernhard, J. Lindtner, J. Collins, H. J. Senn, F. Cavalli, J. Forbes, A. Gudgeon, E. Simoncini, H. Cortes-Funes, A. Veronesi, M. Fey, and A. Goldhirsch. 2000. Burdens and benefits of adjuvant Cyclophosphamide, Methotrexate, and Fluorouracil and Tamoxifen for elderly patients with breast cancer: The International Breast Cancer Study Group Trial VII. *Journal of Clinical Oncology* 18(7):1412-1422.

Crotty, M., D. Rowett, L. Spurling, L. C. Giles, and P. A. Phillips. 2004. Does the addition of a pharmacist transition coordinator improve evidence-based medication management and health outcomes in older adults moving from the hospital to a long-term care facility? Results of a randomized, controlled trial. *American Journal of Geriatric Pharmacotherapy* 2(4):257-264.

Dacal, K., S. M. Sereika, and S. L. Greenspan. 2006. Quality of life in prostate cancer patients taking androgen deprivation therapy. *Journal of the American Geriatrics Society* 54(1):85-90.

Davis, R. G., C. A. Hepfinger, K. A. Sauer, and M. S. Wilhardt. 2007. Retrospective evaluation of medication appropriateness and clinical pharmacist drug therapy recommendations for home-based primary care veterans. *American Journal of Geriatric Pharmacotherapy* 5(1):40-47.

de Moor, J. S., A. B. Mariotto, C. Parry, C. M. Alfano, L. Padgett, E. E. Kent, L. Forsythe, S. Scoppa, M. Hachey, and J. H. Rowland. 2013. Cancer survivors in the United States: Prevalence across the survivorship trajectory and implications for care. *Cancer Epidemiology, Biomarkers & Prevention* 22(4):561-570.

Dees, E. C., S. O'Reilly, S. N. Goodman, S. Sartorius, M. A. Levine, R. J. Jones, L. B. Grochow, R. C. Donehower, and J. H. Fetting. 2000. A prospective pharmacologic evaluation of age-related toxicity of adjuvant chemotherapy in women with breast cancer. *Cancer Investigation* 18(6):521-529.

Dewys, W. D., C. Begg, P. T. Lavin, P. R. Band, J. M. Bennett, J. R. Bertino, M. H. Cohen, H. O. Douglass, Jr., P. F. Engstrom, E. Z. Ezdinli, J. Horton, G. J. Johnson, C. G. Moertel, M. M. Oken, C. Perlia, C. Rosenbaum, M. N. Silverstein, R. T. Skeel, R. W. Sponzo, and D. C. Tormey. 1980. Prognostic effect of weight loss prior to chemotherapy in cancer patients. Eastern Cooperative Oncology Group. *American Journal of Medicine* 69(4):491-497.

Dodge, H. H., T. Kadowaki, T. Hayakawa, M. Yamakawa, A. Sekikawa, and H. Ueshima. 2005. Cognitive impairment as a strong predictor of incident disability in specific ADL-IADL tasks among community-dwelling elders: The Azuchi Study. *Gerontologist* 45(2):222-230.

Duthie, E. H. 2004. Physiology of aging: Relevance to symptoms, perceptions, and treatment tolerance. In *Comprehensive Geriatric Oncology*, 2nd ed., edited by L. Balducci, G. H. Lyman, W. B. Ershler, and M. Extermann. Abingdon, Oxon: Taylor and Francis. Pp. 367-397.

Egger, T., H. Dormann, G. Ahne, U. Runge, A. Neubert, M. Criegee-Rieck, K. G. Gassmann, and K. Brune. 2003. Identification of adverse drug reactions in geriatric inpatients using a computerised drug database. *Drugs and Aging* 20(10):769-776.

Eheman, C., S. J. Henley, R. Ballard-Barbash, E. J. Jacobs, M. J. Schymura, A.-M. Noone, L. Pan, R. N. Anderson, J. E. Fulton, B. A. Kohler, A. Jemal, E. Ward, M. Plescia, L. A. G. Ries, and B. K. Edwards. 2012. Annual report to the nation on the status of cancer, 1975-2008, featuring cancers associated with excess weight and lack of sufficient physical activity. *Cancer* 118(9):2338-2366.

Elkin, E. B., and P. B. Bach. 2010. Cancer's next frontier: Addressing high and increasing costs. *Journal of the American Medical Association* 303(11):1086-1087.

Elkin, E. B., S. H. M. Kim, E. S. Casper, D. W. Kissane, and D. Schrag. 2007. Desire for information and involvement in treatment decisions: Elderly cancer patients' preferences and their physicians' perceptions. *Journal of Clinical Oncology* 25:5275-5280.

Elmer, G. W., W. E. Lafferty, P. T. Tyree, and B. K. Lind. 2007. Potential interactions between complementary/alternative products and conventional medicines in a Medicare population. *Annals of Pharmacotherapy* 41(10):1617-1624.

Emanuel, E. J., and V. R. Fuchs. 2008. Who really pays for health care? The myth of "shared responsibility." *Journal of the American Medical Association* 299(9):1057-1059.

Emanuel, E., N. Tanden, S. Altman, S. Armstrong, D. Berwick, F. de Brantes, M. Calsyn, M. Chernew, J. Colmers, D. Cutler, T. Daschle, P. Egerman, B. Kocher, A. Milstein, E. Oshima Lee, J. D. Podesta, U. Reinhardt, M. Rosenthal, J. Sharfstein, S. Shortell, A. Stern, P. R. Orszag, and T. Spiro. 2012. A systemic approach to containing health care spending. *New England Journal of Medicine* 367(10):949-954.

Emanuel, E., A. P. Abernethy, J. E. Bekelman, O. Brawley, R. L. Erwin, P. A. Ganz, J. S. Goodwin, R. J. Green, J. Gruman, J. R. Hoverman, J. Mendelsohn, L. N. Newcomer, J. M. Peppercorn, S. D. Ramsey, L. E. Schnipper, F. M. Schnell, D. Schrag, Y.-C. T. Shih, J. D. Sprandio, T. J. Smith, A. P. Staddon, and J. S. Temel. 2013. A plan to fix cancer care. *New York Times*, March 23, 2013, SR14.

Espinosa de los Monteros, K., and L. C. Gallo. 2011. The relevance of fatalism in the study of Latinas' cancer screening behavior: A systematic review of the literature. *International Journal of Behavioral Medicine* 18(4):310-318.

Extermann, M., J. Overcash, G. H. Lyman, J. Parr, and L. Balducci. 1998. Comorbidity and functional status are independent in older cancer patients. *Journal of Clinical Oncology* 16(4):1582-1587.

Extermann, M., L. Balducci, and G. H. Lyman. 2000. What threshold for adjuvant therapy in older breast cancer patients? *Journal of Clinical Oncology* 18(8):1709-1717.

Extermann, M., I. Boler, R. R. Reich, G. H. Lyman, R. H. Brown, J. DeFelice, R. M. Levine, E. T. Lubiner, P. Reyes, F. J. Schreiber, 3rd, and L. Balducci. 2012. Predicting the risk of chemotherapy toxicity in older patients: The Chemotherapy Risk Assessment Scale for High-Age Patients (CRASH) score. *Cancer* 118(13):3377-3386.

FDA (Food and Drug Administration). 2012a. *Cancer liaison Program.* http://www.fda.gov/forconsumers/byaudience/forpatientadvocates/cancerliaisonprogram/default.htm (accessed April 26, 2012).

———. 2012b. *About FDA: What we do.* http://www.fda.gov/AboutFDA/WhatWeDo/default.htm (accessed June 27, 2013).

———. 2012c. *Office of Hematology and Oncology Products.* http://www.fda.gov/AboutFDA/CentersOffices/OfficeofMedicalProductsandTobacco/CDER/ucm091745.htm (accessed June 27, 2013).

Fick, D. M., J. W. Cooper, W. E. Wade, J. L. Waller, J. R. Maclean, and M. H. Beers. 2003. Updating the Beers criteria for potentially inappropriate medication use in older adults: Results of a U.S. consensus panel of experts. *Archives of Internal Medicine* 163(22):2716-2724.

Firat, S., M. Bousamra, E. Gore, and R. W. Byhardt. 2002. Comorbidity and KPS are independent prognostic factors in stage I non-small-cell lung cancer. *International Journal of Radiation Oncology, Biology, and Physics* 52(4):1047-1057.

Foster, J. A., G. D. Salinas, D. Mansell, J. C. Williamson, and L. L. Casebeer. 2010. How does older age influence oncologists' cancer management? *Oncologist* 15(6):584-592.

Frasci, G., V. Lorusso, N. Panza, P. Comella, G. Nicolella, A. Bianco, G. De Cataldis, A. Iannelli, D. Bilancia, M. Belli, B. Massidda, F. Piantedosi, G. Comella, and M. De Lena. 2000. Gemcitabine plus Vinorelbine versus Vinorelbine alone in elderly patients with advanced non-small-cell lung cancer. *Journal of Clinical Oncology* 18(13):2529-2536.

Fried, T. R., E. H. Bradley, V. R. Towle, and H. Allore. 2002. Understanding the treatment preferences of seriously ill patients. *New England Journal of Medicine* 346(14):1061-1066.

Fuchs, V. R. 2013. The gross domestic product and health care spending. *New England Journal of Medicine*. DOI: 10.1056/NEJMp1305298 (epub ahead of print).

Goldberg, P. 2013. Paying for cancer drugs: Zaltrap's U.S. price has dropped by nearly half since introduction. *Cancer Letter* 39(26): 1-9.

Goldberg, R. M., I. Tabah-Fisch, H. Bleiberg, A. de Gramont, C. Tournigand, T. Andre, M. L. Rothenberg, E. Green, and D. J. Sargent. 2006. Pooled analysis of safety and efficacy of Oxaliplatin plus Fluorouracil/Leucovorin administered bimonthly in elderly patients with colorectal cancer. *Journal of Clinical Oncology* 24(25):4085-4091.

Gomez, H., M. Hidalgo, L. Casanova, R. Colomer, D. L. Pen, J. Otero, W. Rodriguez, C. Carracedo, H. Cortes-Funes, and C. Vallejos. 1998. Risk factors for treatment-related death in elderly patients with aggressive non-Hodgkin's lymphoma: Results of a multivariate analysis. *Journal of Clinical Oncology* 16(6):2065-2069.

Graham, M. A., G. F. Lockwood, D. Greenslade, S. Brienza, M. Bayssas, and E. Gamelin. 2000. Clinical pharmacokinetics of Oxaliplatin: a critical review. *Clinical Cancer Research* 6(4):1205-1218.

Guidi, T. U. 2013. Going hospital based: Nuts and bolts operational issues. *Journal of Oncology Practice* 9(2):70-72.

Gurwitz, J. H. 2004. Polypharmacy: A new paradigm for quality drug therapy in the elderly? *Archives of Internal Medicine* 164(18):1957-1959.

Hajjar, E. R., A. C. Cafiero, and J. T. Hanlon. 2007. Polypharmacy in elderly patients. *American Journal of Geriatric Pharmacotherapy* 5(4):345-351.

Haller, D. G., P. J. Catalano, J. S. Macdonald, M. A. O'Rourke, M. S. Frontiera, D. V. Jackson, and R. J. Mayer. 2005. Phase III study of Fluorouracil, Leucovorin, and Levamisole in high-risk stage II and III colon cancer: Final report of Intergroup 0089. *Journal of Clinical Oncology* 23(34):8671-8678.

Halpern, M., J. Bian, E. Ward, N. Schrag, and A. Chen. 2007. Insurance status and stage of cancer at diagnosis among women with breast cancer. *Cancer* 110(2):403-411.

Hanlon, J. T., K. E. Schmader, G. P. Samsa, M. Weinberger, K. M. Uttech, I. K. Lewis, H. J. Cohen, and J. R. Feussner. 1992. A method for assessing drug therapy appropriateness. *Journal of Clinical Epidemiology* 45(10):1045-1051.

Hanlon, J. T., M. Weinberger, G. P. Samsa, K. E. Schmader, K. M. Uttech, I. K. Lewis, P. A. Cowper, P. B. Landsman, H. J. Cohen, and J. R. Feussner. 1996. A randomized, controlled trial of a clinical pharmacist intervention to improve inappropriate prescribing in elderly outpatients with polypharmacy. *American Journal of Medicine* 100(4):428-437.

Hanlon, J. T., K. E. Schmader, C. M. Ruby, and M. Weinberger. 2001. Suboptimal prescribing in older inpatients and outpatients. *Journal of the American Geriatrics Society* 49(2):200-209.

Harlan, L., A. Greene, L. Clegg, M. Mooney, J. Stevens, and M. Brown. 2005. Insurance status and the use of guideline therapy in the treatment of selected cancers. *Journal of Clinical Oncology* 23(36):9079-9088.

Hartman, M., A. B. Martin, J. Benson, and A. Catlin. 2013. National health spending in 2011: Overall growth remains low, but some payers and services show signs of acceleration. *Health Affairs (Millwood)* 32(1):87-99.

Holmes, H. M., G. A. Sachs, J. W. Shega, G. W. Hougham, D. Cox Hayley, and W. Dale. 2008. Integrating palliative medicine into the care of persons with advanced dementia: Identifying appropriate medication use. *Journal of the American Geriatrics Society* 56(7):1306-1311.

HRSA (Health Resources and Services Administration). 2012. *National Center for Health Workforce Analysis.* http://bhpr.hrsa.gov/healthworkforce/ (accessed April 26, 2012).

———. 2013a. *About HRSA.* http://www.hrsa.gov/about/index.html (accessed June 27, 2013).

———. 2013b. *About the NHSC.* http://nhsc.hrsa.gov/corpsexperience/aboutus/index.html (accessed June 27, 2013).

Hurria, A., A. Hurria, K. Brogan, K. S. Panageas, C. Pearce, L. Norton, A. Jakubowski, J. Howard, and C. Hudis. 2005. Effect of creatinine clearance on patterns of toxicity in older patients receiving adjuvant chemotherapy for breast cancer. *Drugs and Aging* 22(9):785-791.

Hurria, A., A. Hurria, E. Zuckerman, K. S. Panageas, M. Fornier, G. D'Andrea, C. Dang, M. Moasser, M. Robson, A. Seidman, V. Currie, C. VanPoznak, M. Theodoulou, M. S. Lachs, and C. Hudis. 2006. A prospective, longitudinal study of the functional status and quality of life of older patients with breast cancer receiving adjuvant chemotherapy. *Journal of American Geriatrics Society* 54(7):1119-1124.

Hurria, A., F. L. Wong, D. Villaluna, S. Bhatia, C. T. Chung, J. Mortimer, S. Hurvitz, and A. Naeim. 2008. Role of age and health in treatment recommendations for older adults with breast cancer: The perspective of oncologists and primary care providers. *Journal of Clinical Oncology* 26(33):5386-5392.

Hurria, A., D. Li, K. Hansen, S. Patil, R. Gupta, C. Nelson, S. M. Lichtman, W. P. Tew, P. Hamlin, E. Zuckerman, J. Gardes, S. Limaye, M. Lachs, and E. Kelly. 2009. Distress in older patients with cancer. *Journal of Clinical Oncology* 27(26):4346-4351.

Hurria, A., C. T. Cirrincione, H. B. Muss, A. B. Kornblith, W. Barry, A. S. Artz, L. Schmieder, R. Ansari, W. P. Tew, D. Weckstein, J. Kirshner, K. Togawa, K. Hansen, V. Katheria, R. Stone, I. Galinsky, J. Postiglione, and H. J. Cohen. 2011a. Implementing a geriatric assessment in cooperative group clinical cancer trials: CALGB 360401. *Journal of Clinical Oncology* 29(10):1290-1296.

Hurria, A., K. Togawa, S. G. Mohile, C. Owusu, H. D. Klepin, C. P. Gross, S. M. Lichtman, A. Gajra, S. Bhatia, V. Katheria, S. Klapper, K. Hansen, R. Ramani, M. Lachs, F. L. Wong, and W. P. Tew. 2011b. Predicting chemotherapy toxicity in older adults with cancer: A prospective multicenter study. *Journal of Clinical Oncology* 29(25):3457-3465.

Hutchins, L. F., J. M. Unger, J. J. Crowley, J. Charles, A. Coltman, and K. S. Albain. 1999. Underrepresentation of Patients 65 Years of Age or Older in Cancer-Treatment Trials. *New England Journal of Medicine* 341:2061-2067.

Inouye, S. K., P. N. Peduzzi, J. T. Robison, J. S. Hughes, R. I. Horwitz, and J. Concato. 1998. Importance of functional measures in predicting mortality among older hospitalized patients. *Journal of the American Medical Association* 279(15):1187-1193.

IOM (Institute of Medicine). 1999. *The unequal burden of cancer: An assessment of NIH research and programs for ethnic minorities and the medically underserved.* Washington, DC: National Academy Press.

————. 2003. *Unequal treatment: Confronting racial and ethnic disparities in health care.* Washington, DC: The National Academies Press.

————. 2008. *Knowing what works in health care: A roadmap for the nation.* Washington, DC: The National Academies Press.

————. 2010. *Policy issues in the development of personalized medicine in oncology: Workshop summary.* Washington, DC: The National Academies Press.

————. 2012a. *Best care at lower cost: The path to continuously learning health care in America.* Washington, DC: The National Academies Press.

————. 2012b. *Evolution of translational omics: Lessons learned and the path forward.* Washington, DC: The National Academies Press.

————. 2013. *Delivering affordable cancer care in the 21st century: Workshop summary.* Washington, DC: The National Academies Press.

IOM and NRC (National Research Council). 2005. *From cancer patient to cancer survivor: Lost in transition.* Washington, DC: The National Academies Press.

Kantarjian, H., and experts in chronic myeloid leukemia. 2013. The price of drugs for chronic myeloid leukemia (CML); A reflection of the unsustainable prices of cancer drugs: From the perspective of a large group of CML experts. *Blood* 121(22):4439-4442.

Keating, N. L., M. Norredam, M. B. Landrum, H. A. Huskamp, and E. Meara. 2005. Physical and mental health status of older long-term cancer survivors. *Journal of the American Geriatrics Society* 53(12):2145-2152.

KFF (Kaiser Family Foundation). 2012. *Medicare at a glance: Fact sheet*. http://www.kff.org/medicare/upload/1066-14.pdf (accessed May 1, 2012).

————. 2013a. *Medicaid: A primer—key information on the nation's health coverage program for low-income people*. http://kff.org/medicaid/issue-brief/medicaid-a-primer (accessed August 5, 2013).

————. 2013b. *Overweight and obesity rates for adults by gender*. http://kff.org/other/state-indicator/adult-overweightobesity-rate-by-gender (accessed June 7, 2013).

————. 2013c. *Status of state action on the Medicaid expansion decision, as of June 20, 2013*. http://kff.org/medicaid/state-indicator/state-activity-around-expanding-medicaid-under-the-affordable-care-act/# (accessed June 26, 2013).

————. 2013d. *State decisions for creating health care exchanges, as of May 28, 2013*. http://kff.org/health-reform/state-indicator/health-insurance-exchanges (accessed June 26, 2013).

Kolata, G. 2012. Knotty challenges in health care costs. *The New York Times*, March 6. http://www.nytimes.com/2012/03/06/health/policy/an-interview-with-victor-fuchs-on-health-care-costs.html (accessed December 16, 2012).

Kornblith, A. B., J. E. Herndon, 2nd, E. Zuckerman, C. M. Viscoli, R. I. Horwitz, M. R. Cooper, L. Harris, K. H. Tkaczuk, M. C. Perry, D. Budman, L. C. Norton, and J. Holland. 2001. Social support as a buffer to the psychological impact of stressful life events in women with breast cancer. *Cancer* 91(2):443-454.

Kornblith, A. B., J. E. Herndon, 2nd, R. B. Weiss, C. Zhang, E. L. Zuckerman, S. Rosenberg, M. Mertz, D. Payne, M. Jane Massie, J. F. Holland, P. Wingate, L. Norton, and J. C. Holland. 2003. Long-term adjustment of survivors of early-stage breast carcinoma, 20 years after adjuvant chemotherapy. *Cancer* 98(4):679-689.

Kroenke, C. H., L. D. Kubzansky, E. S. Schernhammer, M. D. Holmes, and I. Kawachi. 2006. Social networks, social support, and survival after breast cancer diagnosis. *Journal of Clinical Oncology* 24(7):1105-1111.

Landi, F., G. Onder, G. Gambassi, C. Pedone, P. Carbonin, and R. Bernabei. 2000. Body mass index and mortality among hospitalized patients. *Archives of Internal Medicine* 160(17):2641-2644.

Lee, S. J., K. Lindquist, M. R. Segal, and K. E. Covinsky. 2006. Development and validation of a prognostic index for 4-year mortality in older adults. *Journal of the American Medical Association* 295(7):801-808.

Leighl, N. B., H. L. Shepherd, P. N. Butow, S. J. Clarke, M. McJannett, P. J. Beale, N. R. Wilcken, M. J. Moore, E. X. Chen, D. Goldstein, L. Horvath, J. J. Knox, M. Krzyzanowska, A. M. Oza, R. Feld, D. Hedley, W. Xu, and M. H. Tattersall. 2011. Supporting treatment decision making in advanced cancer: A randomized trial of a decision aid for patients with advanced colorectal cancer considering chemotherapy. *Journal of Clinical Oncology* 29(15):2077-2084.

The Lewin Group, Inc. 2007. *Cost-effectiveness considerations in the approval and adoption of new health technologies. Final report and case studies*. http://aspe.hhs.gov/sp/reports/2007/CECHT (accessed August 2, 2013).

Maciosek, M. V., A. B. Coffield, T. J. Flottemesch, N. M. Edwards, and L. I. Solberg. 2010. Greater use of preventive services in U.S. health care could save lives at little or no cost. *Health Affairs (Millwood)* 29(9):1656-1660.

Maione, P., F. Perrone, C. Gallo, L. Manzione, F. Piantedosi, S. Barbera, S. Cigolari, F. Rosetti, E. Piazza, S. F. Robbiati, O. Bertetto, S. Novello, M. R. Migliorino, A. Favaretto, M. Spatafora, F. Ferrau, L. Frontini, A. Bearz, L. Repetto, C. Gridelli, E. Barletta, M. L. Barzelloni, R. V. Iaffaioli, E. De Maio, M. Di Maio, G. De Feo, G. Sigoriello, P. Chiodini, A. Cioffi, V. Guardasole, V. Angelini, A. Rossi, D. Bilancia, D. Germano, A. Lamberti, V. Pontillo, L. Brancaccio, F. Renda, F. Romano, G. Esani, A. Gambaro, O. Vinante, G. Azzarello, M. Clerici, R. Bollina, P. Belloni, M. Sannicolo, L. Ciuffreda, G. Parello, M. Cabiddu, C. Sacco, A. Sibau, G. Porcile, F. Castiglione, O. Ostellino, S. Monfardini, M. Stefani, G. Scagliotti, G. Selvaggi, F. De Marinis, O. Martelli, G. Gasparini, A. Morabito, D. Gattuso, G. Colucci, D. Galetta, F. Giotta, V. Gebbia, N. Borsellino, A. Testa, E. Malaponte, M. A. Capuano, M. Angiolillo, F. Sollitto, U. Tirelli, S. Spazzapan, V. Adamo, G. Altavilla, A. Scimone, M. R. Hopps, F. Tartamella, G. P. Ianniello, V. Tinessa, G. Failla, R. Bordonaro, N. Gebbia, M. R. Valerio, M. D'Aprile, E. Veltri, M. Tonato, S. Darwish, S. Romito, F. Carrozza, S. Barni, A. Ardizzoia, G. M. Corradini, G. Pavia, M. Belli, G. Colantuoni, E. Galligioni, O. Caffo, R. Labianca, A. Quadri, E. Cortesi, G. D'Auria, S. Fava, A. Calcagno, G. Luporini, M. C. Locatelli, F. Di Costanzo, S. Gasperoni, L. Isa, P. Candido, F. Gaion, G. Palazzolo, G. Nettis, A. Annamaria, M. Rinaldi, M. Lopez, R. Felletti, G. B. Di Negro, N. Rossi, A. Calandriello, L. Maiorino, R. Mattioli, A. Celano, S. Schiavon, A. Illiano, C. A. Raucci, M. Caruso, P. Foa, G. Tonini, C. Curcio, and M. Cazzaniga. 2005. Pretreatment quality of life and functional status assessment significantly predict survival of elderly patients with advanced non-small-cell lung cancer receiving chemotherapy: A prognostic analysis of the multicenter Italian lung cancer in the elderly study. *Journal of Clinical Oncology* 23(28):6865-6872.

Mandelblatt, J. S., L. A. Faul, G. Luta, S. B. Makgoeng, C. Isaacs, K. Taylor, V. B. Sheppard, M. Tallarico, W. T. Barry, and H. J. Cohen. 2012. Patient and physician decision styles and breast cancer chemotherapy use in older women: Cancer and Leukemia Group B Protocol 369901. *Journal of Clinical Oncology* 30(21):2609-2614.

Margolis, M., J. Christie, G. Silvestri, L. Kaiser, S. Santiago, and J. Hansen-Flaschen. 2003. Racial differences pertaining to a belief about lung cancer surgery: Results of a multicenter survey. *Archives of Internal Medicine* 139(7):558-563.

Mariotto, A. B., K. R. Yabroff, Y. Shao, E. J. Feuer, and M. L. Brown. 2011. Projections of the cost of cancer care in the United States: 2010-2020. *Journal of the National Cancer Institute* 103(2):117-128.

Mather, M. 2012. *What's driving the decline in U.S. population growth?* http://www.prb.org/Articles/2012/us-population-growth-decline.aspx (accessed August 7, 2012).

Meropol, N. J., and K. A. Schulman. 2007. Cost of cancer care: Issues and implications. *Journal of Clinical Oncology* 25(2):180-186.

Milstein, A. 2012. Code red and blue: Safely limiting health care's GDP footprint. *New England Journal of Medicine.*

Mor, V., V. Wilcox, W. Rakowski, and J. Hiris. 1994. Functional transitions among the elderly: Patterns, predictors, and related hospital use. *American Journal of Public Health* 84(8):1274-1280.

Muss, H. B., D. A. Berry, C. Cirrincione, D. R. Budman, I. C. Henderson, M. L. Citron, L. Norton, E. P. Winer, C. A. Hudis, and Cancer and Leukemia Group B Experience. 2007. Toxicity of older and younger patients treated with adjuvant chemotherapy for node-positive breast cancer: The Cancer and Leukemia Group B experience. *Journal of Clinical Oncology* 25(24):3699-3704.

NCI (National Cancer Institute). 2007. *Cancer trends progress report—2007 update: Costs of cancer care.* http://progressreport.cancer.gov/2007/doc_detail.asp?pid=1&did=2007&chid=75&coid=726&mid= (accessed May 13, 2013).

————. 2008. *National Cancer Institute fact sheet. Cancer health disparities.* http://www.cancer. gov/cancertopics/factsheet/disparities/cancer-health-disparities (accessed December 18, 2012).

————. 2012a. *The National Cancer Act of 1971.* http://legislative.cancer.gov/history/ phsa/1971 (accessed August 7, 2012).

————. 2012b. *NCI mission statement.* http://www.cancer.gov/aboutnci/overview/mission (accessed June 27, 2013).

————. 2012d. *SEER cancer statistics review, 1975-2009.* http://seer.cancer.gov/csr/1975_2009_ pops09/results_single/sect_01_table.20_2pgs.pdf (accessed December 18, 2012).

————. 2013a. *SEER stat fact sheets: All sites.* http://seer.cancer.gov/statfacts/html/all. html#incidence-mortality (accessed June 7, 2013).

————. 2013b. *A snapshot of adolescent and young adult cancers.* http://www.cancer.gov/ researchandfunding/snapshots/adolescent-young-adult (accessed June 26, 2013).

NIA (National Institute on Aging). 2012. *About NIA.* http://www.nia.nih.gov/about/ mission (accessed June 27, 2013).

NRC (National Research Council). 2011. *Toward precision medicine: Building a knowledge network for biomedical research and a new taxonomy of disease.* Washington, DC: The National Academies Press.

————. 2012. *Aging and the macroeconomy. Long-term implications of an older population.* Washington, DC: The National Academies Press.

OECD (Organisation for Economic Co-operation and Development). 2013. *Health at a glance 2011: OECD indicators.* http://www.oecd.org/els/health-systems/49105858.pdf (accessed March 12, 2011).

OMH (Office of Minority Health). 2010. *OMB standards for data on race and ethnicity.* http:// minorityhealth.hhs.gov/templates/browse.aspx?lvl=2&lvlID=172 (accessed June 7, 2013).

————. 2012. *Cancer and Asians/Pacific Islanders.* http://minorityhealth.hhs.gov/templates/ content.aspx?ID=3055 (accessed December 18, 2012).

Parry, C., E. E. Kent, A. B. Mariotto, C. M. Alfano, and J. H. Rowland. 2011. Cancer survivors: A booming population. *Cancer Epidemiology, Biomarkers & Prevention* 20(10):1996-2005.

PCORI (Patient-Centered Outcomes Research Institute). 2013. *Mission and vision.* http:// www.pcori.org/about/mission-and-vision (accessed March 26, 2013).

Penninx, B. W., J. M. Guralnik, L. Ferrucci, E. M. Simonsick, D. J. Deeg, and R. B. Wallace. 1998. Depressive symptoms and physical decline in community-dwelling older persons. *Journal of the American Medical Association* 279(21):1720-1726.

Piccirillo, J. F., R. M. Tierney, I. Costas, L. Grove, and E. L. Spitznagel, Jr. 2004. Prognostic importance of comorbidity in a hospital-based cancer registry. *Journal of the American Medical Association* 291(20):2441-2447.

Pollack, A. 2012. Sanofi halves price of cancer drug Zaltrap after Sloan-Kettering rejection. *New York Times,* November 9, B3.

Qato, D. M., G. C. Alexander, R. M. Conti, M. Johnson, P. Schumm, and S. T. Lindau. 2008. Use of prescription and over-the-counter medications and dietary supplements among older adults in the United States. *Journal of the American Medical Association* 300(24):2867-2878.

Repetto, L., I. Carreca, D. Maraninchi, M. Aapro, P. Calabresi, and L. Balducci. 2003. Use of growth factors in the elderly patient with cancer: A report from the Second International Society for Geriatric Oncology 2001 meeting. *Critical Reviews in Oncology/ Hematology* 45(2):123-128.

Reuben, D. B., L. V. Rubenstein, S. H. Hirsch, and R. D. Hays. 1992. Value of functional status as a predictor of mortality: Results of a prospective study. *American Journal of Medicine* 93(6):663-669.

Riechelmann, R., and A. Del Giglio. 2009. Drug interactions in oncology: How common are they? *Annals of Oncology* 20(12):1907.

Rigler, S. K., S. Studenski, D. Wallace, D. M. Reker, and P. W. Duncan. 2002. Co-morbidity adjustment for functional outcomes in community-dwelling older adults. *Clinical Rehabilitation* 16(4):420-428.

Rolita, L., and M. Freedman. 2008. Over-the-counter medication use in older adults. *Journal of Gerontological Nursing* 34(4):8-17.

Ryu, A. J., T. B. Gibson, M. R. McKellar, and M. E. Chernew. 2013. The slowdown in health care spending in 2009-11 reflected factors other than the weak economy and thus may persist. *Health Affairs (Millwood)* 32(5):835-840.

Safran, D. G., P. Neuman, C. Schoen, M. S. Kitchman, I. B. Wilson, B. Cooper, A. Li, H. Chang, and W. H. Rogers. 2005. Prescription drug coverage and seniors: Findings from a 2003 national survey. *Health Affairs (Millwood)* Suppl Web Exclusives:W5-152-W155-166.

Satariano, W. A., and D. R. Ragland. 1994. The effect of comorbidity on 3-year survival of women with primary breast cancer. *Annals of Internal Medicine* 120(2):104-110.

Sauvaget, C., M. Yamada, S. Fujiwara, H. Sasaki, and Y. Mimori. 2002. Dementia as a predictor of functional disability: A four-year follow-up study. *Gerontology* 48(4):226-233.

Sawhney, R., M. Sehl, and A. Naeim. 2005. Physiologic aspects of aging: Impact on cancer management and decision making, part I. *Cancer Journal* 11(6):449-460.

Seeman, T. E., G. A. Kaplan, L. Knudsen, R. Cohen, and J. Guralnik. 1987. Social network ties and mortality among the elderly in the Alameda County Study. *American Journal of Epidemiology* 126(4):714-723.

Seeman, T. E., L. F. Berkman, F. Kohout, A. Lacroix, R. Glynn, and D. Blazer. 1993. Intercommunity variations in the association between social ties and mortality in the elderly. A comparative analysis of three communities. *Annals of Epidemiology* 3(4):325-335.

Sehl, M., R. Sawhney, and A. Naeim. 2005. Physiologic aspects of aging: Impact on cancer management and decision making, part II. *Cancer Journal* 11(6):461-473.

Shrestha, L. B., and E. J. Heisler. 2009. *The changing demographic profile of the United States.* http://aging.senate.gov/crs/aging4.pdf (accessed September 13, 2012).

———. 2011. *The changing demographic profile of the United States.* http://www.fas.org/sgp/crs/misc/RL32701.pdf (accessed August 7, 2012).

Sleiman, I., R. Rozzini, P. Barbisoni, A. Morandi, A. Ricci, A. Giordano, and M. Trabucchi. 2009. Functional trajectories during hospitalization: A prognostic sign for elderly patients. *The Journals of Gerontology: Series A, Biological Sciences and Medical Sciences* 64(6):659-663.

Smith, B. D., G. L. Smith, A. Hurria, G. N. Hortobagyi, and T. A. Buchholz. 2009. Future of cancer incidence in the United States: Burdens upon an aging, changing nation. *Journal of Clinical Oncology* 27(17):2758-2765.

Sommers, B. D., T. Buchmueller, S. L. Decker, C. Carey, and R. Kronick. 2013. The Affordable Care Act has led to significant gains in health insurance and access to care for young adults. *Health Affairs (Millwood)* 32(1):165-174.

Spinewine, A., C. Swine, S. Dhillon, P. Lambert, J. B. Nachega, L. Wilmotte, and P. M. Tulkens. 2007. Effect of a collaborative approach on the quality of prescribing for geriatric inpatients: A randomized, controlled trial. *Journal of the American Geriatrics Society* 55(5):658-665.

Stafford, R. S., and P. L. Cyr. 1997. The impact of cancer on the physical function of the elderly and their utilization of health care. *Cancer* 80(10):1973-1980.

Stein, K., L. Zhao, C. Crammer, and T. Gansler. 2007. Prevalence and sociodemographic correlates of beliefs regarding cancer risks. *Cancer* 110(5):1139-1148.

Steyerberg, E. W., B. A. Neville, L. B. Koppert, V. E. Lemmens, H. W. Tilanus, J. W. Coebergh, J. C. Weeks, and C. C. Earle. 2006. Surgical mortality in patients with esophageal cancer: Development and validation of a simple risk score. *Journal of Clinical Oncology* 24(26):4277-4284.

Studenski, S. A., S. M. Lai, P. W. Duncan, and S. K. Rigler. 2004. The impact of self-reported cumulative comorbidity on stroke recovery. *Age and Ageing* 33(2):195-198.

Stuijt, C. C., E. J. Franssen, A. C. Egberts, and S. A. Hudson. 2008. Appropriateness of pre-scribing among elderly patients in a Dutch residential home: Observational study of outcomes after a pharmacist-led medication review. *Drugs and Aging* 25(11):947-954.

Sullivan, R., J. Peppercorn, K. Sikora, J. Zalcberg, N. J. Meropol, E. Amir, D. Khayat, P. Boyle, P. Autier, I. F. Tannock, T. Fojo, J. Siderov, S. Williamson, S. Camporesi, J. G. McVie, A. D. Purushotham, P. Naredi, A. Eggermont, M. F. Brennan, M. L. Steinberg, M. De Ridder, S. A. McCloskey, D. Verellen, T. Roberts, G. Storme, R. J. Hicks, P. J. Ell, B. R. Hirsch, D. P. Carbone, K. A. Schulman, P. Catchpole, D. Taylor, J. Geissler, N. G. Brinker, D. Meltzer, D. Kerr, and M. Aapro. 2011. Delivering affordable cancer care in high-income countries. *Lancet Oncology* 12(10):933-980.

Talarico, L., G. Chen, and R. Pazdur. 2004. Enrollment of elderly patients in clinical trials for cancer drug registration: A 7-year experience by the US Food and Drug Administration. *Journal of Clinical Oncology* 22(22):4626-4631.

Tangka, F. K., J. G. Trogdon, L. C. Richardson, D. Howard, S. A. Sabatino, and E. A. Finkelstein. 2010. Cancer treatment cost in the United States: Has the burden shifted over time? *Cancer* 116(14):3477-3484.

Toffoli, G., G. Corona, R. Sorio, I. Robieux, B. Basso, A. M. Colussi, and M. Boiocchi. 2001. Population pharmacokinetics and pharmacodynamics of oral etoposide. *British Journal of Clinical Pharmacology* 52(5):511-519.

Tulner, L. R., S. V. Frankfort, G. J. Gijsen, J. P. van Campen, C. H. Koks, and J. H. Beijnen. 2008. Drug-drug interactions in a geriatric outpatient cohort: Prevalence and relevance. *Drugs and Aging* 25(4):343-355.

Unger, J. M., J. C. A. Coltman, J. J. Crowley, L. F. Hutchins, S. Martino, R. B. Livingston, J. S. Macdonald, C. D. Blanke, D. R. Gandara, E. D. Crawford, and K. S. Albain. 2006. Impact of the year 2000 Medicare policy change on older patient enrollment to cancer clinical trials. *Journal of Clinical Oncology* 24(1):141-144.

U.S. Census Bureau. 2013. *U.S. and world population clock.* http://www.census.gov/popclock (accessed June 10, 2013).

Vestal, R. E. 1997. Aging and pharmacology. *Cancer* 80(7):1302-1310.

Vincent, G. K., and V. A. Velkoff. 2010. *The next four decades. The older population in the United States: 2010 to 2050. Population estimates and projections.* http://www.census.gov/prod/2010pubs/p25-1138.pdf (accessed August 7, 2012).

Vinks, T. H., T. C. Egberts, T. M. de Lange, and F. H. de Koning. 2009. Pharmacist-based medication review reduces potential drug-related problems in the elderly: The SMOG controlled trial. *Drugs and Aging* 26(2):123-133.

Wadley, V. G., O. Okonkwo, M. Crowe, and L. A. Ross-Meadows. 2008. Mild cognitive impairment and everyday function: evidence of reduced speed in performing instru-mental activities of daily living. *American Journal of Geriatric Psychiatry* 16(5):416-424.

Walter, L. C., R. J. Brand, S. R. Counsell, R. M. Palmer, C. S. Landefeld, R. H. Fortinsky, and K. E. Covinsky. 2001. Development and validation of a prognostic index for 1-year mortality in older adults after hospitalization. *Journal of the American Medical Associa-tion* 285(23):2987-2994.

Ward, E., A. Jemal, V. Cokkinides, G. K. Singh, C. Cardinez, A. Ghafoor, and M. Thun. 2004. Cancer disparities by race/ethnicity and socioeconomic status. *CA: A Cancer Journal for Clinicians* 54(2):78-93.

Waxler-Morrison, N., T. G. Hislop, B. Mears, and L. Kan. 1991. Effects of social relationships on survival for women with breast cancer: A prospective study. *Social Science and Medicine* 33(2):177-183.

Weber, V., A. White, and R. McIlvried. 2008. An electronic medical record (EMR)-based intervention to reduce polypharmacy and falls in an ambulatory rural elderly population. *Journal of General Internal Medicine* 23(4):399-404.

Weinberger, M. I., A. J. Roth, and C. J. Nelson. 2009. Untangling the complexities of depression diagnosis in older cancer patients. *Oncologist* 14(1):60-66.

Yabroff, K. R., J. Lund, D. Kepka, and A. Mariotto. 2011. Economic burden of cancer in the United States: Estimates, projections, and future research. *Cancer Epidemiology, Biomarkers & Prevention* 20(10):2006-2014.

Yancik, R. 1997. Cancer burden in the aged: An epidemiologic and demographic overview. *Cancer* 80(7):1273-1283.

Yancik, R., W. Ershler, W. Satariano, W. Hazzard, H. J. Cohen, and L. Ferrucci. 2007. Report of the National Institute on Aging Task Force on Comorbidity. *Journals of Gerontology: Series A, Biological Sciences and Medical Sciences* 62(3):275-280.

Yee, K. W. L., J. L. Pater, L. Pho, B. Zee, and L. L. Siu. 2003. Enrollment of older patients in cancer treatment trials in Canada: Why is age a barrier? *Journal of Clinical Oncology* 21(8):1618-1623.

Yoon, S. L., and S. D. Schaffer. 2006. Herbal, prescribed, and over-the-counter drug use in older women: Prevalence of drug interactions. *Geriatric Nursing* 27(2):118-129.

Yuen, G. J. 1990. Altered pharmacokinetics in the elderly. *Clinics in Geriatric Medicine* 6(2):257-267.

Zhan, C., J. Sangl, A. S. Bierman, M. R. Miller, B. Friedman, S. W. Wickizer, and G. S. Meyer. 2001. Potentially inappropriate medication use in the community-dwelling elderly: Findings from the 1996 Medical Expenditure Panel Survey. *Journal of the American Medical Association* 286(22):2823-2829.

ANNEX 2-1 RELEVANT PROVISIONS OF
THE AFFORDABLE CARE ACT

Provision	Description
Access to Care and Health Disparities	

Coverage for Participation in Clinical Trials	• New rule for insurers (exempts grandfathered plans)
	• Prohibits insurers from dropping or limiting coverage for individuals participating in clinical trials
	  o Applicable to clinical trials that treat cancer or other life-threatening conditions
	  o Provides routine care costs for approved clinical trials only

Essential Health Benefits (EHB) Package	• Health insurance mandate • Requires all health plans sold to individuals and small businesses to cover a minimum set of services, including chronic disease management • Each state selects one plan to serve as the benchmark plan in their state
Health Professional Opportunity Grants	• Human service grant program • Provides comprehensive health care training and employment-related public services (e.g., transportation) to low-income workers
Health Resources and Services Administration (HRSA) Community Health Center Program	• Established a fund to expand the existing program • Provides access to primary health care for vulnerable populations
Medicaid Expansion	• States can choose to extend Medicaid eligibility to all U.S. citizens under the age of 65 with incomes less than 133 percent of federal poverty level • Provides EHB to newly eligible individuals through "benchmark" coverage plans • Requires participating hospitals to make presumptive eligibility determinations for Medicaid patients
National Health Service Corps	• Expansion of existing program • Funds and places health professionals in areas with workforce shortages

Prescription Drug Discounts	• Relief to seniors in the Centers for Medicare & Medicaid Services (CMS) prescription drug benefit coverage gap (i.e., the "donut hole")
	  o Provides a 50 percent discount on covered brand-name prescription drugs
	  o The discount reduces by a certain percentage each year, until the gap closes in 2020

continued

Provision	Description
State Option to Provide Health Homes for Enrollees with Chronic Conditions	• Optional amendment to state Medicaid programs • Allows beneficiaries with chronic conditions to be enrolled into a health home
Tobacco Cessation Services for Pregnant Women with Medicaid	• Requires Medicaid to cover, without cost sharing, counseling and pharmacotherapy services for tobacco cessation for pregnant women
Understanding Health Disparities	• Data collecting and reporting requirement • All federally funded health care or public health programs, activities, or surveys must collect and report standardized data on race, ethnicity, sex, primary language, and disability status • National Coordinator for Health Information Technology to develop national standards for management of the data collected

Coordination and Organization of Care

Community Health Teams to Support the Patient-Centered Medical Home (PCMH)	• Grant program • Supports states in establishing community health teams that can staff PCMH
Medication Management Services in Treatment of Chronic Disease	• Grant program • Aids clinicians in delivering medication management services for the treatment of chronic diseases
National Center for Health Workforce Analysis	• New section of HRSA • Collects health workforce data and intelligence
National Health Care Workforce Commission	• Commission of 15 members appointed by the Comptroller General • Coordinates federal efforts to monitor and address challenges faced by the nation's health care workforce
Patient Navigator System	• Reauthorization of a patient navigator program • Connects patients with health care service coordinators to diagnose, treat, and manage chronic disease(s)
Program to Facilitate Shared Decision Making	• Program to develop, test, and disseminate educational tools to aid in health decision making • Agency for Healthcare Research and Quality (AHRQ) to issue contract with an entity to develop patient decision aids • U.S. Department of Health and Human Services (HHS) to disperse grants for the establishment and support of Shared Decision Making Resource Centers

Provision	Description
Prevention	
Clinical and Community Preventive Services	• Creates the Community Preventive Services Task Force; an independent, nonfederal panel of public health and prevention experts • Provides Congress with a yearly report of findings and recommendations on community preventive services, programs, and policies
Community Transformation Grant Program	• Grant program funded through the Prevention and Public Health Fund • Supports community-driven interventions focused on reducing chronic conditions, preventing the development of secondary conditions, addressing health care disparities, and developing stronger evidence for community-level prevention programming
Coverage of Preventive Health Services	• New rule for insurers • Requires insurers to provide a minimum level of preventive health services without cost sharing o Services include those rated "A" or "B" by the U.S. Preventive Services Task Force (USPSTF), screening and mammography recommended by the USPSTF, immunizations recommended by the Advisory Committee on Immunization Practices, and preventive care and screenings for youth and women recommended by HRSA
Education and Outreach Campaign Regarding Preventive Benefits	• National public-private partnership campaign • Funded through the Prevention and Public Health Fund • Raises awareness of the importance of prevention • Educates public and health care clinicians about preventive health services recommended by the USPSTF and covered by exchange programs
National Prevention Strategy	• Product of the National Prevention, Health Promotion and Public Health Council • Comprehensive plan to improve the health of the nation through preventive efforts
Prevention and Public Health Fund	• Fund within HHS • Makes investments in prevention and public health programs

continued

Provision	Description
Reimbursement and Incentives	

Advanced Payment ACO Model	• Incentive program in the CMS Innovation Center
	• Encourages participation in the Shared Savings Program
	   o Provides ACOs with a pre-payment of a portion of their future shared savings
	   o This money is to be invested in infrastructure and staff for care coordination

Community Care Transitions Program	• Five-year program in the CMS Innovation Center • Tests models for improving care transitions from the hospital to other settings and avoiding unnecessary hospital readmissions
CMS Innovation Center	• A new center in CMS • Tests innovative payment and service delivery models intended to reduce program expenditures, while preserving or enhancing the quality of care • HHS Secretary has the authority to scale successful delivery models up to the national level
Hospital Readmissions Reduction Program	• CMS program • Reduces Medicare payment to hospitals with high readmissions for specific conditions • Excludes hospitals providing primarily rehabilitative, psychiatric, or long-term care; children's hospitals; critical access hospitals; and certain cancer and research centers
Hospital Value-Based Purchasing (VBP) Program	• Incentive program in CMS • Hospitals are reimbursed for inpatient acute care services based on the quality of the care they provide, not the quantity of services • Hospitals publicly report performance on a set of quality measures
Independent Payment Advisory Board	• Independent 15-member panel of appointed experts • Recommends cost-saving measures for Medicare should it exceed an established targeted growth rate
Medicare Advantage Quality Bonus Payment Demonstration	• Reward program in CMS • Bonuses paid to Medicare Advantage plans that meet certain standards

Medicare's Shared Savings Program	• Incentive program in the CMS Innovation Center
	• Encourages the formation of accountable care organizations (ACOs) by allowing these organizations to
	   o Receive traditional Medicare fee-for-service payments
	   o Be eligible for additional payments if they meet predetermined quality and savings targets

Provision	Description
Pioneer ACO Model	• Incentive program in the CMS Innovation Center • Encourages health care clinicians already experienced with providing coordinated care to become ACOs • Uses a shared savings payment model with higher levels of shared savings and risk
Quality Metrics	
Medicare Prospective Payment System Exempt Cancer Hospitals	• CMS cancer-focused quality reporting program • Applies to 11 cancer centers whose federal reimbursement is not based on traditional payment system and are exempt from existing federal reporting programs (e.g., CMS core measures) • Mandates reporting of process, structure, outcomes, efficiency, costs of care, and patients' perspective on care measures • Measure rates will be posted on a federal website (i.e., Hospital Compare)
Medicare Qualified Entities Data Release Program	• CMS program • Makes Medicare claims data available to qualifed entities to measure health care provider and supplier performance
National Quality Strategy	• National quality improvement strategy • HHS Secretary will annually update the strategy and identify priorities to improve the delivery of health care services, patient outcomes, and population health
Public Reporting of Provider Performance Information	• HHS strategic framework for publicly reporting provider performance information • Performance information available on a website, tailored to different viewers' perspectives

Quality Measure Development	• Component of National Quality Strategy
	• Requires HHS Secretary to select an entity to convene stakeholders and provide input on the selection of quality measures
	• Provides grants to entities for further improving, updating, or expanding quality measures
	• HHS Secretary to develop and periodically update outcome measures for hospital providers and physicians, including at least
	   o 10 measurements for acute and chronic diseases; and
	   o 10 measurements for primary and preventive care

Provision	Description
Rapid Learning Health Care/Information Technology/Infrastructure for Research	

Patient-Centered Outcomes Research Institute (PCORI)	• Nonprofit corporation
	• Assists patients, clinicians, policy makers, and purchasers in making informed health decisions by assessing
	   o National clinical research priorities
	   o New clinical evidence and gaps in evidence
	   o Relevance of clinical evidence and economic impact

3

Patient-Centered Communication and Shared Decision Making

The committee's conceptual framework for a high-quality cancer care delivery system highlights the critical importance of engaged patients. Patients are at the center of the framework (see Figure S-2), which conveys the most important goal of a high-quality cancer care delivery system: meeting the needs of patients with cancer and their families. Such a system should support all patients and families in making informed health care decisions that are consistent with their needs, values, and preferences. This will require a delivery system and workforce oriented to the provision of patient-centered care, defined as "providing care that is respectful of and responsive to individual patient preferences, needs, and values and ensuring that patient values guide all clinical decisions" (IOM, 2001, p. 40). Patient-centered care includes fostering good communication between patients and their cancer care team; developing and disseminating evidence-based information to inform patients, caregivers, and the cancer care team about treatment options; and practicing shared decision making. Although patient-centered communication and shared decision making were not a major focus of the Institute of Medicine's (IOM's) *Ensuring Quality Cancer Care* report (IOM and NRC, 1999), several concepts from that report are relevant to the committee's recommendations on both topics: the importance of developing a cancer care plan; managing pain, other symptoms, and side effects; as well as the timely referral to hospice care at the end of life.

Currently, patient-centered communication and shared decision making in oncology are suboptimal (Aiello Bowles et al., 2008; Ayanian et al., 2005, 2010; Wagner et al., 2010). In a study of 1,057 patient encounters with

3,552 clinical decisions, only 9 percent resulted in what was defined as an informed medical decision (Braddock et al., 1999). More recently, studies have found that clinicians ask for patient preferences in medical decisions only about half the time (Lee et al., 2012; Zikmund-Fisher et al., 2010). A number of obstacles prevent patient-centered communication and shared decision making among patients, their family, caregivers, and the cancer care team. The emotional, financial, and logistical repercussions of a cancer diagnosis and the complexity of treatment options, together with patients' limitations in health literacy and lack of experience with the health care system, can make it difficult for patients and their families to actively engage in making health care decisions. The current reimbursement system does not incentivize clinicians to engage in patient-centered communication and shared decision making. In addition, clinicians often lack training in communication, leading to difficulties in recognizing and responding to patients' informational and emotional needs. A lack of understandable and easily available information on prognosis, treatment options, likelihood of treatment responses, palliative care, psychosocial support, and the costs of cancer care contribute to communication problems, which are exacerbated in patients with advanced cancer.[1]

This chapter describes the benefits, challenges, and characteristics of patient-centered communication and shared decision making; presents approaches and tools to facilitate patient-centered communication and shared decision making; and discusses the importance of advance care planning, the provision of palliative care and psychosocial support across the cancer continuum, and timely referral to hospice when patients near the end of life. The evidence base for this chapter is primarily derived from the National Cancer Policy Forum's workshop summaries on *Patient-Centered Cancer Treatment Planning: Improving the Quality of Oncology Care, Assessing and Improving Value in Cancer Care*, and *Delivering Affordable Cancer Care in the 21st Century*, and the National Cancer Institute's (NCI's) monograph *Patient-Centered Communication in Cancer Care* (Epstein and Street, 2007; IOM, 2009a, 2011b, 2013). The committee identifies two recommendations to improve patient-centered communication and shared decision making.

DEFINING PATIENT-CENTERED COMMUNICATION AND SHARED DECISION MAKING

The concept of patient-centeredness as an important attribute of high-quality health care gained national prominence with the IOM report

---

[1] Cancer that has spread to other places in the body and usually cannot be cured or controlled with treatment (NCI, 2013b).

Crossing the Quality Chasm: A New Health System for the 21st Century (IOM, 2001). The IOM defines patient-centeredness as "providing care that is respectful of and responsive to individual patient preferences, needs, and values and ensuring that patient values guide all clinical decisions" (IOM, 2001, p. 40).[2] Over time, other organizations and individuals have elaborated on the attributes of patient-centered care (Bechtel and Ness, 2010; Berwick, 2009; Epstein et al., 2010; Picker Institute, 2013). In the cancer setting, some of the attributes of patient-centered care highlighted at an IOM National Cancer Policy Forum workshop included (IOM, 2011a)

- patient education and empowerment;
- patient-centered communication, which involves the patient, family, and friends; explains treatment options; and includes patients in treatment decisions to reflect patients' values, preferences, and needs;
- coordination and integration of care; and
- provision of emotional support as needed, such as relieving fear and anxiety and addressing mental health issues.

Effective patient-clinician communication and shared decision making are key components of patient-centered care. These components require that informed, activated, and participatory patients and family members interact with a patient-centered care team that has effective communication skills and is supported by an accessible, well-organized, and responsive health care system (see Figure 3-1) (Epstein and Street, 2007). As described by the NCI's monograph *Patient-Centered Communication in Cancer Care*, the primary functions of patient-centered communication are to (1) foster healing relationships, (2) exchange information, (3) respond to emotions, (4) manage uncertainty, (5) make decisions, and (6) enable patient self-management (see Table 3-1) (Epstein and Street, 2007). These six functions dynamically interact to influence the quality of patient-clinician interactions and may ultimately influence patients' health outcomes (Epstein and Street, 2007). They are skills that need to be developed, utilized, and maintained across the cancer care continuum.

Sepucha and colleagues (2004, p. 57) argued that the "quality of a clinical decision, or its patient-centeredness, is the extent to which it reflects the considered needs, values, and expressed preferences of a well-informed patient and is thus implemented." Rather than relying on clinician-directed decision making, over the past few decades patients

---

[2] Needs generally refer to a patient's physical or emotional requirements. Values and preferences represent a patient's concerns, expectations, and choices regarding health care, based on a full and accurate understanding of care options (adapted from IOM, 2001, 2003).

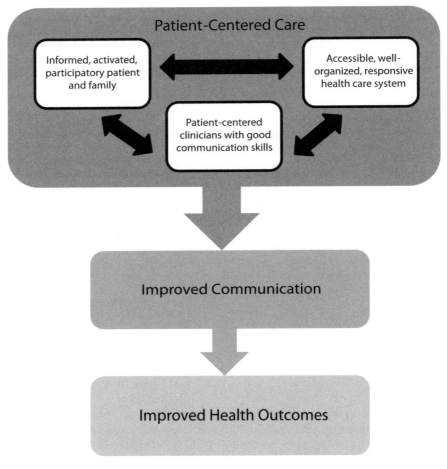

FIGURE 3-1 Model of patient-centered care. The patient, clinicians, and health care system dynamically interact to influence patient-centered care. The delivery of patient-centered care has the potential to improve communication and health outcomes.
SOURCE: Adapted from Epstein and Street, 2007.

have individually and collectively pushed for a greater role in medical decision making (Clancy, 2008) (see Figure 3-2). Health researchers, advocacy organizations, and the Agency for Healthcare Research and Quality (AHRQ) have also encouraged patients to play a larger role in making medical decisions. Research indicates that when patients are involved in their own care, they are more satisfied with the care they receive and

TABLE 3-1 Important Functions of Patient-Clinician Communication

Function	Description
Fostering Healing Relationships	Developing a patient-clinician relationship that is characterized by trust and rapport is critical to patient-centered communication and shared decision making. This involves mutual understanding of patient and clinician roles, as well as clinician self-awareness and provision of emotional support, guidance, and understanding.
Exchanging Information	The cancer care team should ascertain patients' informational needs. Conveying information to patients can be facilitated through the ask-tell-ask method, an approach described in the section on prioritizing clinician training in communication. The exchange includes the cancer care team's provision of accurate prognostic information and treatment options, realistic expectations for response to treatment, and the cost of cancer care to inform patients' decisions.
Responding to Emotions	The cancer care team should recognize and respond to patients' emotions, which involves verbally expressing understanding, legitimizing feelings, and providing empathy and support. This also includes the development of a psychosocial care plan and linking patients to psychosocial care if they experience high levels of emotional distress, anxiety, and depressive symptoms.
Managing Uncertainty	Clinicians play an important role in reducing and managing the uncertainty associated with cancer care. This can include cognitive-behavioral interventions to help patients cope with this uncertainty and, if possible, improve understanding.
Making Decisions	Shared decision making involves three processes—information exchange, deliberation, and reaching a final decision. A patient's decision often extends beyond medical issues, and includes factors such as finances and the expense of treatment, and impact on employment and family. The logistics of scheduling and receiving cancer treatment can be an enormous strain for patients, families, and caregivers; disrupt family life; and require negotiations with employers for time off or flexible work schedules.
Enabling Patient Self-Management	The cancer care team should provide individuals with resources to be proactive in their care. Examples of self-management tools and enablers include cancer care plans, survivorship care plans, and patient navigators who assist patients to overcome health care system barriers and facilitate timely access to health care services.

SOURCES: C-Change, 2005; Epstein and Street, 2007; Lauria et al., 2001.

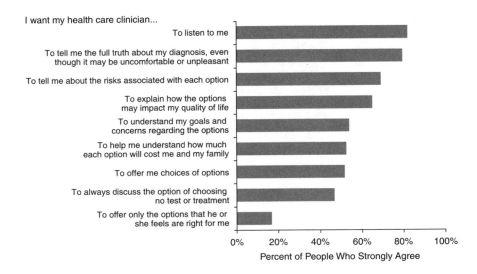

FIGURE 3-2 People want to be involved in understanding evidence and making decisions about their care. The IOM surveyed a nationally representative sample of 1,068 U.S. adults who had seen at least one health care clinician in the previous year. The majority of adults strongly agreed that they should be actively involved in understanding and making decisions about their care.
SOURCE: Alston et al., 2012.

often experience better health outcomes (Alston et al., 2012; CFAH, 2010; Hibbard and Greene, 2013; Lantz et al., 2005; Maurer et al., 2012; Roseman et al., 2013). Thus, shared decision making is a critical feature of patient-centered communication, and is defined as "the process of negotiation by which physicians and patients arrive at a specific course of action, based on a common understanding of the goals of treatment, the risks and benefits of the chosen treatment versus reasonable alternatives, and each other's values and preferences" (IOM, 2011a, p. 8; adapted from Sheridan et al., 2004).

Patients with cancer and their families are often required to manage greater portions of their cancer care due to advances in cancer treatment, as well as changes in the practice of health care, such as earlier discharge from the hospital (CFAH, 2010; McCorkle et al., 2011). These duties may include drug management, wound care, rehabilitation, and lifestyle changes (CFAH, 2010). Clinicians help patients engage in self-management, which involves managing the medical and psychological aspects of cancer care, as well as adapting to changes in roles that result from cancer diagnosis (McCorkle et al., 2011). Promoting patient self-management can facilitate shared decision making and improve cancer care.

THE IMPORTANCE OF PATIENT-CENTERED COMMUNICATION AND SHARED DECISION MAKING IN CANCER

A number of factors related to cancer care necessitate a patient-centered approach to communication: (1) cancer care is extremely complex and patients' treatment choices have serious implications for their health outcomes and quality of life; (2) the evidence supporting many decisions in cancer care is limited or incomplete; and (3) trade-offs in the risks and benefits of cancer treatment choices may be weighed differently by individual patients, and clinicians need to elicit patient needs, values, and preferences in these circumstances. Each of these factors is discussed below.

Complexity of Cancer Care

Cancer care is complex. It may involve multiple treatment modalities, including chemotherapy, radiation, and surgery, all of which need to be coordinated among different cancer care specialists. Treatment regimens can also be time intensive, debilitating, and often result in serious and sometimes long-term complications (IOM, 2011a). In addition, patients must often choose from multiple cancer treatment options, requiring patients and their families to decide on the goals of treatment (e.g., prioritizing survival time vs. maximizing quality of life), whether to participate in clinical trials, and to weigh evidence of the risks and benefits of different treatment approaches. These decisions often need to be revisited at various points along the cancer care continuum. A patient's goals or preferences at the time of initial diagnosis, for example, may be very different from a patient who has advanced cancer.

Limitations in the Evidence Base

As described in Chapter 5, the committee recommends that researchers improve the breadth and depth of information collected in clinical research. Studies indicate that there is a lack of evidence to support many medical decisions (El Dib et al., 2007; IOM, 2008b, 2012; Villas Boas et al., 2012). Evidence supporting patients' medical decisions can be especially limited for older adults and individuals with comorbidities, as these individuals are often underrepresented or excluded from clinical trials (IOM, 2009b, 2010). While comparative effectiveness research (CER) and learning health care systems aim to fill these evidence gaps, they have limitations. Clinicians should fully communicate gaps in the evidence base to their patients during the medical decision-making process. When evidence is sparse, patient preferences should be a particularly important consideration in the health care decision-making process.

Preference-Sensitive Decisions

Some decisions in cancer care are particularly sensitive to patient preferences. For example, women with breast cancer can often choose from different courses of treatment—mastectomy versus lumpectomy followed by radiation—and expect equivalent survival outcomes (Fisher et al., 2002). Women may choose mastectomy, or the removal of the entire breast, for peace of mind or to avoid radiation therapy, while women who choose lumpectomy followed by radiation may do so to conserve their breasts (Collins et al., 2009). Women with *BRCA 1* and *2* gene mutations are at higher risk for developing breast and ovarian cancer, and may face difficult decisions about breast cancer screening, as well as consideration of prophylactic mastectomy or oophorectomy to reduce the risk of cancer[3] (Jolie, 2013; Schwartz et al., 2009). These decisions can have a major impact on an individual's future. Thus, patients' preferences need to inform medical decisions. Patients' preferences are also particularly important when they consider their treatment goals, such as choosing a less aggressive treatment strategy in order to maintain a high quality of life (Berman, 2012; Epstein and Street, 2007; Gruman, 2013). Preferences may also change over time and clinicians need to revisit these throughout the cancer care continuum. For example, women considering second line chemotherapy may prefer to take a more active role in decision making compared to women who are considering first line chemotherapy (Grunfeld et al., 2006).

CHALLENGES TO PATIENT-CENTERED COMMUNICATION AND SHARED DECISION MAKING IN CANCER

There are a number of challenges to patient-centered communication and shared decision making. This section discusses patient, clinician, and health care system challenges.

Challenges for Patients

A cancer diagnosis can lead to a state of crisis for an individual and his or her family because most people are not immediately equipped to understand their diagnosis or how to identify options for moving forward (NCCS, 2012a). Because treatment and its side effects, as well as recovery

---

[3] Oophrectomy is surgery to remove one or both ovaries (NCI, 2013b).

and the worry about recurrence, can result in a series of crises for a patient, the crisis does not end once the shock of initial diagnosis wears off (NCCS, 2012a).

The emotional repercussions of a cancer diagnosis can prevent patients from engaging in effective communication with their clinicians about their diagnosis and treatment. Patients can become anxious; feel vulnerable, alone, and fearful; and experience feelings of losing control when receiving a cancer diagnosis. Given these emotions, patients may be unable to retain important information regarding their treatment when speaking with their care team (IOM, 2011a).

Patients' lack of assertiveness may also create communication challenges. Ideally, patients are active communicators, asking questions, assertively stating their opinions, introducing new topics of conversation, and discussing their concerns, feelings, or preferences when communicating with their clinicians (Epstein and Street, 2007). Patients' lack of experience with the health care delivery system and illness, however, can impede their active participation (IOM, 2011a).

Research indicates that the average patient asks five or fewer questions during a 15-minute doctor's visit (IOM, 2008a), and an AHRQ public service announcement noted that people ask more questions when buying a cell phone or ordering a meal than they do during medical appointments. Patients may refrain from asking questions because some clinicians are not receptive or because patients fear they will be considered difficult and receive worse care (Frosch et al., 2012; Gruman, 2013).

Patients who only participate in their care on a limited basis risk poor health outcomes because they may fail to express their needs, fears, expectations, and preferences, which are important to their health care decisions. These patients may also feel dissatisfied when interacting with their clinicians (Epstein and Street, 2007), a problem exacerbated by patients' awe of their clinicians or lack of self-confidence (Hoffman, 2004). Older adults may be more reluctant to question their clinicians' authority because they may think it is impolite or inappropriate to ask questions or make decisions about their own care (Busari, 2013; Hoffman, 2004; IOM, 2008a). Research has also linked patients' level of participation in clinical encounters with their level of education, ethnicity, gender, personality, and the orientation of patient-clinician relationships (shared control versus physician control) (Epstein and Street, 2007). Box 3-1 lists a number of questions that patients with cancer can discuss with their clinicians.

In addition, a patient's level of health literacy and numeracy can affect patient-centered communication and shared decision making (Peters et al., 2007). More than 90 million adults in the United States have poor reading and writing skills and only 38 percent of high school seniors are proficient in reading (Kutner et al., 2007; NAEP, 2010; NRC, 2012).

BOX 3-1
Questions That Patients with Cancer Can
Discuss with Their Clinicians

Questions About Prognosis

- What is the goal of treatment? Is it directly treating the cancer or improving my symptoms, or both?
- How long does the average person with this cancer live? (ask for a window and the most likely scenario)
- How will I feel?
- What is my likelihood of a cure?
- If I cannot be cured, will I live longer with treatment? How much longer?
- Will I feel better or worse?
- Can I receive palliative care focused on maintaining the quality of my and my family's life during my cancer treatment?
- What options do I have if I don't want to continue my cancer treatment?
- When should I think about hospice? Can I meet with hospice now, when I am well?
- How often should we check in about my care plan?

Questions About Treatment

- What are my treatment options?
- Why do I need this treatment?
- How does this treatment compare with other treatment options?
- What things are likely to happen to me?
- Am I healthy enough to undergo the treatment?
- What are the risks and benefits of treatment?
- Are there any side effects?

Furthermore, many individuals have inadequate health literacy, which is defined as "the degree to which individuals have the capacity to obtain, process, and understand basic health information and services needed to make appropriate health decisions" (IOM, 2004a, p. 32; Ratzan and Parker, 2000). AHRQ estimated that 36 percent of the adult population, or approximately 80 million individuals, have poor health literacy, with low health literacy more prevalent in certain subgroups, including older adults, racial and ethnic minority populations, adults who spoke a language other than English prior to starting school, individuals who have not completed high school, and people living in poverty (Berkman et al., 2011). Poor health literacy can hinder patients' ability to receive health care, including their ability to communicate with their clinicians and man-

- Will treatment make me feel better or worse?
- How many times have you done this procedure?
- What is the cost of this treatment?
- What clinical trials are available?
  - o What are the potential benefits of clinical trials?
  - o Am I eligible to participate?
  - o How do I enroll?
- Which hospital is best for my needs?
- Which clinician(s) will coordinate my care?
- How do you spell the name of that drug?
- Will this medicine interact with medicines that I'm already taking?

Questions About Advance Care Planning

- Are there things I should be doing to plan ahead?
  - o Draft a will?
  - o Participate in advance care planning and decide on my advance directives?
  - o Choose a health care proxy who can speak for me if I am unable?
  - o Address financial or family legal issues?
  - o Appoint a durable power of attorney for financial affairs?
  - o Write notes or create DVDs for loved ones?

Questions About Family, Psychosocial, and Spiritual Needs

- Will you help me talk with my children?
- Who is available to help me cope with this situation?

SOURCES: Adapted from AHRQ, 2013b; ASCO and Cancer.Net, 2012; Harrington and Smith, 2008.

age chronic illnesses (IOM, 2011b). Poor health literacy is associated with increased hospitalizations, greater use of emergency room services, and lower probability of receiving preventive care (Berkman et al., 2011). Poor health literacy is especially concerning for older adults, as Berkman and colleagues (2011) found that lower health literacy in this group was associated with a higher risk of mortality and a worse overall health status.

Even if a patient has good health literacy, he or she may experience information overload when interacting with clinicians, which can be exacerbated by clinicians' use of unfamiliar terminology or jargon (Hoffman, 2004; IOM, 2011a). Patients may not retain important information if they feel overwhelmed with new terminology while grappling with all of the information clinicians are trying to impart. Moreover, patients have very different expectations regarding the amount of information they need in order to make shared decisions about their care; while many patients want to know as much as possible, some patients do not want information (Epstein and Street, 2007; IOM, 2011a). Additionally, a patient's informational needs may vary substantially from those of the patient's family and caregivers.

There are a number of special considerations when the cancer care team communicates with older adults who have cancer. Older patients may be less technologically savvy and may need alternate options for communicating (such as large print brochures, plain language, and more repetition). Likewise, family members may have to make medical decisions for some older patients with cancer due to a patient's' cognitive status, further complicating the communication and shared decision-making processes. In addition, it may be more difficult for the care team to communicate treatment options to older adults, as multiple comorbid chronic diseases are more prevalent in this population, making the options for cancer treatment especially complex.

Challenges for Clinicians

A number of factors can prevent clinicians from engaging in patient-centered communication and shared decision making, including clinicians' lack of training in communication (see section below on prioritizing clinician training in communication) and insensitivity to patients' informational, cultural, and emotional needs. Clinician characteristics, such as age, gender, and training, may influence the provision of patient-centered communication (Epstein and Street, 2007; Porter-O'Grady and Malloch, 2007). For example, some older clinicians may use authoritative communication styles rather than more collaborative approaches (Busari, 2013; Frosch et al., 2012).

Epstein and Street (2007) noted that some clinicians fail to appreciate the range of patient and family needs, explaining, in part, patients and their families' dissatisfaction with the timing and amount of information given to them by clinicians. As mentioned previously, clinicians need to be aware of the differing informational needs of patients and adapt their communication approach accordingly (Epstein and Street, 2007; IOM, 2011a). A clinician's level of comfort discussing specific aspects of cancer care can also impede patient-centered communication and shared decision making. Research shows that clinicians are often uncomfortable discussing poor prognoses, psychosocial and emotional aspects of care, and sexuality (Epstein and Street, 2007; IOM, 2008a; Mack and Smith, 2012). Furthermore, clinicians may not recognize patients' emotional cues and may be unfamiliar with resources and services designed to meet patients' psychosocial health needs (Epstein and Street, 2007; IOM, 2008a).

Clinicians can also misjudge patient preferences. For example, clinicians may expect women with early stage breast cancer to prefer to keep their breast, given that mastectomy and lumpectomy followed by radiation can be equally effective treatment options for some patients. A study of breast cancer patients who were provided comprehensive information about both treatment options, however, found that approximately one-third of women chose to have a mastectomy (Collins et al., 2009). Other patients may prioritize quality of life rather than length of life as a primary goal (Berman, 2012; IOM, 2011a). In addition, patients with cancer may assess the benefits and risks of chemotherapy differently than their clinicians, and may be more willing to undergo chemotherapy with small benefits and high risks of toxicity (Matsuyama et al., 2006).

Differences between patients' and clinicians' culture and language may influence clinicians' ability to engage in patient-centered communication and shared decision making. Surbone (2010, p. 4) emphasized that language and cultural barriers can be a major source of stress for patients, family members, and clinicians, especially if "linguistic, health literacy, and cultural differences combined render mutual understanding especially difficult." Clinicians' and patients' mutual misunderstanding can result in frustration and mistrust, negatively impacting the care received by patients with cancer (Surbone, 2010). Epstein and Street (2007) noted that cultural beliefs will affect communication between clinicians and patients, influence how patients and clinicians interpret their interaction, and impact communication outcomes. Given the growing diversity of the U.S. population (see Chapter 2), it is imperative for clinicians and the health care system to overcome cultural and language barriers to ensure that all patients with cancer receive patient-centered care. In 2013, the U.S. Department of Health and Human Services (HHS) released a blueprint that aims to ensure culturally and linguistically appropriate health care (HHS, 2013a). To address barriers in language, the American Cancer Society's National Cancer Information Center works with interpreter-services to provide cancer information assistance for the public in 160 languages (see Annex 8-1).

Clinicians' lack of time may also limit the provision of patient-centered communication and shared decision making. The reimbursement system fails to adequately compensate clinicians for the time it takes to facilitate patient-centered care (IOM, 2009a, 2011b). Smith and Hillner (2011) argued that many of the responsibilities of oncologists are reimbursed poorly or not at all. Cognitive care[4]—which can include discussions with patients about prognosis and likely response to treatment, referrals to clinical trials, development of advanced medical directives, and family conferences—is not reimbursed as well as the administration of chemotherapy. Chapter 8 further discusses the perverse incentives of the current reimbursement system and new models of payment that have the potential to improve patient-centered communication and shared decision making in cancer.

System-Level Challenges

The fragmented nature of the cancer care system can prohibit patient-centered communication and shared decision making (IOM and NRC, 1999). Epstein and Street (2007) emphasized that patient-centered communication and shared decision making relies on more than the patient-clinician interactions; it also includes the physical and procedural characteristics of the health care system. Patients who find it difficult to navigate the health care system are likely to experience lower quality patient-clinician communication and shared decision making, which could contribute to underutilization of high-quality care, overuse of care that is unlikely to improve patient outcomes, and higher costs.

Fragmentation of the cancer care delivery system also contributes to communication problems between patients and their care teams. Patients with cancer may need to coordinate care among multiple clinicians on their cancer care team and other care teams. Jessie Gruman, a four-time cancer survivor, pointed out that in 1 year, eight physicians cared for her, and yet only once did two of those physicians communicate directly with each other; she was primarily responsible for sharing her medical information among the different clinicians (Gruman, 2013). It can be especially difficult for care team members to share information and communicate effectively with patients if the care team members' electronic health records (EHRs) are not interoperable (see Chapter 7 on additional information technology challenges). With system problems such as these, it can be unclear to patients and care teams who is responsible for each aspect of care and who needs to be contacted to address a treatment complication (IOM, 2011a). New models of care and reimbursement, such as accountable care organizations (ACOs) or oncology patient-centered medical homes, may address some of these system challenges (see Chapter 8).

---

[4] Cognitive care refers to evaluation and management services, which entails time spent discussing, for example, prognosis and treatment options (Smith and Hillner, 2011).

IMPROVING PATIENT-CENTERED COMMUNICATION AND SHARED DECISION MAKING IN CANCER

This section discusses strategies for improving patient-centered communication and shared decision making, including (1) making more comprehensive and understandable information available to patients and their families; (2) developing decision aids to facilitate patient-centered communication and shared decision making; (3) prioritizing clinician training in communication; (4) preparing cancer care plans; and (5) using new models of payment to incentivize patient-centered communication and shared decision making.

Making More Comprehensive Information Available

The availability of easily understood, accurate information on cancer prognosis, treatment benefits and harms, palliative care, psychosocial support, and likelihood of treatment response can improve patient-centered communication and shared decision making. A number of trusted organizations have developed print, electronic, and social resources to inform patients and their families about cancer, such as the NCI, the American Cancer Society, the Centers for Disease Control and Prevention, the Mayo Clinic, the National Coalition for Cancer Survivorship, American Society of Clinical Oncology, LIVE**STRONG**, and the Susan G. Komen Foundation (see Table 3-2 for examples of patient resources).[5] However, there are some serious limitations with the type of information included in the available resources on cancer. In addition, there are a number of other websites that may contain inaccurate or outdated information. Thus, finding accurate, useful cancer information online can be a major challenge for patients and their families (Chan et al., 2012; IOM, 2011a; Irwin et al., 2011; Lawrentschuk et al., 2012; Quinn et al., 2012; Shah et al., 2013).

Information that is readily available on cancer often does not answer all of the questions that are important to patients. Some organizations do not provide detailed information on prognosis for various cancers or on the likelihood that treatments will cure cancer or prolong life (IOM, 2009a). Without this information, patients may have poorly informed or unrealistic expectations about the benefit of certain interventions or their likelihood of survival (IOM, 2009a, 2013; Smith and Hillner, 2010). These inaccurate perceptions could result in care that is not aligned with a patient's goals, such as futile chemotherapy near the end of life. Around 70 to 80 percent of patients with metastatic lung and colorectal cancer in a

---

[5] See http://www.cancer.gov; http://www.cancer.org; http://www.cdc.gov/cancer; http://www.mayoclinic.com/health-information; http://www.canceradvocacy.org; http://www.cancer.net; http://www.livestrong.org; and http://ww5.komen.org (accessed March 28, 2013).

TABLE 3-2 Examples of Web-Based Information, Resources, and Tools for Patients

Resource	Description
AARP Medicare Starter Kit	This kit provides individuals who are approaching age 65 with information on Medicare, including information on choosing a health insurance plan and a timeline for making decisions. It explains in detail issues related to coverage, costs, options, enrollment deadlines, and eligibility. The kit also identifies resources where individuals can find further information on the program.
American Society of Clinical Oncology's (ASCO's) Advanced Cancer Care Planning Booklet	This booklet offers patients with advanced cancer information about treatment options, clinical trial participation, palliative care and hospice care, the role of family in the decision-making process, and end-of-life planning (e.g., creating an advanced directive, developing a living will, and how to find religious or spiritual support if desired). It includes a blank sheet on which patients can write questions and answers from their clinicians. It also provides additional resources for caregiving, end-of-life care planning, grief and bereavement, cancer treatment, and general patient support.
ASCO's Cancer.Net Mobile	This application helps patients plan and manage their cancer treatment and care, including tools to assemble questions for clinicians and record their responses, track symptoms and side effects during treatment, among other resources.
Cancer Support Community	This organization provides a variety of online support groups and discussion boards. The support groups meet in a chat room for 90 minutes per week and are led by licensed mental health professionals. Support groups are organized based on issues, such as caregiving and dealing with bereavement. The discussion boards allow patients to connect with others in order to receive and offer advice and support from those with similar cancer experiences.
Center for Advancing Health	This organization runs the Prepared Patient Forum, an interactive website where individuals can read about other patients' experiences with the health care system and share their own experiences. It also publishes the latest research related to health care decisions and provides links to trusted and helpful resources.

TABLE 3-2 Continued

Resource	Description
John M. Eisenberg Center for Clinical Decisions and Communications Science	This center translates comparative effectiveness research findings into plain language that patients can understand. It creates a variety of products, ranging from research summaries to decision aids and other materials, for use by patients, clinicians, and policy makers. It also runs a conference series to discuss state-of-the-art in communication and medical decision making.
Leukemia & Lymphoma Society's Acute Myeloid Leukemia (AML) Guide	This guide provides detailed information about the biology of AML, considerations in treatment planning (e.g., choosing a specialist, risks and benefits of various treatment options, clinical trial participation, follow-up care), and general strategies for maintaining health (e.g., maintaining a healthy diet and seeing a doctor regularly). It also includes definitions of medical terms.
National Coalition for Cancer Survivorship's (NCCS's) Cancer Survival Toolbox	This toolbox is a free, self-learning audio program composed of various scenarios cancer patients and survivors commonly face during their cancer journey. The goal of the program is to help patients develop the skills needed to better face and understand the challenges of their illness. It emphasizes developing communication skills, finding information, making decisions, and solving problems. It also includes links to cancer-specific programs that teach patients more about their disease. The NCCS Pocket Cancer Care Guide, a cell phone application, helps patients build question lists, and record and play back office visit conversations, among other features.
Patient Advocate Foundation	This organization has a list of resources to help patients find assistance in addressing a variety of medical-related issues. Resources include the National Financial Resource Directory (provides information on financial relief for all areas in life, such as housing, utilities, and food), the National Uninsured Resource Directory & Financial Resource (provides information on available organizations and resources that may help with access to care), National Underinsured Resource Directory & Financial Resource (provides information for patients whose insurance plan does not provide full coverage), and InsureUStoday (provides information on the Affordable Care Act).

SOURCES: AHRQ, 2012; ASCO, 2011; ASCO and Cancer.Net, 2012; Cancer Support Community, 2012; CFAH, 2012; Finch, 2011; Leukemia & Lymphoma Society, 2012; NCCS, 2012c; Patient Advocate Foundation, 2012.

recent survey, for example, did not understand that their chemotherapy was unlikely to result in a cure (Weeks et al., 2012). In another survey, 64 percent of patients with metastatic lung cancer did not understand that radiation therapy was unlikely to result in a cure (Chen et al., 2013). To inform patients' expectations about therapy, Smith and Hillner suggested that the NCI revise www.cancer.gov to summarize the available information from clinical research on various cancers' curability, average lifespan, average treatment benefit, most common side effects, and available clinical trials (Smith and Hillner, 2010).

There is a dearth of information on the patient experience with cancer and its treatment. Oftentimes, available information focuses on survival but neglects other outcomes that matter to patients and their families (Fleurence et al., 2013). Patients are often interested in how they are going to feel during treatment or how long it will take before they can go back to work (Basch, 2013; IOM, 2008a, 2011a). The concept of providing patients with this type of information is consistent with the aims of the Patient-Centered Outcomes Research Institute (PCORI) to support research that aligns with a patient's experience with treatment (PCORI, 2013b). In its first round of funded projects, PCORI focused largely on addressing questions that are critical to patients and clinicians when making health care decisions (Fleurence et al., 2013). PCORI has also prioritized communication and dissemination of research results, including comparing approaches to disseminate CER, engaging people to ask for information from CER, and supporting shared decision making (PCORI, 2012). In Chapter 5, the committee recommends that the NCI, other federal agencies, PCORI, and researchers work to develop a common set of data elements in research studies that will capture patient-reported outcomes, relevant patient characteristics, and health behaviors to address the need for better clinical information.

Patients and families also lack access to information about the cost of cancer care. In this report, the committee defines the total cost of cancer care as all direct medical costs resulting from the provision of cancer care,[6] including payment reimbursed by insurance companies to hospitals and clinicians as well as out-of-pocket costs. Out-of-pocket costs are expenses for medical care that are paid for by the patient and can include deductibles, coinsurance, and copayments for covered services, as well as services that are not covered by insurance (HealthCare.gov, 2013).

The complexity of calculating costs from the multiple perspectives of cancer care (i.e., society, health care system, payer, or patients) presents a

---

[6] This definition varies from other uses of total cost of care, which factor in direct nonmedical costs (such as transportation and parking associated with the receipt of care) and indirect costs (such as lost productivity due to disease morbidity or premature death).

major challenge to making the cost of cancer care more transparent. The price that a clinician or hospital charges for care is often different from the amount collected for that care. Hospitals and clinician practices, for example, usually have a chargemaster that consists of a comprehensive listing of charges for each billable item associated with the care they provide. This chargemaster serves as a starting point for negotiating reimbursement with payers. Thus, the amount that payers reimburse clinicians and hospitals likely varies by payer and is almost always less than what is listed in the chargemaster. In addition, differences in patients' health insurance benefit plan designs, including variations in the benefits covered and cost-sharing requirements, mean that individual patients can pay different out-of-pocket amounts for the same care. Uninsured patients, who do not have a payer to negotiate the price on their behalf, may pay much more than a well-insured patient for the same care. According to Reinhardt, "this situation has resulted in an opaque system in which payers with market power force weaker payers to cover disproportionate shares of providers' fixed costs—a phenomenon sometimes termed *cost shifting*—or providers simply succeed in charging higher prices when they can" (Reinhardt, 2011, p. 2125).

The system's lack of price transparency is very problematic for patients and clinicians who want to be cost conscious when making decisions about care (Gruman, 2013). A recent study found that only 16 percent of a randomly selected group of U.S. hospitals were able to provide a cost estimate for a hospital stay that included both hospital charges and physician fees for a common surgical procedure (Rosenthal et al., 2013).

A growing number of stakeholders, however, have recognized the importance of price transparency in health care, including state and federal government leaders, private-sector trade groups, and health payers (Rosenthal et al., 2013). The Government Accountability Office concluded that a number of health care and legal factors make it difficult for consumers to obtain price information and recommended that HHS assess the feasibility of estimating complete costs of health care available to consumers through its ongoing and future price transparency efforts (GAO, 2011).

The Patient Protection and Affordable Care Act (ACA)[7] requires hospitals to annually publish and update a list of standard charges for their services. In 2014, Health Insurance Marketplaces will require participating health plans to create communication tools where patients can research anticipated out-of-pocket costs for specific services. Private companies are also utilizing proprietary software that analyzes claims data to estimate the costs of common medical procedures (Hostetter and Klein, 2012). As

---

[7] Patient Protection and Affordable Care Act, Public Law 111-148, 111th Congress, 2nd Sess. (March 23, 2010).

of February 2013, at least 30 states had signed laws or proposed legislation focusing on health care price transparency (NCSL, 2013). Several states have also created all-payer claims databases, which collect health insurance claims information from all payers into a single database, including information on charges and payments, the clinicians/hospitals receiving payment, clinical diagnosis and procedure codes, and patient demographics (APCD, 2013; NCSL, 2013).

As depicted in the committee's conceptual framework (see Figure S-2), publicly reported quality measurement will facilitate better information about the cost of cancer care. The Centers for Medicare & Medicaid Services (CMS) may be in the best position to provide this information. In 2013, HHS released average Medicare charges for 100 common inpatient hospital procedures and 30 outpatient procedures in an effort to improve the affordability and accountability of the health care system (CMS, 2013b; HHS, 2013b). In addition, a U.S. federal judge has lifted an injunction preventing public access to a database that provides information on Medicare insurance claims by individual clinicians (Tamman, 2013). Clinical practice guidelines could also include cost information for different chemotherapy regimens (IOM, 2013; Ramsey and Shankaran, 2012). One study found that when cost information was included in laboratory test ordering forms, it led to a decrease in the number of tests clinicians ordered and reduced hospital charges by more than $400,000 over the 6-month intervention (Feldman et al., 2013). In addition, the decision-support software eviti® provides clinicians with cost data based on average wholesale price for more than 1,100 different cancer care regimens (Licking, 2012). Although one study found that eviti® reduced nonstandard treatment in lung cancer, its impact on the cost of care was not assessed (Ganz, 2013; Grund et al., 2012).

Given patients' needs for more comprehensive information about cancer care, the committee recommends that the **NCI, CMS, PCORI, as well as patient advocacy organizations, professional organizations, and other public and private stakeholders, improve the development of clinical and cost information and make it available through print, electronic, and social media.** This information should be easily accessible to patients and their families. Access to more comprehensive information on cancer care will enable patients to make better informed decisions about their care.

Improving Shared Decision Making Using Decision Aids

One of the important functions of communication in cancer care is ensuring that patients make decisions that are consistent with their needs, preferences, and values. Clinicians have an important role in improving patient-centered communication and shared decision making by listening actively, assessing a patient's understanding of treatment options, validating a patient's participation in the decision-making process, and communicating empathy both verbally and nonverbally (Epstein and Street, 2007). In addition, decision making can be improved through use of decision aids that facilitate patient understanding of treatment options and enable patients to take a more active role in decision making. A decision aid is a "tool that provides patients with evidence-based, objective information on all treatment options for a given condition. Decision aids present the risks and benefits of all options and help patients understand how likely it is that those benefits or harms will affect them" (MedPAC, 2010, p. 195). Decision aids can include written material, Web-based tools, videos, and multimedia programs (MedPAC, 2010). Some decision aids are designed for patient use and others are designed for clinicians to use with patients.

Decision aids have rapidly been developed by organizations such as AHRQ, the NCI, the Informed Medical Decisions Foundation, Healthwise, and many others (MedPAC, 2010). Estimates suggest that there are more than 500 decision aids currently available (Elwyn et al., 2006; OHRI, 2013). In the cancer setting, one of the most recognized decision aids is Adjuvant! Online. Clinicians and patients use Adjuvant! Online to assess the risk of an individual patient developing a recurrence and/or dying from breast cancer within 10 years of their diagnosis in order to guide decisions about adjuvant treatment for breast cancer (chemotherapy, endocrine therapy, or none) (Gribbin and Dewis, 2009). The Informed Medical Decisions Foundation's website includes a number of decision aids relevant to cancer, including those for breast cancer, prostate cancer, and end-of-life decisions, as well as screening aids for colorectal cancer and prostate cancer (Informed Medical Decisions Foundation, 2012b). PCORI also supports research on decision aids (PCORI, 2013a). Oshima Lee and Emanuel (2013) have suggested that PCORI's research on the effectiveness of shared decision-making techniques could be broadly disseminated to improve the development of future decision aids.

There are a number of ongoing efforts to improve shared decision making. The University of California, San Francisco, and the Dartmouth-Hitchcock Medical Center, for example, offer decision support programs for patients with breast cancer (see Box 3-2), and in 2007, Washington state became the first state to enact legislation promoting the use of shared decision making and decision aids in practice (Armstron and Arterburn, 2013). Group Health recently implemented a demonstration project using 12 video-based decision aids for elective surgical procedures and has since distributed more than 31,000 decision aids to participating patients. More

---

BOX 3-2
Examples of Decision Support Programs

University of California, San Francisco, Carol Franc Buck Breast Care Center
   This program provides patients with information packets and decision aids to review prior to their medical appointments, as well as an intern who accompanies them throughout their consultation and treatment planning process. The interns generate a prioritized list of questions for the patients to ask their clinicians. They may also accompany patients to their medical appointments to record the discussion and write down answers doctors provide to their questions. The written answers are reviewed by the clinicians, put in the medical chart, and sent home with the patient, along with an audio recording of the visit.

Dartmouth-Hitchcock Medical Center
   At this center, every breast cancer patient is referred to the Center for Shared Decision Making when first diagnosed. Patients complete online surveys to capture their medical and family history, how important it is to them to keep their breasts and avoid radiation, and other personal treatment-related preferences. The patients also watch a video with a decision aid that is appropriate for their situation. Following the video, patients are asked what treatment they prefer, how certain they are in their decision, and if they understand the survival and recurrence rates associated with their various treatment options. The collected information is entered into a clinical decision support system, which will alert the center's clinicians to different actions based on the patients' responses.

SOURCES: Informed Medical Decisions Foundation, 2012a; IOM, 2011a; UCSF Carol Franc Buck Breast Cancer Center, 2012.

---

than 65 percent of patients who undergo elective surgery at Group Health now use a decision aid (Armstron and Arterburn, 2013).

A Cochrane systematic review of 86 studies found that individuals who used decision aids had improved knowledge about their care options and more accurate expectations about potential benefits and harms, made decisions more consistent with their values, and were more engaged in their care compared to individuals who did not use decision aids (Stacey et al., 2011). In cancer care, a systematic review of 23 randomized clinical trials of cancer decision aids found that decision aids improved patient participation in decision making and resulted in higher-quality medical decisions (Stacey et al., 2008). For example, a randomized controlled trial found that Adjuvant! Online made a difference in patients' decisions on whether or not to take adjuvant therapy and resulted in treatment decisions that were more tailored to patient preferences (Siminoff et al., 2006). Video decision aids have also been effective in the cancer setting in promoting patients' understanding of end-of-life care options (El-Jawahri et al., 2010; Volandes et al., 2013). Decision aids that provide information on prognosis are acceptable and desired among patients with metastatic cancer (Chiew et al., 2008; Smith et al., 2011), and these decision aids improve knowledge without creating anxiety (Leighl et al., 2011) or diminishing hope (Smith et al., 2010).

In addition, decision aids may reduce the cost of care (The Commonwealth Fund, 2007; Oshima Lee and Emanuel, 2013). One study found that individuals who used decision aids had 5.3 percent lower overall medical costs compared to individuals who had received standard of care (Veroff et al., 2013). Some savings from shared decision making could result from patients opting for less aggressive interventions that are more aligned with their needs, values, and preferences (Covinsky et al., 2000; El-Jawahri et al., 2010; Oshima Lee and Emanuel, 2013; Veroff et al., 2013). Because of these benefits, the committee recommends that the **NCI, CMS, PCORI, as well as patient advocacy organizations, professional organizations, and other public and private stakeholders, improve the development of decision aids and make them available through print, electronic, and social media.**

To ensure the development and dissemination of high-quality decision aids, it may be beneficial to have a mechanism for quality control. Oshima Lee and Emanuel (2013) called upon CMS to begin certifying patient decision aids in order to (1) promote an ideal approach to patient-clinician decision making, (2) improve the quality of health care decisions, and (3) reduce the cost of health care. Other groups have also developed criteria to evaluate decision aids (Elwyn et al., 2006). This mechanism for quality control may be met by Section 3506 of the ACA, which calls for HHS to establish a program that would facilitate shared decision making. Although this program would be responsible for developing, certifying, and disseminating patient decision aids, it has not yet been funded (Informed Medical Decisions Foundation, 2013).

The cancer community could also promote more widespread use of high-quality decision aids by addressing barriers in uptake among patients and clinicians. Clinicians lack incentives to use decision aids in their practices and have limited training in their use (Lin et al., 2013). King and Moulton (2013) noted that the Group Health demonstration project overcame clinician reluctance to using decision aids by changing institutional culture, presenting patient satisfaction data to clinicians, and providing decision aid training. Additional research on patient use of decision aids could inform interventions designed to broaden the reach of these decision aids (Belkora et al., 2011; Partin et al., 2006).

Prioritizing Clinician Training in Communication

Communication is a core responsibility for clinicians and the Accreditation Council for Graduate Medical Education expects medical residents to demonstrate competency in communication (ACGME, 2008; Moore et al., 2013). As discussed previously, clinicians need to communicate effectively with patients to build patient-clinician relationships focused on trust and rapport, as well as to exchange information, respond to patient emotions, manage the uncertainty associated with a cancer diagnosis and treatment, participate in shared decision making, and enable patient self-management (Epstein and Street, 2007). Effective communication is associated with patients experiencing faster recovery, improved pain control, and better psychological functioning; ineffective communication is associated with patient anxiety, uncertainty, and dissatisfaction with cancer care (reviewed in Moore et al., 2013). In addition, the availability of clinical and cost information is insufficient to assist patients in making decisions consistent with their needs, preferences, and values. It is also critically important for clinicians to provide patients with the opportunity to discuss this information in real time with members of the cancer care team. Technology-enabled approaches, such as telemedicine, may increase the opportunity for patients to have these interactions (see Chapter 4).

Many clinicians, however, are not trained to communicate well and many patients with cancer have unmet communication needs (Hack, 2005). Kissane et al. (2012) noted that medical schools teach generic communication skills, but the cancer setting requires specialty communication skills training, including breaking bad news, discussing prognosis and risk, using shared decision making to make care plans, responding to emotions, dealing with recurrence, changing treatment goals, running a family meeting, and discussing death and dying. Because cancer is a life-threatening condition, giving bad news, such as discussing a poor prognosis, recurrence, or progression, is a common clinician task. But clinicians are rarely trained to have these difficult conversations with patients (Baile et al., 2000; Oncotalk, 2002; Orlander et al., 2002; Quill and Townsend, 1991; Wittenberg-Lyles et al., 2013). A survey of oncologists found that less than 10 percent reported formal training in breaking bad news and only 32 percent had the opportunity during training to regularly observe other clinicians break bad news to patients (Baile et al., 2000).

Given the importance of communication in the cancer setting, the committee recommends that professional educational programs for members of the cancer care team should provide comprehensive and formal training in communication. A Cochrane systematic review assessing communication skills training in cancer found that this training is effective and improves clinician empathy and use of open-ended questions

(Moore et al., 2013). Additional research will be needed to understand the link between clinician communication training and improved patient outcomes (Moore et al., 2013; Uitterhoeve et al., 2010). However, there is some evidence on how to train clinicians most effectively.

Many clinicians learn communication skills by watching mentors communicate with patients or through didactic approaches, but research indicates that there are more effective methods of improving communication skills (Back et al., 2009a, 2010; Berkhof et al., 2010). Key attributes of effective communication skills training include (1) recognition and definition of the essential skills in communication (for example, demonstrating empathy, using open-ended questions, and assessing psychosocial care needs); (2) opportunities for clinicians to practice communication skills through role-playing; (3) thoughtful feedback from skilled communicators; (4) self-reflection through video and audio recordings; and (5) continued practice of communication skills (Back et al., 2009a; Moore et al., 2013).

Communication skills training has been delivered in a number of formats, including sessions integrated into a degree program, as well as multi-day workshops (Moore et al., 2013). Epstein and Street (2007) suggested that communication training should be introduced as early as possible in medical and nursing education, because clinicians immediately start establishing routines for interacting with patients. Additional research is necessary to assess the duration of effectiveness of this training (Moore et al., 2013).

There are a number of challenges to implementing communication skills training. Compared to other types of clinician training that test knowledge to assess improvement, it is more difficult to measure improvements in communication skills. The diversity of settings in which communication skills training occurs (i.e., medical and nursing schools, residency programs, and clinical practice), along with the various levels of exposure that clinicians have to communication skills training, may also make it difficult to implement. In addition, communication skills training needs to be reinforced over time, but there is a lack of information regarding how often this should occur. There is also uncertainty regarding the scalability of current communication programs, given the resources needed to establish a communication skills training program, measure performance, and evaluate outcomes. Additional communication training could be supported through the NCI R25 mechanism (NCI, 2013a), but Kissane et al. (2012) argued that this funding is unlikely to sustain these programs over time. The importance of communication to new models of payment, however, may spur investment in communication skills training (see Chapter 8).

In addition, a number programs and models are available to improve clinician communication skills in the cancer setting. Oncotalk®8 uses a series of learning modules (e.g., fundamental communication skills, giving bad news, discussing treatment options, and informed consent, etc.) to teach clinicians about specific communication tasks, provide suggestions for implementing these skills, and review recommended sources for more information. One of the communication approaches advocated by Oncotalk is the ask-tell-ask method, which has clinicians ask their patients to describe their understanding of an issue by using prompts such as, "to make sure we are on the same page, can you tell me what your understanding of your disease is?" The process of asking for this information can improve the patient-clinician relationship, demonstrate a clinician's willingness to listen, and help direct the conversation. Next, clinicians tell their patients the information that needs to be conveyed in straightforward language, breaking down the information so that it is not overwhelming to the patient. In the final step, clinicians ask patients if they understand the information, which acts as a check to see if patients received the information the clinician tried to impart and provides an opportunity for patients to ask questions (Back et al., 2009b). An evaluation of Oncotalk found that the program was a successful teaching model for improving communication skills in postgraduate medical trainees (Back et al., 2007).

Another approach to communication emphasized in the palliative care setting for nurses is the COMFORT model (Communicate, Orientation and opportunity, Mindful presence, Family, Openings, Relating, and Team) (Goldsmith et al., 2013; Wittenberg-Lyles et al., 2013). This approach builds a number of communication skills, including practicing empathy, engaging in interdisciplinary collaboration, gauging health literacy, and recognizing the patient and family in palliative care interactions.

Communicating Information and Preparing Cancer Care Plans

To achieve high-quality cancer care, the cancer care team needs to effectively communicate and engage in shared decision making with patients to ensure that patients understand their disease, know their care options, and develop a plan for care. **The committee recommends that the cancer care team provide patients and their families with understandable information on cancer prognosis, treatment benefits and harms, palliative care, psychosocial support, and estimates of the total and out-of-pocket costs of cancer care. The cancer care team should communicate and personalize this information for their patients at key decision points along the continuum of cancer care, using decision aids**

---

[8] See http://depts.washington.edu/oncotalk (accessed January 3, 2013).

when available. The American Board of Internal Medicine's (ABIM's) Charter for medical professionalism highlights the fundamental importance of communication with patients such that "patients are completely and honestly informed . . . [and] empowered to decide on the course of therapy" (ABIM, 2013).

The cancer care team personalizes this information for patients by ensuring that the communication approach takes into account a patient's language, health literacy, and informational and emotional needs. Health literacy toolkits may help clinicians more effectively convey understandable information to their patients (AMA, 2013; DeWalt et al., 2010; LINCS, 2013). In addition, several IOM workshops highlighted some methods that clinicians could use to present complicated information to patients in a format that facilitates comprehension (see Table 3-3).

Patient-clinician communication is especially important when patients and their families need to make specific decisions about their care. This includes key decision points, such as at the time of initial diagnosis, when patients experience cancer progression or recurrence, following treatment, or when the goals of care or patient preferences change.

Cancer care plans facilitate clinicians' communication of this information because they provide patients and their families with a roadmap to navigate their cancer care. They can also facilitate coordinated care by summarizing all relevant information into a single location that can be shared among members of the cancer care team, the primary care/ geriatrics care team, and other clinicians involved in a patient's care. Additionally, cancer care plans can encourage patient participation in decisions about their care and help patients retain important information by providing a summary of key information (IOM, 2011a).

The IOM report *Ensuring Quality Cancer Care* recommended that patients with cancer have "an agreed-upon care plan that outlines the goals of care" (IOM and NRC, 1999, p. 7). The IOM also recommended care plans for cancer survivors completing primary treatment (IOM and NRC, 2005). More recently, an IOM workshop highlighted the importance of care planning for promoting patient-centered communication and shared decision making (IOM, 2011a). **Thus, the committee recommends that the cancer care team collaborate with their patients to develop a care plan that reflects their patients' needs, values, and preferences, and considers palliative care needs and psychosocial support across the cancer care continuum.** Involvement of patients' primary/geriatrics and specialist care teams may also be helpful in developing a care plan, especially for patients with comorbidities.

Currently, the evidence base for care plans is limited and primarily related to survivorship care plans rather than care plans for ongoing cancer care. The IOM report *From Cancer Patient to Cancer Survivor: Lost in Transi-*

TABLE 3-3 Examples of Communication Strategies Clinicians Can Use to Present Complicated Information to Patients

Strategy	Description
Absolute risk	Patients and caregivers are better at comprehending absolute risk than relative risk. Relative risk compares risk in two different populations. For example, people who smoke are about 15 to 30 times more likely to develop lung cancer or die from lung cancer compared to people who do not smoke. In contrast, absolute risk represents an individual's overall risk. For example, the risk that a woman who is 40 years old will be diagnosed with breast cancer during the next 10 years is 1.47 percent (or 1 in 68 women).
Graphical formats	Graphs can help patients and caregivers comprehend risk. Some graphical formats are easier for patients and caregivers to interpret. For example, pictographs (or diagrams representing statistical data in pictorial form) improve patients' and caregivers' comprehension compared to bar graphs or pie charts.
Rare events	Comparing the likelihood of a medical event to the likelihood of a commonly understood rare event can help patients and caregivers understand risk. For example, "an individual has a 1 in 10,000,000 chance of getting struck by lightning, and about a 1 in 100 chance of dying if they smoke 10 cigarettes a day for one year."
Multiple formats	Presenting patients and caregivers with complicated information in multiple formats improves comprehension. For example, clinicians can present information as both percentages and as frequencies, and numerical information can be presented both orally and visually (e.g., in a graph).
Read back	When clinicians ask their patients to repeat back the information they heard, rather than just ask whether they understood the information, comprehension improves. Repetition requires patients to demonstrate to the clinicians that they understand the information. It also gives clinicians the opportunity to clarify information or emphasize necessary details.
Videos	Clinicians can use videos to provide realistic visual images of various treatment options and outcomes. For example, a study evaluating the effect of a video on the cardiopulmonary resuscitation (CPR) preferences of patients with advanced cancer found that patients who watched the video had improved knowledge of CPR and more confidence in their health care decisions, compared to patients who did not watch the video.

SOURCES: CDC, 2013; El-Jawahri et al., 2010; Gigerenzer and Edwards, 2003; IOM, 2009a, 2011b; NCI, 2012; Peters et al., 2007; Volandes et al., 2013.

tion argues that even though there is limited evidence to support survivor-ship care plans, "some elements of care simply make sense—that is, they have strong face validity and can reasonably be assumed to improve care" (IOM and NRC, 2005). Only one randomized clinical trial on survivorship care planning has been published (Grunfeld et al., 2011), which found that survivorship care plans were not beneficial for improving patient-reported outcomes. However, the validity and generalizability of this study has been questioned (Parry et al., 2013). Moreover, the relevance of this finding on care plans in the treatment setting is unknown. CMS rec-ognizes the promise of care planning and is in the process of implement-ing a new Medicare payment policy to reward care planning delivered in the context of a patient-centered medical home for patients with complex chronic conditions (Bindman et al., 2013). Bindman and colleagues note that the "care plan is based on a physical, mental, cognitive, psychosocial, and functional and environmental (re)assessment of the patient and on an inventory of resources and supports available to the patient." The need to consider multiple treatment modalities, facilitate shared decision mak-ing, and coordinate care in the cancer treatment setting suggests that care plans may prove especially beneficial there.

Documenting information in a patient's care plan is insufficient to en-sure patient-centered communication and shared decision making. Parry and colleagues (2013) noted that "much like electronic health records, care plans are vehicles for communication and coordination of care, nothing more. We cannot expect a document to do the work of a process, and we certainly cannot expect it to fix a flawed process" (p. 2651). The care plan is a tool to facilitate communication and shared decision making, care co-ordination, and retention of the path of care. Equally important to the care plan itself are the conversations that a patient and clinician have regard-ing a patient's cancer care. Improving clinician training in communication will be essential to implementing the committee's recommendation on cancer care planning.

Progress on implementing cancer care planning is under way. CMS has established two new Healthcare Common Procedure Coding System codes for cancer treatment planning and care coordination related to initial treatment and change of treatment (NCCS, 2012b). In June 2013, the Planning Actively for Cancer Treatment (PACT) Act of 2013 was in-troduced in the U.S. House of Representatives.[9] This bill would provide Medicare coverage for cancer care planning and coordination services, including the development of a written plan for cancer treatment. A number of cancer organizations have endorsed the PACT Act of 2013,

---

[9] H.R. 2477. Planning Actively for Cancer Treatment (PACT) Act of 2013. 113th Cong. 1st. sess. (June 25, 2013).

including the American Cancer Society Cancer Action Network, ASCO, LIVE**STRONG**, the National Coalition for Cancer Survivorship, and the National Comprehensive Cancer Network (NCCS, 2013).

Care Plan Components

Cancer care plans document information about a patient's diagnosis and prognosis, the planned path of care, and who is responsible for each portion of that care. Box 3-3 lists examples of typical features of cancer care plans, and the section below elaborates on a number of critical fea-

---

BOX 3-3
Information in a Cancer Care Plan

Utilizing patient-centered communication and shared decision making, the cancer care team should collaborate with patients to develop a cancer care plan. Examples of components in a patient-specific cancer care plan include

- Patient information (e.g., name, date of birth, medication list, and allergies)
- Diagnosis, including specific tissue information, relevant biomarkers, and stage
- Prognosis
- Treatment goals (curative, life-prolonging, symptom control, palliative care)
- Initial plan for treatment and proposed duration, including specific chemo-therapy drug names, doses, and schedule as well as surgery and radiation therapy (if applicable)
- Expected response to treatment
- Treatment benefits and harms, including common and rare toxicities and how to manage these toxicities, as well as short-term and late effects of treatment
- Information on quality of life and a patient's likely experience with treatment
- Who will take responsibility for specific aspects of a patient's care (e.g., the cancer care team, the primary care/geriatrics care team, or other care teams)
- Advance care plans, including advanced directives and other legal documents
- Estimated total and out-of-pocket costs of cancer treatment
- A plan for addressing a patient's psychosocial health needs, including psychological, vocational, disability, legal, or financial concerns and their management
- Survivorship plan, including a summary of treatment and information on recommended follow-up activities and surveillance, as well as risk reduction and health promotion activities

SOURCES: IOM, 2011a; IOM and NRC, 2005.

tures, including clinical and cost information, palliative care, psychosocial support, and advance care planning. Care plans should be updated when new information becomes relevant, such as changes in treatment response or patient preferences. Further research on care plans will also be needed, including the optimal presentation of this information and the relationship between care plans and patient-clinician communication and shared decision making, among other topics. Table 3-4 illustrates an example of a care plan for cancer, which could be imported into electronic health records (EHRs) and shared with patients.

Clinical information. The clinical information that the cancer care team discusses with patients should include all relevant information for patients to make decisions about their care options, including cancer prognosis, likelihood of treatment response, treatment benefits and harms, and likely experience with a treatment. The prognostic information should include specifics about curability, response rates for various treatment options, and a treatment's impact on survival as well as quality of life.

Palliative care. Palliative care is defined as "patient- and family-centered care that optimizes quality of life by anticipating, preventing, and treating suffering. Palliative care throughout the continuum of illness involves addressing physical, intellectual, emotional, social, and spiritual needs and facilitating patient autonomy, access to information, and choice" (NQF, 2006, p. 3).

Palliative care has the following characteristics:

- Care is provided and services are coordinated by an interdisciplinary team;
- Patients, families, and palliative and non-palliative health care clinicians collaborate and communicate about care needs;
- Services are available concurrently with or independent of curative or life-prolonging care; and
- Clinicians respect their patients and families' dignity throughout the course of illness, during the dying process, and after death.

Despite the importance of palliative care in improving the quality of patients' lives, clinicians often fail to address patients' palliative care needs in their care plans. Clinicians often equate palliative care with end-of-life care and consider it an alternative, rather than a complement, to curative or life-extending treatment (see Box 3-4). However, palliative care services may be introduced at any point along the continuum of cancer care as a critical layer of support that is delivered concurrently

TABLE 3-4 Example of a Written Plan for Communication

Plan component	Purpose
Name_____	Lets the cancer care team personalize each patient's plan; make a copy for the medical record.
Medical Record No._____	
Date_____	
1. Diagnosis:_____	Gives the disease a name so the patient can look it up.
2. Stage (where it has spread):_____ (list all areas)	Allows discussion of prognosis. Showing metastases to the brain and liver quickly points out the seriousness of the illness.
3. Prognosis:_____ List whether curable or not curable and expected average lifespan	Allows the cancer care team to ask first if patients want to know the full details of their illness! Allows open communication about goals, rest-of-life planning. Some patients will persist in denial, but this allows open dialogue with the family.
4. Treatment Goals:_____ List cure, long- or short-term control, pain relief, hospice care	Makes explicit what the cancer care team can and cannot do; for curable disease, this reinforces the patient's goal, and that cure is possible. The cancer care team can use this to bring up do-not-resuscitate and cardiopulmonary resuscitation issues. Allows the cancer care team to emphasize that hospice care does not mean "no treatment," but a different set of treatment goals.
5. Treatment Options:_____ List all that apply	The cancer care team should list treatments, response rates, and common toxicities. The cancer team should specifically mention vomiting and hair loss, the two most feared symptoms. If the cancer care team cannot define a real benefit then there is no justification for treatment.
6. Call the doctor if:_____ List the threshold for fever, pain, and other symptoms	Gives patients explicit reasons to call their cancer care team and gives explicit permission to call.
7. How to reach me:_____ List the phone numbers during office and off-hours	The cancer care team should tell patients to keep this handy. They will call, and for real events. Emails for nonemergency purposes work well for prescription refills, questions about new drugs, encouragement, etc.
8. Signed:_____, MD	Personalizes the plan as well as making it a part of the medical record.

SOURCE: Adapted from Smith, T.: *J Clin Oncol* 21(9 Suppl), 2003: 12s-16s. Reprinted with permission. © 2003 American Society of Clinical Oncology. All rights reserved.

BOX 3-4
Challenges to the Delivery of Palliative Care
Across the Cancer Care Continuum

In this report, the committee utilizes the term palliative care and adopts the National Quality Forum's definition: "patient- and family-centered care that optimizes quality of life by anticipating, preventing, and treating suffering. Palliative care throughout the continuum of illness involves addressing physical, intellectual, emotional, social, and spiritual needs and facilitating patient autonomy, access to information, and choice" (NQF, 2006, p. 3). The committee conceptualizes palliative care as an added layer of support that can be delivered concurrently with other therapeutic treatment modalities to improve quality of life for cancer patients.

A lack of awareness about palliative care and definitional challenges reduce patients' access to palliative care across the cancer care continuum. A recent survey found that 70 percent of the public had no knowledge about palliative care, but once informed, 95 percent of respondents agreed that patients with serious illness should be informed about palliative care (Center to Advance Palliative Care, 2011).

Although the general public has little knowledge about palliative care, clinicians often conflate palliative care with hospice care (Center to Advance Palliative Care, 2011; Meier, 2012). Thus, clinicians often neglect recommending palliative care until late in the cancer care continuum. Studies suggest that some oncology clinicians prefer the term supportive care as opposed to palliative care, and if the name were changed, clinicians would be more likely to refer patients earlier in the cancer care continuum (Dalal et al., 2011; Hui et al., 2013; Wentlandt et al., 2012). However, others have asserted that changing the name risks even more confusion: "Rather than changing the name from 'palliative care,' risking ambiguity and confusion, we believe that improved communication is key to appropriate engagement with palliative care services" (Milne et al., 2013).

---

with therapeutic treatment modalities to improve quality of life for cancer patients (Ferris et al., 2009; Hennessy et al., 2013; Spinks et al., 2012). In a provisional clinical opinion, ASCO endorsed the provision of palliative care concurrent with usual cancer care (Smith et al., 2012). This concept is illustrated in Figure 3-3, showing palliative and life-prolonging care being delivered simultaneously. Generally, the majority of a patient's care is initially focused on life-prolonging therapy, but as a patient's disease progresses, palliative care takes on a more prominent role. However, individuals' need for palliative care may vary throughout their disease trajectory. For example, a patient may require more palliative care early in treatment (during chemotherapy or following surgery or radiation treatment) and then have lower palliative care needs during periods of remission.

Provision of Palliative Care
Exclusively at End of Life

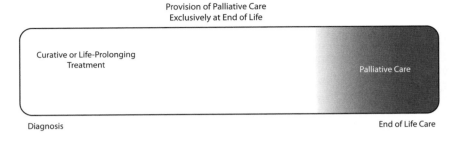

Diagnosis   End of Life Care

Incorporation of Palliative Care
Throughout the Cancer Care Continuum

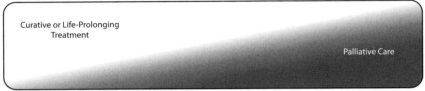

FIGURE 3-3 Relationship of curative or life-prolonging treatment to palliative care for cancer. In current practice, there is often a single focus on curative or life-prolonging treatment, with palliative care provided only near the end of life. The committee's framework of high-quality cancer care incorporates palliative care throughout the cancer continuum, becoming more intensive toward the end of life.
SOURCE: Adapted from IOM, 1997.

There is strong evidence to support the provision of palliative care throughout the cancer care continuum. Early palliative care referral has been associated with improved symptom management (Bandieri et al., 2012; Temel et al., 2010), increased survival time (Temel et al., 2010), lower utilization of aggressive end-of-life care (Greer et al., 2012; Temel et al., 2010), and more accurate patient expectations regarding long-term prognoses (Temel et al., 2011). Despite these benefits, clinicians often do not refer their patients to palliative care until the last 2 months of life (Cheng et al., 2005; Osta et al., 2008). At one comprehensive cancer center, fewer than half of patients received a palliative care consultation before they died, and palliative care consultations occurred late in the disease process (Hui et al., 2012).

Inclusion of palliative care in the cancer care plan will help improve patient access to palliative care across the cancer continuum. Addressing palliative care needs is also critical for high-quality end-of-life care. This is discussed in greater depth in the sections below on Emphasizing Palliative Care and Psychosocial Support and Providing Timely Referred Hospice Care.

Psychosocial support. Care plans should address a patient's psychosocial health needs (see Table 3-5). Many patients with cancer have unmet psychosocial needs, and patients with cancer report that their clinicians often do not understand their psychosocial needs; do not consider psychological support as a component of cancer care; and fail to recognize, treat, or refer patients to psychosocial services (IOM, 2008a). The committee endorses the recommendations in the IOM report *Cancer Care for the Whole Patient*, which stated that the cancer care team should identify each patient's psychosocial health needs and design and implement a care plan that (1) links the patient and family with psychosocial services; (2) coordinates biomedical and psychosocial care; and (3) engages and supports patients in managing their illness and health (IOM, 2008a).The psychosocial care plan should be revisited across the cancer care continuum, as these needs are likely to change depending on a patient's circumstances. Meeting psychosocial health needs in end-of-life care is especially important, as discussed below. Chapter 4 elaborates on the workforce providing psychosocial support to patients with cancer.

Cost. The cancer care team should discuss the total and out-of-pocket cost of cancer care with patients. There is a growing recognition of the role of care teams in discussing cost with their patients as a critical aspect of patient-centered communication and shared decision making (Moriates, et al., 2013). The American Society of Clinical Oncology's (ASCO's) policy statement states that "communication with patients about the cost of care is a key component of high quality care" (Meropol et al., 2009, p. 3871). Discussing costs "openly, in a way that allows patients an opportunity to hear the justification for cost-conscious decisions and to be active agents in thinking through treatment choices when feasible, is consistent with physicians' ethical duties to be transparent with patients and provide patient-centered care" (Sommers et al., 2013, p. 344). Additional experts have asserted that "'financial toxicity' as a result of disease or treatment decisions might be considered analogous to physical toxicity and might be considered a relevant variable in guiding cancer management" (Zafar et al., 2013, p. 381).

Because cancer treatment can be a large financial burden, cost is an important issue for many patients and families (Bernard et al., 2011; IOM, 2013; Stump et al., 2013). A survey found that more than a third of individuals reported that medical problems were the reason for bankruptcy, even though three out of four families studied had insurance at the onset of illness (Himmelstein et al., 2009). Cancer patients, especially those under 65 years, have a higher bankruptcy rate compared to people who do not have cancer (Ramsey et al., 2013). Another study of patients undergoing adjuvant treatment for regional colon cancer found that 38

TABLE 3-5 Psychosocial Needs and Formal[a] Services to Address Them

Psychosocial Need	Health Services
Information about illness, treatments, health, and services	• Provision of information (e.g., on illness, treatments, effects on health, and psychosocial services) and help to patients/families in understanding and using the information
Help in coping with emotions accompanying illness and treatment	• Peer support programs • Counseling/psychotherapy to individuals or groups • Pharmacological management of mental symptoms
Help in managing illness	• Comprehensive illness self-management/self-care programs

Assistance in changing behaviors to minimize impact of disease	• Behavioral/health promotion interventions, such as:
	  o clinician assessment/monitoring of health behaviors (e.g., smoking, exercise)
	  o brief clinician counseling
	  o patient education (e.g., in cancer-related health risks and risk reduction measures)

Material and logistical resources, such as transportation	• Provision of resources
Help in managing disruptions in work, school, and family life	• Family caregiver education • Assistance with activities of daily living (ADLs), instrumental ADLs, chores • Legal protections and services (e.g., under Americans with Disabilities Act and Family and Medical Leave Act) • Cognitive testing and educational assistance
Financial advice and/or assistance	• Financial planning/counseling, including management of day-to-day activities such as bill paying • Insurance (e.g., health, disability) counseling • Eligibility assessment/counseling for other benefits (e.g., Supplemental Security Income, Social Security Disability Income) • Supplemental financial grants

[a]Family members and friends and other informal sources of support are key providers of psychosocial health services. This table includes only formal sources of psychosocial support—those that must be secured through the assistance of an organization or agency that in some way enables the provision of needed services (sometimes at no cost or through volunteers).
SOURCE: Adapted from IOM, 2008a.

percent of patients reported at least one treatment-related financial hardship (Shankaran et al., 2012).

The committee recognizes that there are a number of challenges to discussing the cost of care. Both clinicians and patients can be reluctant to broach the subject of cancer care costs (Neumann et al., 2010; Sommers et al., 2013). For example, a survey of oncologists found that only 43 percent always or frequently discuss the cost of cancer care with patients (Neumann et al., 2010). Clinicians may not explain the potential cost implications for different cancer care options because these discussions are time consuming and not prioritized under the current reimbursement system (see Chapter 8). In addition, some clinicians may not know the total costs involved in cancer care or the out-of-pocket costs for which patients may be responsible, given the variable insurance plans with differing benefit packages. However, a recent survey found that 76 percent of physicians were "aware of the costs of the tests/treatments [they] recommend" (Tilburt et al., 2013), and oncologists have reported that their incomes increase when they administer chemotherapy and growth factors (Malin et al., 2013). Because exact information may not always be available, the cancer care team should provide patients with estimates of the total and out-of-pocket costs of cancer care.

Another challenge to discussing cost information with patients is the possibility that some patients may reject potentially beneficial cancer care due to cost concerns. However, this information is important for patients to make informed decisions about their care. Patients may not be aware of their out-of-pocket costs until after care is provided, but discussing these costs prior to cancer care could facilitate more fully informed decisions. If patients have multiple treatment options to consider, the cancer care team should provide patients with information that compares the relative costs of these different options. In addition, providing information on the total cost of care can enable cost-conscious patients to consider equally effective, lower cost cancer care options.

Given time constraints for clinicians, nonclinician practice staff, such as financial counselors or other administrative practice staff, may be helpful in communicating with patients about the cost of cancer care. Some oncology practices have already started employing financial counselors who inform patients about the total costs of cancer treatment, their insurance benefits, and anticipated out-of-pocket costs for treatment (Gesme and Wiseman, 2011). New models of payment may also help facilitate this change.

Advance care planning. Advance care planning is defined by the National Hospice and Palliative Care Organization as "making decisions about the care you would want to receive if you happen to become unable to speak for yourself" (NHPCO, 2013, p. 1). The cancer care team should discuss advance care planning with patients and document these preferences in the care plan. Advance care planning should begin early in the cancer care continuum and be revisited under changing circumstances, such as when patients' cancers progress, or they change their preferences. It may be helpful for the cancer care team to work with the primary care/geriatrics care team in advance care planning, because the primary care/geriatrics care team may have a more established relationship with a patient and be better suited to eliciting their patients' preferences. The cancer care team should then implement their patients' advance care plans if their patients lose decisional capacity at any point in the course of illness. (Also see the section below on "Implementing Advance Care Planning.")

Advancing New Payment Models

The committee recommends that CMS and other payers design, implement, and evaluate innovative payment models that incentivize the cancer care team to discuss information on cancer prognosis, treatment benefits and harms, palliative care, psychosocial support, and estimates of the total and out-of-pocket costs of cancer care with their patients and document their discussions in each patient's care plan. As mentioned previously, the current fee-for-service reimbursement system does not compensate the cancer care team well for providing cognitive care to their patients, such as having conversations about prognosis, likelihood of treatment responses, and support services for patients. Because it can result in care that is misaligned with their preferences and contribute to unnecessary or harmful interventions, the current reimbursement system is detrimental to the quality of care that patients with cancer receive. In Chapter 8, the committee elaborates on new delivery and payment models that could incentivize better patient-clinician communication and shared decision making, including oncology patient-centered medical homes, ACOs, and bundled payments. These models reward the cancer care team for the quality, patient-centeredness, and efficiency of care they provide. Effective patient-clinician communication will be necessary in these models to avert potentially costly complications. In addition, these models are designed to disincentivize clinicians from using more (or more costly) interventions when they are unlikely to benefit a patient.

Financial incentives in fee-for-service reimbursement can also hinder the provision of palliative care and psychosocial support across the cancer continuum. The current system incentivizes clinicians to provide highly interventional care, because interventional care is reimbursed more generously than palliative care and psychosocial support. A previous IOM committee highlighted the deficiencies of fee-for-service reimbursement in the provision of palliative care and recommended that new payment models be considered (IOM, 1997). This committee makes a similar recommendation.

IMPROVING PATIENT-CENTERED COMMUNICATION AND SHARED DECISION MAKING AT THE END OF LIFE

Patients with advanced cancer confront "complex physical, psychological, social, and spiritual consequences of disease and its treatment" (Peppercorn et al., 2011, p. 755). And, too often, patients with advanced cancer receive suboptimal care. This section describes challenges and opportunities to improve cancer care for individuals approaching the end of life, including the importance of palliative care, psychosocial support, advance care planning, end-of-life communication, and timely referral to hospice.

A related activity is an IOM consensus committee on transforming end-of-life care. That committee is currently examining issues in end-of-life care, including advance care planning, patient-clinician communication of values and preferences, and health care financing and reimbursement. The report is expected to be released in 2014.

Implementing Advance Care Planning

Advance care planning is "making decisions about the care you would want to receive if you happen to become unable to speak for yourself" (NHPCO, 2013, p. 1). Ideally, all patients should have an advance care plan in place, prior to diagnosis, as a routine part of medical care. Advance care planning is also a part of a patient's care plan. The cancer care team should discuss advance care planning early in the course of a patient's care and implement the plan when needed. The ASCO policy statement on advanced cancer recommends that "[a]ll patients must have a regular opportunity to make their preferences about how to live their final weeks and months clear to their oncologist. Only through these discussions do we have an opportunity to match patients' goals with the actual care delivered" (Peppercorn et al., 2011, p. 757).

Components of advance care planning include consideration of what types of life-sustaining treatments align with a patient's preferences, preparation of advance directives, and identification of a health care proxy. Advance directives are "formal legal documents specifically authorized by state laws that allow patients to continue their personal autonomy and that provide instructions for care in case they become incapacitated and cannot make decisions" (AHRQ, 2013a, p. 1). A health care proxy is a document that "allows the patient to designate a surrogate, a person who will make treatment decisions for the patient if the patient becomes too incapacitated to make such decisions" (AHRQ, 2013a, p. 1).

Advance care planning is an opportunity for cancer care teams to engage with their patients to make more informed decisions about care that is aligned with a patient's needs, values, and preferences and can help maximize quality of life for the time a patient has left (IOM, 2011a). Patients who discuss advance care planning with their clinicians are more likely to receive end-of-life care that is consistent with their preferences (Detering et al., 2010; Mack et al., 2010; Silveira et al., 2010).

Advance care planning, however, is currently underutilized. Many discussions with patients about advance care planning occur during acute hospital care with clinicians other than oncologists late in the course of disease (Mack et al., 2012a). In addition, estimates suggest that only around half of individuals have an advance directive in their medical record (reviewed in AHRQ, 2003; Wilson et al., 2013; Yung et al., 2010). As a result, clinicians may provide end-of-life care that is not aligned with their patients' preferences. For example, 70 percent of people say they want to die at home, but 70 percent of people die in hospitals or nursing homes (Goodman, 2012). A study found that the patients' expressed preferences for end-of-life care and documentation of this information in the medical record matched only 30 percent of the time (Heyland et al., 2013). Surveys also suggest that many patients, particularly older patients, would prefer care focused on comfort over life-extending care (see the sections below on Emphasizing Palliative Care and Psychosocial Support and Providing Timely Referred Hospice Care) (Barnato et al., 2007; Maida et al., 2010; Rose et al., 2004), but end-of-life care for cancer patients is often intensive (Morden et al., 2012). Allison and Sudore (2013) assert that failure to discuss and document patient preferences for end-of-life care is tantamount to a medical error. **Thus, the committee recommends that in the setting of advanced cancer, the cancer care team should revisit and implement their patients' advance care plans to provide patients with end-of-life care consistent with their needs, values, and preferences (Recommendation 2).**

Many efforts to improve advance care planning are under way. In 2013, the Personalize Your Care Act was introduced in the U.S. House of Representatives.[10] This act would provide Medicare and Medicaid patients with coverage for voluntary advance care planning consultations. It would also direct the Secretary of HHS to develop standards for EHR documentation of the result of advance care planning discussions. Currently, EHRs often do not record patients' decisions made during advance care planning in an actionable format (Tai-Seale et al., 2012). Although this

---

[10] Personalize Your Care Act of 2013, H.R. 1173, 113th Cong., 1st Sess. (March 14, 2013).

act would greatly improve the availability of advance care planning, its likelihood of passing Congress is unknown. Previous Congressional efforts to improve advance care planning have been very controversial and failed to become law (Tinetti, 2012).

The most evidence-based and widespread model of advance care planning is *Respecting Choices*®, which was developed by health care organizations in La Crosse, Wisconsin. This model incorporates six goals into routine care: (1) patients are invited to understand and discuss plans for future health care; (2) patients are supported by trained nonclinicians in the planning process; (3) patients develop plans that are specific and understandable to all stakeholders; (4) plans are accessible wherever a patient is treated; (5) plans are updated and become more specific as a patient's illness progresses, and (6) clinicians review and honor plans at the right time (Hammes et al., 2010). After 2 years of implementation, a retrospective analysis found that 85 percent of all adult decedents in La Crosse had an advance directive; 95 percent of the advance directives were in the patient's medical record; and in 98 percent of the cases, instructions in the advance directive were consistent with care near the end of life (Hammes and Rooney, 1998). More recent data from La Crosse found even greater prevalence and accessibility of advance directives (Hammes et al., 2010).

There are also a number of grassroots educational campaigns, such as the Conversation Project and Honoring Choices Minnesota®, which are encouraging people to have honest conversations about their preferences for end-of-life care with their families (Bisognano and Goodman, 2013; Wilson and Schettle, 2013). The Conversation Project is also collaborating with the Institute for Healthcare Improvement to ensure that the health care delivery system is well prepared to elicit and respect patient preferences for end-of-life care (Bisognano and Goodman, 2013). Similarly, ASCO and Cancer.Net have prepared a booklet for patients and families about advance care planning for people with cancer (ASCO and Cancer. Net, 2012). As mentioned previously, videos may also assist patients in making more informed decisions about their care options at the end of life. For example, Volandes et al. (2013) found that patients with advanced cancer who viewed a video of cardiopulmonary resuscitation (CPR) were less likely to opt for CPR than those who listened to a verbal description of CPR.

Improving Clinician Training in End-of-Life Communication

The advanced cancer care setting presents a number of added challenges to patient-centered communication and shared decision making, particularly because conversations about the end of life are understandably difficult for both clinicians and patients (Harrington and Smith,

2008; IOM, 2009a; The et al., 2000). Clinicians, concerned that patients will become depressed or lose hope, are often reluctant to discuss realistic prognostic information with patients, despite evidence that patients want their clinicians to be honest and truthful (IOM, 2011a; Mack and Smith, 2012; Smith and Longo, 2012). Good communication about prognosis is especially important because a patient's understanding of his or her illness is strongly linked to the treatment choices the patient makes. Patients with advanced cancer who understand that their disease is incurable are more likely to prefer symptom-directed care, while patients who overestimate their prognosis are more likely to receive disease-focused care with unclear benefit (Greer et al., 2013). The ASCO policy statement on advanced cancer care estimated that clinicians have realistic conversations with fewer than 40 percent of their patients with advanced cancer (Peppercorn et al., 2011). Clinicians often delay conversations about advance directives until there are no longer any curative or life-prolonging treatment options available to patients (Keating et al., 2010). One study found that as many as half of all non-small-cell lung cancer patients had not discussed hospice with any of their doctors 2 months prior to their deaths (Huskamp et al., 2009).

Given the need for better communication at the end of life and the effectiveness of communication training programs, the committee recommends that professional educational programs for members of the cancer care team provide comprehensive and formal training in end-of-life communication. These professional education programs need to be available both during initial training as well as for clinicians currently practicing. All clinicians working in oncology should be proficient at discussing these difficult issues.

Aligned with this recommendation, the IOM report *Approaching Death: Improving Care at the End of Life* (1997) recommended that educators and health professionals make changes to undergraduate, graduate, and continuing education programs to ensure that clinicians are well equipped to provide high-quality end-of-life care. The committee emphasized a number of interpersonal skills and attitudes that clinicians should develop, including listening to patients, families, and other members of the care team; conveying difficult news; understanding and managing patient and family responses to illness; providing information and guidance on prognosis and care options; practicing shared decision making and conflict resolution; recognizing and understanding the clinician's own feelings and anxieties about dying and death; and demonstrating empathy and sensitivity to religious, ethnic, and other personal characteristics.

Emphasizing Palliative Care and Psychosocial Support

As discussed previously, high-quality cancer care includes the provision of palliative care and psychosocial support throughout the cancer continuum. **In addition, the committee recommends that in the setting of advanced cancer, the cancer care team should place a primary emphasis on providing cancer patients with palliative care and psychosocial support for end-of-life care.** Palliative care can be provided by a number of clinicians in a variety of settings, including the outpatient setting and inpatient hospital units (GPC, 2013a). Given the limited supply of palliative care clinicians and recognition that some palliative care tasks are routine aspects of care (see Chapter 4), Quill and Abernethy (2013) suggested a model of care that includes primary and specialty palliative care. In this model, the cancer care team would provide primary palliative care, including basic management of pain, symptoms, depression, and anxiety, as well as basic discussions about prognosis, goals of treatment, suffering, and advance directives. If patients require more complex palliative care needs, the cancer care team would refer patients to palliative care specialists, who would manage refractory pain, more complex psychosocial needs, and conflict resolution regarding the goals or methods of treatment (Quill and Abernethy, 2013).

Patients with advanced cancer and their families may have a number of psychosocial health needs (see Table 3-5). Compared to patients with earlier stage disease, patients with advanced cancer may have different needs, such as greater concern about religion and spirituality, as well as coping with existential suffering (Balboni et al., 2007; IOM, 2004b; Kissane, 2012). They are also more likely to experience distress. Estimates suggest that one-third to one-half of patients with cancer experience considerable distress, and those who are diagnosed with cancers associated with poorer prognoses experience greater distress (Zabora et al., 2001). Family caregivers also report considerable distress that may interfere with their ability to provide emotional or logistical support and exacerbate patients' emotional distress (Braun et al., 2007; IOM, 2008a; Siegel et al., 1996). Thus, in the advanced cancer setting, it is especially important for the cancer care team to identify the psychosocial health needs of patients and their families, and to develop a care plan that addresses these needs.

Providing Timely Referral to Hospice Care

Hospice care is a form of palliative care and occurs at the end of life. It is defined by the National Quality Forum as "a service delivery system that provides palliative care for patients who have a limited life expectancy and require comprehensive biomedical, psychosocial, and spiritual support as they enter the terminal stage of an illness or condition. It also supports family members coping with the complex consequences of illness, disability, and aging as death nears. Hospice care further addresses the bereavement needs of the family following the death of the patient" (NQF, 2006, p. 3). The Medicare hospice benefit is available for patients who have 6 months or less to live (prognosis must be agreed upon by two physicians) and who agree to forgo Medicare-covered benefits to treat their terminal illness (Medicare will still pay for covered benefits for any health problems that are not related to the terminal illness) (CMS, 2013a). Hospice care is often provided to patients in their homes, but it can also be delivered in freestanding hospice facilities, hospitals, nursing homes, and other long-term care facilities (GPC, 2013b).

The benefits of hospice care have been well documented in terms of improved quality of life, reductions in symptom distress, better outcomes for family caregivers, and patient and family satisfaction with care (Black et al., 2011; Shepperd et al., 2011; Teno et al., 2004; Wright et al., 2010). Unfortunately, these services are often underutilized by patients and their cancer care teams. In 2011, the median length of hospice care for patients in the United States was only 19.1 days and the average length of hospice care for patients was 69.1 days (NHPCO, 2012). More than one-third of patients with hospice care had a length of stay less than 7 days (NHPCO, 2012). **Because access to hospice care improves the quality of cancer care, the committee recommends that the cancer care team provide cancer patients with timely referral to hospice care for end-of-life care.**

Not all patients will opt for hospice care (Goodman, 2012; Matsuyama et al., 2006). The majority of patients with advanced cancer, however, would likely choose to transition to hospice care if a clinician or knowledgeable person had an honest conversation with them about their prognosis at the end of life. However, patients with advanced cancer are often treated aggressively near the end of their lives (Earle et al., 2004; Morden et al., 2012). In an analysis of Medicare claims data, more than 15 percent of cancer patients who received chemotherapy were treated within 2 weeks of their deaths (Earle et al., 2004).

Several studies have found that when a physician discusses a prognosis and end-of-life care preferences with the patient, that patient is less likely to want aggressive measures; for example, they are three times more likely to complete "do not resuscitate" forms and twice as likely to choose hospice care than are patients who do not have this discussion (Mack et al., 2012b; Wright et al., 2008). In a randomized clinical trial, Casarett and colleagues (2005) conducted structured interviews with nursing home residents to identify residents whose goals for care, treatment preferences, and palliative care needs indicated that hospice care would be the preferred course. They then notified these residents' physicians and asked them to authorize a hospice informational visit. The result of this intervention was a 20-fold increase in the number of patients choosing hospice care. Similarly, at the Ireland Cancer Center in Cleveland, all patients with advanced lung cancer met with a chaplain, a social worker, and an advanced practice nurse from a nearby hospice facility to discuss their care needs and goals. These conversations increased hospice use from 13 percent to 80 percent and the length of stay in hospice from an average of 10 to 44 days (Ford Pitorak et al., 2003). Thus, it is important that these services be discussed with and be accessible to patients.

Advancing New Payment Models

The current fee-for-service reimbursement system can impede high-quality communication and care for patients with advanced cancer. The ASCO statement on advanced cancer highlights time as a major barrier to clinicians' provision of high-quality advanced cancer care, noting that discussions of prognosis, treatment options, and the patient's goals and preferences require substantially more time than a standard follow-up visit (Peppercorn et al., 2011). Thus, ASCO recommends that payers reimburse clinicians for care planning to support the time and effort required to provide individualized care for individuals with advanced cancer (Peppercorn et al., 2011). **The committee endorses this concept and recommends that CMS and other payers design, implement, and evaluate innovative payment models that incentivize the cancer care team to counsel their patients about advance care planning.** As discussed previously, new models of payment may better support clinicians for having these important conversations compared to fee-for-service reimbursement.

In addition, insurance policies that prevent the dual use of hospice services and active treatment are a challenge to clinicians' delivery of hospice care. Patients who use the Medicare hospice benefit must agree to forgo disease-directed treatment (MedPAC, 2012). The Medicare Payment Advisory Commission (MedPAC) has said that shorter hospice stays are not the result of benefit design but, rather, reluctance among clinicians, patients, and families to recognize that a patient's condition is incurable and clinicians' financial incentives to continue to treat a patient with active therapy (MedPAC, 2009). A number of stakeholders in oncology have suggested, however, that the requirement to forgo anti-cancer treatment when entering hospice care is problematic for patients with cancer (Harrington and Smith, 2008; Peppercorn et al., 2011). The ASCO statement on advanced cancer recommended that pilot programs evaluate the potential for providing concurrent anti-cancer treatment with hospice care (Peppercorn et al., 2011).

The committee recommends that in the setting of advanced cancer, CMS and other payers design, implement, and evaluate innovative payment models that incentivize the cancer care team to provide cancer patients with timely referral to hospice care for end-of-life care. A number of innovative palliative and hospice care models can inform payers in implementing this recommendation (see Table 3-6). In addition, the ACA directed the Secretary of HHS to establish a demonstration program that evaluates whether hospice care provided concurrently with disease-

TABLE 3-6 Examples of Hospice Care Models

Program	Description
Aetna's Compassionate Care Program	A care management program involving nurses trained in managing the care of terminally ill patients. Care managers identify patients' needs through a comprehensive assessment and through consults with the patient, family, and clinicians involved with the patient's care. Care managers provide patients and their families with education, support, and assistance with pain medications, psychosocial needs, and advance directives. An "enhanced hospice access" arm of this program has expanded patients' access to hospice care by changing the definition of terminal illness to 12 months of life expectancy and allowing patients to access both hospice benefits and disease-directed therapy simultaneously. In this program, hospice election has been associated with patient satisfaction and a decrease in the use of acute care, intensive care, and emergency services. In the commercially insured population, patients' hospice election has resulted in a net medical cost decrease of approximately 22 percent.
Sutter's Advanced Illness Management (AIM) Program	The AIM program is an integrated system of care for individuals with advanced disease that provides home-based transitional and palliative care services. The AIM program provides patients and families with counseling with the goal of increasing hospice use and decreasing the use of unwanted acute care. Preliminary data suggest that AIM improves patient, family, and clinician satisfaction with care and increases use of hospice. AIM is associated with decreased hospitalizations and an average savings of $2,000 per patient a month.

SOURCES: Aetna, 2013; Krakauer et al., 2009; Meyer, 2011.

directed care improves patient care, quality of life, and cost-effectiveness for Medicare beneficiaries. CMS has not yet initiated the demonstration project (Rau, 2013). Chapter 8 discusses different payment models that may offer improved care for patients with advanced cancer, including patient-centered medical homes, ACOs, and bundled payments.

SUMMARY AND RECOMMENDATIONS

Patients are at the center of the committee's conceptual framework (see Figure S-2), which conveys the most important goal of a high-quality cancer care delivery system: meeting the needs of patients with cancer and their families. Such a system should support all patients in making informed medical decisions that are consistent with their needs, values, and preferences. In the current system, information to help patients understand their cancer prognoses, treatment benefits and harms, palliative care, psychosocial support, and costs of care is often unavailable or not regularly communicated. Additionally, patient-clinician communication and shared decision making is often less than optimal, impeding the delivery of patient-centered, high-quality cancer care. For example, several recent studies found that approximately 65 to 80 percent of cancer patients with poor prognoses incorrectly believed their treatments could result in a cure.

Recommendation 1: Engaged Patients

Goal: The cancer care team should provide patients and their families with understandable information on cancer prognosis, treatment benefits and harms, palliative care, psychosocial support, and estimates of the total and out-of-pocket costs of cancer care.

To accomplish this:

- **The National Cancer Institute, the Centers for Medicare & Medicaid Services, the Patient-Centered Outcomes Research Institute, as well as patient advocacy organizations, professional organizations, and other public and private stakeholders should improve the development of this information and decision aids and make them available through print, electronic, and social media.**
- **Professional educational programs for members of the cancer care team should provide comprehensive and formal training in communication.**

- The cancer care team should communicate and personalize this information for their patients at key decision points along the continuum of cancer care, using decision aids when available.
- The cancer care team should collaborate with their patients to develop a care plan that reflects their patients' needs, values, and preferences, and considers palliative care needs and psychosocial support across the cancer care continuum.
- The Centers for Medicare & Medicaid Services and other payers should design, implement, and evaluate innovative payment models that incentivize the cancer care team to discuss this information with their patients and document their discussions in each patient's care plan.

Patients with advanced cancer face specific communication and decision-making needs. Clinicians should discuss these patients' options, such as implementing advance care plans, emphasizing palliative care, and psychosocial support, and maximizing quality of life by providing timely use of hospice care. These difficult conversations do not occur as frequently or as timely as they should, resulting in care that may not be aligned with patient preferences.

Recommendation 2: Engaged Patients

Goal: In the setting of advanced cancer, the cancer care team should provide patients with end-of-life care consistent with their needs, values, and preferences.

To accomplish this:

- Professional educational programs for members of the cancer care team should provide comprehensive and formal training in end-of-life communication.
- The cancer care team should revisit and implement their patients' advance care plans.
- The cancer care team should place a primary emphasis on providing cancer patients with palliative care, psychosocial support, and timely referral to hospice care for end-of-life care.
- The Centers for Medicare & Medicaid Services and other payers should design, implement, and evaluate innovative payment models that incentivize the cancer care team to counsel their patients about advance care planning and timely referral to hospice care for end-of-life care.

REFERENCES

ABIM (American Board of Internal Medicine). 2013. *Physician charter.* http://www.abim foundation.org/Professionalism/Physician-Charter.aspx (accessed July 31, 2013).

ACGME (Accreditation Council for Graduate Medical Education). 2008. *Educational program.* http://www.acgme.org/acgmeweb/Portals/0/PDFs/commonguide/IVA5d_ EducationalProgram_ACGMECompetencies_IPCS_Documentation.pdf (accessed August 7, 2013).

Aetna. 2013. *Aetna Compassionate Care SM Program.* http://www.aetna.com/individuals-families-health-insurance/sas/compassionate-care/program-description.html (accessed June 20, 2013).

AHRQ (Agency for Healthcare Research and Quality). 2003. *Advance care planning, preferences for care at the end of life: Research in action.* www.ahrq.gov/research/findings/factsheets/ aging/endliferia/index.html (accessed June 20, 2013).

———. 2012. *About the Eisenberg Center.* http://effectivehealthcare.ahrq.gov/index.cfm/ who-is-involved-in-the-effective-health-care-program1/about-the-eisenberg-center (accessed January 4, 2013).

———. 2013a. *Advance care planning, preferences for care at the end of life.* http://www.ahrq. gov/research/findings/factsheets/aging/endliferia/index.html (accessed April 1, 2013).

———. 2013b. *Questions are the answer. Better communication. Better care.* http://www.ahrq. gov/legacy/questions/index.html (accessed April 1, 2013).

Aiello Bowles, E. J., L. Tuzzio, C. J. Wiese, B. Kirlin, S. M. Greene, S. B. Clauser, and E. H. Wagner. 2008. Understanding high-quality cancer care: a summary of expert perspectives. *Cancer* 112(4):934-942.

Allison, T. A., and R. L. Sudore. 2013. Disregard of patients' preferences is a medical error. *JAMA Internal Medicine* 173(9):787-788.

Alston, C., L. Paget, G. C. Halvorson, B. Novelli, J. Guest, P. McCabe, K. Hoffman, C. Koepke, M. Simon, S. Sutton, S. Okun, P. Wicks, T. Undem, V. Rohrbach, and I. V. Kohorn. 2012. *Communicating with patients on health care evidence: Discussion paper.* http://www.iom. edu/~/media/Files/Perspectives-Files/2012/Discussion-Papers/VSRT-Evidence.pdf (accessed March 28, 2013).

AMA (American Medical Association). 2013. *Health literacy resources.* http://www.ama-assn. org/ama/pub/about-ama/ama-foundation/our-programs/public-health/health-literacy-program/health-literacy-kit.page? (Accessed August 7, 2013).

APCD (All-Payer Claims Database). 2013. *Interactive state report map.* http://www.apcdcouncil. org/state/map (accessed April 30, 2013).

Armstron, S., and D. Arterburn. 2013. *Creating a culture to promote shared decision making at Group Health.* http://www.iom.edu/Global/Perspectives/2013/SharedDecision Making.aspx (accessed May 2, 2013).

ASCO (American Society of Clinical Oncology). 2011. *ASCO launches cancer.net mobile, a new app for iPhone, iPad, and iPod Touch that puts cancer care in the hands of patients and caregivers.* http://www.asco.org/press-center/asco-launches-cancernet-mobile-new-app-iphone-ipad-and-ipod-touch-puts-cancer-care (accessed May 2, 2013).

ASCO and Cancer.Net. 2012. *Advanced cancer care planning: What patients and families need to know about their choices when facing serious illness.* http://www.cancer.net/patient/ Coping/Advanced%20Cancer%20Care%20Planning/Advanced_Cancer_Care_ Planning.pdf (accessed May 2, 2012).

Ayanian, J. Z., A. M. Zaslavsky, E. Guadagnoli, C. S. Fuchs, K. J. Yost, C. M. Creech, R. D. Cress, L. C. O'Connor, D. W. West, and W. E. Wright. 2005. Patients' perceptions of quality of care for colorectal cancer by race, ethnicity, and language. *Journal of Clinical Oncology* 23(27):6576-6586.

Ayanian, J. Z., A. M. Zaslavsky, N. K. Arora, K. L. Kahn, J. L. Malin, P. A. Ganz, M. van Ryn, M. C. Hornbrook, C. I. Kiefe, Y. He, J. M. Urmie, J. C. Weeks, and D. P. Harrington. 2010. Patients' experiences with care for lung cancer and colorectal cancer: findings from the Cancer Care Outcomes Research and Surveillance Consortium. *Journal of Clinical Oncology* 28(27):4154-4161.

Back, A. L., R. M. Arnold, W. F. Baile, K. A. Fryer-Edwards, S. C. Alexander, G. E. Barley, T. A. Gooley, and J. A. Tulsky. 2007. Efficacy of communication skills training for giving bad news and discussing transitions to palliative care. *Archives of Internal Medicine* 167(5):453-460.

Back, A. L., R. M. Arnold, W. F. Baile, J. A. Tulsky, G. E. Barley, R. D. Pea, and K. A. Fryer-Edwards. 2009a. Faculty development to change the paradigm of communication skills teaching in oncology. *Journal of Clinical Oncology* 27(7):1137-1141.

Back, A. L., R. M. Arnold, W. F. Baile, J. A. Tulsky, and K. A. Fryer-Edwards. 2009b. Approaching difficult communication tasks in oncology. *CA: A Cancer Journal for Clinicians* 55(3):164-177.

Back, A. L., R. M. Arnold, J. A. Tulsky, W. F. Baile, and K. Fryer-Edwards. 2010. "Could I add something?" Teaching communication by intervening in real time during a clinical encounter. *Academic Medicine* 85(6): 1048-1051.

Baile, W. F., R. Buckman, R. Lenzi, G. Glober, E. A. Beale, and A. P. Kudelka. 2000. SPIKES— A six-step protocol for delivering bad news: Application to the patient with cancer. *Oncologist* 5(4):302-311.

Balboni, T. A., L. C. Vanderwerker, S. D. Block, M. E. Paulk, C. S. Lathan, J. R. Peteet, and H. G. Prigerson. 2007. Religiousness and spiritual support among advanced cancer patients and associations with end-of-life treatment preferences and quality of life. *Journal of Clinical Oncology* 25(5):555-560.

Bandieri, E., D. Sichetti, M. Romero, C. Fanizza, M. Belfiglio, L. Buonaccorso, F. Artioli, F. Campione, G. Tognoni, and M. Luppi. 2012. Impact of early access to a palliative/supportive care intervention on pain management in patients with cancer. *Annals of Oncology* 23(8):2016-2020.

Barnato, A. E., M. B. Herndon, D. L. Anthony, P. M. Gallagher, J. S. Skinner, J. P. Bynum, and E. S. Fisher. 2007. Are regional variations in end-of-life care intensity explained by patient preferences?: A study of the U.S. Medicare population. *Medical Care* 45(5):386-393.

Basch, E. 2013. Toward patient-centered drug development in oncology. *New England Journal of Medicine* 369(5):397-400.

Bechtel, C., and D. L. Ness. 2010. If you build it, will they come? Designing truly patient-centered health care. *Health Affairs (Millwood)* 29(5):914-920.

Belkora, J. K., A. Teng, S. Volz, M. K. Loth, L. J. Esserman. 2011. Expanding the reach of decision and communication aids in a breast care center: A quality improvement study. *Patient Education and Counseling* 83(2):234-239.

Berkhof, M., H. J. van Rijssen, A. J. M. Schellart, J. R. Anema, and A. J. van der Beek. 2010. Effective training strategies for teaching communication skills to physicians: An overview of systematic reviews. *Patient Education and Counseling* 84(2):152-162.

Berkman, N. D., S. L. Sheridan, K. E. Donahue, D. J. Halpern, A. Viera, K. Crotty, A. Holland, M. Brasure, K. N. Lohr, E. Harden, E. Tant, I. Wallace, and M. Viswanathan. 2011. *Health literacy interventions and outcomes: An updated systematic review, Evidence Report/Technology Assessment: Number 199.* Rockville, MD: Agency for Healthcare Research and Quality.

Berman, A. 2012. Living life in my own way—and dying that way as well. *Health Affairs (Millwood)* 31(4):871-874.

Bernard, D. S., S. L. Farr, and Z. Fang. 2011. National estimates of out-of-pocket health care expenditure burdens among nonelderly adults with cancer: 2001 to 2008. *Journal of Clinical Oncology* 29(20):2821-2826.

Berwick, D. M. 2009. What "patient-centered" should mean: Confessions of an extremist. *Health Affairs (Millwood)* 28(4):w555-w565.

Bindman, A. B., J. D. Blum, and R. Kronick. 2013. Medicare payment for chronic care delivered in a patient-centered medical home. *Journal of the American Medical Association.* (epub ahead of print).

Bisognano, M., and E. Goodman. 2013. Engaging patients and their loved ones in the ultimate conversation. *Health Affairs (Millwood)* 32(2):203-206.

Black, B., K. Herr, P. Fine, S. Sanders, X. Tang, K. Bergen-Jackson, M. Titler, and C. Forcucci. 2011. The relationships among pain, nonpain symptoms, and quality of life measures in older adults with cancer receiving hospice care. *Pain Medicine* 12(6):880-889.

Braddock, C. H., 3rd, K. A. Edwards, N. M. Hasenberg, T. L. Laidley, and W. Levinson. 1999. Informed decision making in outpatient practice: Time to get back to basics. *Journal of the American Medical Association* 282(24):2313-2320.

Braun, M., M. Mikulincer, A. Rydall, A. Walsh, and G. Rodin. 2007. Hidden morbidity in cancer: spouse caregivers. *Journal of Clinical Oncology* 25(30):4829-4834.

Busari, J. O. 2013. The discourse of generational segmentation and the implications for postgraduate medical education. *Perspectives on Medical Education.* (epub ahead of print).

Cancer Support Community. 2012. *Online Support.* http://www.cancersupportcommunity.org/MainMenu/Cancer-Support/Online-Support-Groups.html (accessed January 4, 2013).

Casarett, D., J. Karlawish, K. Morales, R. Crowley, T. Mirsch, and D. A. Asch. 2005. Improving the use of hospice services in nursing homes: A randomized controlled trial. *Journal of the American Medical Association* 294(2):211-217.

C-Change. 2005. *Cancer patient navigation overview.* http://cancerpatientnavigation.org (accessed September 26, 2012).

CDC (Centers for Disease Control and Prevention). 2013. *Lung cancer risk factors.* http://www.cdc.gov/cancer/lung/basic_info/risk_factors.htm (accessed April 24, 2013).

Center to Advance Palliative Care. 2011. *2011 public opinion research on palliative care: A report based on research by Public Opinion Strategies.* New York: Center to Advance Palliative Care.

CFAH (Center for Advancing Health). 2010. *Snapshot of people's engagement in their health care.* http://www.cfah.org/file/CFAH_Snapshot_2010_Full.pdf (accessed September 25, 2012).

———. 2012. *Prepared Patient Forum.* http://www.preparedpatientforum.org/prepared patient/index.cfm (accessed January 4, 2013).

Chan, D. S., A. Willicombe, T. D. Reid, C. Beaton, D. Arnold, J. Ward, I. L. Davies, and W. G. Lewis. 2012. Relative quality of internet-derived gastrointestinal cancer information. *Journal of Cancer Education* 27(4):676-679.

Chen, A,. B., A. Cronin, J. C. Weeks, E. A. Chrischilles, J. Malin, J. A. Hayman, and D. Schrag. 2013. Expectations about the effectiveness of radiation therapy among patients with incurable lung cancer. *Journal of Clinical Oncology* 31(21):2730-2735.

Cheng, W. W., J. Willey, J. L. Palmer, T. Zhang, and E. Bruera. 2005. Interval between palliative care referral and death among patients treated at a comprehensive cancer center. *Journal of Palliative Medicine* 8(5):1025-1032.

Chiew, K. S., H. Shepherd, J. Vardy, M. H. Tattersall, P. N. Butow, and N. B. Leighl. 2008. Development and evaluation of a decision aid for patients considering first-line chemotherapy for metastatic breast cancer. *Health Expectations* 11(1):35-45.

Clancy, C. M. 2008. *How patient-centered healthcare can improve quality.* http://www.psqh. com/marapr08/ahrq.html (accessed September 25, 2012).

CMS (Centers for Medicare & Medicaid Services). 2013a. *Medicare hospice benefits.* http:// www.medicare.gov/Pubs/pdf/02154.pdf (accessed May 2, 2013).

———. 2013b. *Medicare provider charge data.* http://www.cms.gov/Research-Statistics-Data-and-Systems/Statistics-Trends-and-Reports/Medicare-Provider-Charge-Data (accessed July 31, 2013).

Collins, E. D., C. P. Moore, K. F. Clay, S. A. Kearing, A. M. O'Connor, H. A. Llewellyn-Thomas, J. R. J. Barth, and K. R. Sepucha. 2009. Can women with early-stage breast cancer make an informed decision for mastectomy? *Journal of Clinical Oncology* 27(4):519-525.

The Commonwealth Fund. 2007. *Bending the curve: Options for achieving savings and improving value in U.S. health spending.* New York: The Commonwealth Fund.

Covinsky, K. E., J. D. Fuller, K. Yaffe, C. B. Johnston, M. B. Hamel, J. Lynn, J. M. Teno, and R. S. Phillips. 2000. Communication and decision-making in seriously ill patients: Findings of the SUPPORT project. The Study to Understand Prognoses and Preferences for Outcomes and Risks of Treatments. *Journal of the American Geriatrics Society* 48(5 Suppl):S187-S193.

Dalal, S., S. Palla, D. Hui, L. Nguyen, R. Chacko, Z. Li, N. Fadul, C. Scott, V. Thornton, B. Coldman, Y. Amin, and E. Bruera. 2011. Association between a name change from palliative to supportive care and the timing of patient referrals at a comprehensive cancer center. *Oncologist* 16(1):105-111.

Detering, K. M., A. D. Hancock, M. C. Reade, and W. Silvester. 2010. The impact of advance care planning on end of life care in elderly patients: Randomized controlled trial. *British Medical Journal* 340:c1345.

DeWalt, D. A., L. F. Callahan, V. H. Hawk, K. A. Broucksou, A. Hink, R. Rudd, and C. Brach. 2010. *Health literacy universal precautions toolkit. AHRQ Publication No. 10-0046-EF.* Rockville, MD: Agency for Healthcare Research and Quality.

Earle, C. C., B. A. Neville, M. B. Landrum, J. Z. Ayanian, S. D. Block, and J. C. Weeks. 2004. Trends in the aggressiveness of cancer care near the end of life. *Journal of Clinical Oncology* 22(2):315-321.

El Dib, R. P., A. N. Atallah, and R. B. Andriolo. 2007. Mapping the Cochrane evidence for decision making in health care. *Journal of Evaluation in Clinical Practice* 13:689-692.

El-Jawahri, A., L. M. Podgurski, A. F. Eichler, S. R. Plotkin, J. S. Temel, S. L. Mitchell, Y. Chang, M. J. Barry, and A. E. Volandes. 2010. Use of video to facilitate end-of-life discussions with patients with cancer: A randomized controlled trial. *Journal of Clinical Oncology* 28(2):305-310.

Elwyn, G., A. O'Connor, D. Stacey, R. Volk, A. Edwards, A. Coulter, R. Thomson, A. Barratt, M. Barry, S. Bernstein, P. Butow, A. Clarke, V. Entwistle, D. Feldman-Stewart, M. Holmes-Rovner, H. Llewellyn-Thomas, N. Moumjid, A. Mulley, C. Ruland, K. Sepucha, A. Sykes, and T. Whelan. 2006. Developing a quality criteria framework for patient decision aids: Online international Delphi consensus process. *BMJ* 333(7565):417.

Epstein, R. M., and R. L. Street, Jr. 2007. *Patient-centered communication in cancer care: Promoting healing and reducing suffering. National Cancer Institute, NIH Publication No. 07-6225.* Bethesda, MD: National Cancer Institute.

Epstein, R. M., K. Fiscella, C. S. Lesser, and K. C. Stange. 2010. Why the nation needs a policy push on patient-centered health care. *Health Affairs (Millwood)* 29(8):1489-1495.

Feldman, L. S., H. M. Shihab, D. Thiemann, H. C. Yeh, M. Ardolino, S. Mandell, and D. J. Brotman. 2013. Impact of providing fee data on laboratory test ordering: A controlled clinical trial. *Journal of the American Medical Association Internal Medicine* 1-6. doi: 10.1001./jamainternmed.2013.232. (epub ahead of print).

Ferris, F. D., E. Bruera, N. Cherny, C. Cummings, D. Currow, D. Dudgeon, N. Janjan, F. Strasser, C. F. von Gunten, and J. H. Von Roenn. 2009. Palliative cancer care a decade later: accomplishments, the need, next steps—from the American Society of Clinical Oncology. *Journal of Clinical Oncology* 27(18):3052-3058.

Finch, C. 2011. AARP Launches Free Medicare Starter Kit Guide for Boomers. *Suite101*, http://suite101.com/article/aarp-launches-free-medicare-starter-kit-guide-for-boomers-a363274 (accessed January 4, 2013).

Fisher, B., S. Anderson, J. Bryant, R. G. Margolese, M. Deutsch, E. R. Fisher, J.-H. Jeong, and N. Wolmark. 2002. Twenty-year follow-up of a randomized trial comparing total mastectomy, lumpectomy, and lumpectomy plus irradiation for the treatment of invasive breast cancer. *New England Journal of Medicine* 347(16):567-575.

Fleurence, R., J. V. Selby, K. Odom-Walker, G. Hunt, D. Meltzer, J. R. Slutsky, and C. Yancy. 2013. How the Patient-Centered Outcomes Research Institute is engaging patients and others in shaping its research agenda. *Health Affairs (Millwood)* 32(2):393-400.

Ford Pitorak, E., M. Beckham Armour, and H. D. Sivec. 2003. Project safe conduct integrates palliative goals into comprehensive cancer care. *Journal of Palliative Medicine* 6(4):645-655.

Frosch, D. L., S. G. May, K. A. Rendle, C. Tietbohl, and G. Elwyn. 2012. Authoritarian physicians and patients' fear of being labeled "difficult" among key obstacles to shared decision making. *Health Affairs (Millwood)* 31(5):1030-1038.

Ganz, P. A. 2013. Identifying tools and strategies to provide quality oncology care. *Journal of Oncology Practice* 9(3):125-127.

GAO (Government Accountability Office). 2011. *Meaningful price information is difficult for consumers to obtain prior to receiving care.* http://www.gao.gov/products/GAO-11-791 (accessed March 29, 2013).

Gesme, D. H., and M. Wiseman. 2011. A financial counselor on the practice staff: A win-win. *Journal of Oncology Practice* 7(4):273-275.

Gigerenzer, G., and A. Edwards. 2003. Simple tools for understanding risks: From innumeracy to insight. *BMJ* 327(7417):741-744.

Goldsmith, J., B. Ferrell, E. Wittenberg-Lyles, and S. L. Ragan. 2013. Palliative care communication in oncology nursing. *Clinical Journal of Oncology Nursing* 17(2):163-167.

Goodman, E. 2012. Die the way you want to. *Harvard Business Review* January-February 2012., http://hbr.org/2012/01/tackling-social-problems/ar/1 (accessed April 25, 2013).

GPC (Get Palliative Care). 2013a. *Frequently asked questions.* http://www.getpalliativecare.org/whatis/faq/#who-provides-palliative-care (accessed August 8, 2013).

———. 2013b. *Glossary.* http://www.getpalliativecare.org/whatis/glossary (accessed August 8, 2013).

Greer, J. A., W. F. Pirl, V. A. Jackson, A. Muzikansky, I. T. Lennes, R. S. Heist, E. R. Gallagher, and J. S. Temel. 2012. Effect of early palliative care on chemotherapy use and end-of-life care in patients with metastatic non-small-cell lung cancer. *Journal of Clinical Oncology* 30(4):394-400.

Greer, J. A., V. A. Jackson, D. E. Meier, and J. S. Temel. 2013. Early integration of palliative care services with standard oncology care for patients with advanced cancer. *CA: A Cancer Journal for Clinicians.* (epub ahead of print).

Gribbin, J., and R. Dewis. 2009. Appendix 1 Adjuvant! Online: Review of evidence concerning its validity, and other considerations relating to its use in the NHS. In *NICE treatment guidelines, No. 80.* Cardiff, UK: National Collaborating Centre for Cancer.

Gruman, J. C. 2013. An accidental tourist finds her way in the dangerous land of serious illness. *Health Affairs (Millwood)* 32(2):427-431.

Grund, S. H., A. A. Forastiere, W. A. Flood, E. Whyler, V. Kozlovski, and Y.-N. Wong. 2012. A Web-based decision support platform to reduce non-evidence-based treatment of non-small cell lung cancer. *Journal of Clinical Oncology* 30(Suppl 34):abstr 71.

Grunfeld, E. A., E. J. Maher, S. Browne, P. Ward, T. Young, B. Vivat, G. Walker, C. Wilson, H. W. Potts, A. M. Westcombe, M. A. Richards, and A. J. Ramirez. 2006. Advanced breast cancer patients' perceptions of decision making for palliative chemotherapy. *Journal of Clinical Oncology* 24(7):1090-1098.

Grunfeld, E., J. A. Julian, G. Pond, E. Maunsell, D. Coyle, A. Folkes, A. A. Joy, L. Provencher, D. Rayson, D. E. Rheaume, G. A. Porter, L. F. Paszat, K. I. Pritchard, A. Robidoux, S. Smith, J. Sussman, S. Dent, J. Sisler, J. Wiernikowski, and M. N. Levine. 2011. Evaluating survivorship care plans: results of a randomized, clinical trial of patients with breast cancer. *Journal of Clinical Oncology* 29(36):4755-4762.

Hack, T. F., L. F. Degner, P. A. Parker, and SCRN Communication Team. 2005. The communication goals and needs of cancer patients: A review. *Psychooncology* 14(10):831-845.

Hammes, B. J., and B. L. Rooney. 1998. Death and end-of-life planning in one midwestern community. *Archives of Internal Medicine* 158(4):383-390.

Hammes, B. J., B. L. Rooney, and J. D. Goodman. 2010. A comparative, retrospective, observational study of the prevalence, availability, and specificity of advance care plans in a county that implemented an advance care planning microsystem. *Journal of the American Geriatrics Society* 58(7):1249-1255.

Harrington, S. E., and T. J. Smith. 2008. The role of chemotherapy at the end of life: "When is enough, enough?" *Journal of the American Medical Association* 299(22):2667-2678.

HealthCare.gov. 2013. *Out-of-pocket costs*. http://www.healthcare.gov/glossary/O/oop-costs.html (accessed April 22, 2013).

Hennessy, J. E., B. A. Lown, L. Landzaat, and K. Porter-Williamson. 2013. Practical issues in palliative and quality-of-life care. *Journal of Oncology Practice* 9(2):78-80.

Heyland, D. K., D. Barwich, D. Pichora, P. Dodek, F. Lamontagne, J. J. You, C. Tayler, P. Porterfield, T. Sinuff, and J. Simon. 2013. Failure to engage hospitalized elderly patients and their families in advance care planning. *JAMA Internal Medicine*: 1-10. doi: 10.1001/jamainternmed.2013.180. (epub ahead of print).

HHS (U.S. Department of Health and Human Services). 2013a. *National standards for culturally and linguistically appropriate services in health and health care: A blueprint for advancing and sustaining CLAS policy and practice*. Washington, DC: Office of Minority Health.

———. 2013b. *Administration offers consumers an unprecedented look at hospital charges*. http://www.hhs.gov/news/press/2013pres/05/20130508a.html (accessed July 31, 2013).

Hibbard, J. H., and J. Greene. 2013. What the evidence shows about patient activation: Better health outcomes and care experiences; fewer data on costs. *Health Affairs (Millwood)* 32(2):207-214.

Himmelstein, D. U., D. Thorne, E. Warren, and S. Woolhandler. 2009. Medical bankruptcy in the United States, 2007: results of a national study. *American Journal of Medicine* 122(8):741-746.

Hoffman, B., ed. 2004. *A cancer survivor's almanac: Charting your journey*. Hoboken, NJ: John Wiley & Sons, Inc.

Hostetter, M., and S. Klein. 2012. *Quality matters. Health care price transparency: Can it promote high-value care?* http://www.commonwealthfund.org/Newsletters/Quality-Matters/2012/April-May/In-Focus.aspx (accessed March 29, 2013).

Hui, D., S. H. Kim, J. H. Kwon, K. C. Tanco, T. Zhang, J. H. Kang, W. Rhondali, G. Chisholm, and E. Bruera. 2012. Access to palliative care among patients treated at a comprehensive cancer center. *Oncologist* 17(12):1574-1580.

Hui, D., M. De La Cruz, M. Mori, H. A. Parsons, J. H. Kwon, I. Torres-Vigil, S. H. Kim, R. Dev, R. Hutchins, C. Liem, D. H. Kang, and E. Bruera. 2013. Concepts and definitions for "supportive care," "best supportive care," "palliative care," and "hospice care" in the published literature, dictionaries, and textbooks. *Supportive Care Cancer* 21(3):659-685.

Huskamp, H. A., N. L. Keating, J. L. Malin, A. M. Zaslavsky, J. C. Weeks, C. C. Earle, J. M. Teno, B. A. Virnig, K. L. Kahn, Y. He, and J. Z. Ayanian. 2009. Discussions with physicians about hospice among patients with metastatic lung cancer. *Archives of Internal Medicine* 169(10):954-962.

Informed Medical Decisions Foundation. 2012a. *Dartmouth-Hitchcock Medical Center.* http://informedmedicaldecisions.org/imdf_demo_site/dartmouth-hitchcock-medical-center/ (accessed January 4, 2013).

———. 2012b. *How the foundation develops decision aids.* http://informedmedicaldecisions.org/shared-decision-making-in-practice/decision-aids (accessed January 4, 2013).

———. 2013. *Affordable Care Act.* http://informedmedicaldecisions.org/shared-decision-making-policy/federal-legislation/affordable-care-act (accessed March 20, 2013).

IOM (Institute of Medicine). 1997. *Approaching death: Improving care at the end of life.* Washington, DC: National Academy Press.

———. 2001. *Crossing the quality chasm: A new health system for the 21st century.* Washington, DC: National Academy Press.

———. 2003. *Unequal treatment: Confronting racial and ethnic disparities in health care.* Washington, DC: The National Academies Press.

———. 2004a. *Health literacy: A prescription to end confusion.* Washington, DC: The National Academies Press.

———. 2004b. *Meeting psychosocial needs of women with breast cancer.* Washington, DC: The National Academies Press.

———. 2008a. *Cancer care for the whole patient: Meeting psychosocial health needs.* Washington, DC: The National Academies Press.

———. 2008b. *Knowing what works in health care: A roadmap for the nation.* Washington, DC: The National Academies Press.

———. 2009a. *Assessing and improving value in cancer care.* Washington, DC: The National Academies Press.

———. 2009b. *Initial national priorities for comparative effectiveness research.* Washington, DC: The National Academies Press.

———. 2010. *A national cancer clinical trials system for the 21st century: Reinvigorating the NCI Cooperative Group Program.* Washington, DC: The National Academies Press.

———. 2011a. *Patient-centered cancer treatment planning: Improving the quality of oncology care: Workshop summary.* Washington, DC: The National Academies Press.

———. 2011b. *Promoting health literacy to encourage prevention and wellness: Workshop summary.* Washington, DC: The National Academies Press.

———. 2012. *Best care at lower cost: The path to continuously learning health care in America.* Washington, DC: The National Academies Press.

———. 2013. *Delivering affordable cancer care in the 21st century: Workshop summary.* Washington, DC: The National Academies Press.

IOM and NRC (National Research Council). 1999. *Ensuring quality cancer care.* Washington, DC: National Academy Press.

———. 2005. *From cancer patient to cancer survivor: Lost in transition.* Washington, DC: The National Academies Press.

Irwin, J. Y., T. Thyvalikakath, H. Spallek, T. Wali, A. R. Kerr, and T. Schleyer. 2011. English and Spanish oral cancer information on the internet: a pilot surface quality and content evaluation of oral cancer web sites. *Journal of Public Health Dentistry* 71(2):106-116.

Jolie, A. 2013. My medical choice. *New York Times*, May 14, A25.

Keating, N. L., M. B. Landrum, S. O. Rogers, Jr., S. K. Baum, B. A. Virnig, H. A. Huskamp, C. C. Earle, and K. L. Kahn. 2010. Physician factors associated with discussions about end-of-life care. *Cancer* 116(4):998-1006.

King, J., and B. Moulton. 2013. Group Health's participation in a shared decision-making demonstration yielded lessons, such as role of culture change. *Health Affairs (Millwood)* 32(2):294-302.

Kissane, D. W. 2012. The relief of existential suffering. *Archives of Internal Medicine* 172(19): 1501-1505.

Krakauer, R., C. M. Spettell, L. Reisman, and M. J. Wade. 2009. Opportunities to improve the quality of care for advanced illness. *Health Affairs (Millwood)* 28(5):1357-1359.

Kutner, M., E. Greenberg, Y. Jin, B. Boyle, Y. Hsu, and E. Dunleavy. 2007. *Literacy in everday life: Results from the 2003 National Assessment of Adult Literacy (NCES 2007-480)*. Washington, DC: National Center for Education Statistics.

Lantz, P. M., N. K. Janz, A. Fagerlin, K. Schwartz, L. Liu, I. Lakhani, B. Salem, and S. J. Katz. 2005. Satisfaction with surgery outcomes and the decision process in a population-based sample of women with breast cancer. *Health Services Research* 40(3):745-767.

Lauria, M. M., E. J. Clark, J. F. Hermann, and N. M. Stearns, eds. 2001. *Social work in oncology: Supporting survivors, families, and caregivers*. Atlanta, GA: American Cancer Society.

Lawrentschuk, N., D. Sasges, R. Tasevski, R. Abouassaly, A. M. Scott, and I. D. Davis. 2012. Oncology health information quality on the Internet: A multilingual evaluation. *Annals of Surgical Oncology* 19(3):706-713.

Lee, C. N., Y. Chang, N. Adimorah, J. K. Belkora, B. Moy, A. H. Partridge, D. W. Ollila, and K. R. Sepucha. 2012. Decision making about surgery for early-stage breast cancer. *Journal of the American College of Surgeons* 214(1):1-10.

Leighl, N. B., H. L. Shepherd, P. N. Butow, S. J. Clarke, M. McJannett, P. J. Beale, N. R. Wilcken, M. J. Moore, E. X. Chen, D. Goldstein, L. Horvath, J. J. Knox, M. Krzyzanowska, A. M. Oza, R. Feld, D. Hedley, W. Xu, and M. H. Tattersall. 2011. Supporting treatment decision making in advanced cancer: A randomized trial of a decision aid for patients with advanced colorectal cancer considering chemotherapy. *Journal of Clinical Oncology* 29(15):2077-2084.

Leukemia & Lymphoma Society. 2012. *The AML guide: Information for patients and caregivers acute myeloid leukemia*. http://www.lls.org/content/nationalcontent/resourcecenter/freeeducationmaterials/leukemia/pdf/amlguide.pdf (accessed January 4, 2013).

Licking, E. 2012. *As new tools offer explicit cost data on cancer treatments, will payers push for their use?* http://realendpoints.com/2012/02/as-new-tools-offer-explicit-cost-data-on-cancer-treatments-will-payers-push-for-their-use (accessed April 22, 2013).

Lin, G. A., M. Halley, K. A. Rendle, C. Tietbohl, S. G. May, L. Trujillo, and D. L. Frosch. 2013. An effort to spread decision aids in five California primary care practices yielded low distribution, highlighting hurdles. *Health Affairs (Millwood)* 32(2):311-320.

LINCS (Literacy Information and Communication System). 2013. *Resource collection topics*. http://lincs.ed.gov/professional-development/resource-collections (accessed August 7, 2013).

Mack, J. W., and T. J. Smith. 2012. Reasons why physicians do not have discussions about poor prognosis, why it matters, and what can be improved. *Journal of Clinical Oncology* 30(22):2715-2117.

Mack, J. W., J. C. Weeks, A. A. Wright, S. D. Block, and H. G. Prigerson. 2010. End-of-life discussions, goal attainment, and distress at the end of life: Predictors and outcomes of receipt of care consistent with preferences. *Journal of Clinical Oncology* 28(7):1203-1208.

Mack, J. W., A. Cronin, N. Taback, H. A. Huskamp, N. L. Keating, J. L. Malin, C. C. Earle, and J. C. Weeks. 2012a. End-of-life care discussions among patients with advanced cancer: A cohort study. *Annals of Internal Medicine* 156(3):204-210.

Mack, J. W., A. Cronin, N. L. Keating, N. Taback, H. A. Huskamp, J. L. Malin, C. C. Earle, and J. C. Weeks. 2012b. Associations between end-of-life discussion characteristics and care received near death: A prospective cohort study. *Journal of Clinical Oncology* 30(35):4387-4395.

Maida, V., J. Peck, M. Ennis, N. Brar, and A. R. Maida. 2010. Preferences for active and aggressive intervention among patients with advanced cancer. *BMC Cancer* 10:592.

Malin, J. L., J. C. Weeks, A. L. Potosky, M. C. Hornbrook, and N. L. Keating. 2013. Medical oncologists' perceptions of financial incentives in cancer care. *Journal of Clinical Oncology* 31(5)L530-535.

Matsuyama, R., S. Reddy, and T. J. Smith. 2006. Why do patients choose chemotherapy near the end of life? A review of the perspective of those facing death from cancer. *Journal of Clinical Oncology* 24(21):3490-3496.

Maurer, M., P. Dardess, K. L. Carman, K. Frazier, and L. Smeeding. 2012. *Guide to patient and family engagement: Environmental scan report. (Prepared by American Institutes for Research under contract HHSA 290-200-600019). AHRQ Publication No. 12-0042-EF*. Rockville, MD: Agency for Healthcare Research and Quality.

McCorkle, R., E. Ercolano, M. Lazenby, D. Schulman-Green, L. S. Schilling, K. Lorig, and E. H. Wagner. 2011. Self-management: Enabling and empowering patients living with cancer as a chronic illness. *CA: A Cancer Journal for Clinicians* 6(1):50-62.

MedPAC (Medicare Payment Advisory Commission). 2009. *Report to the Congress: Medicare payment policy*. http://www.medpac.gov/documents/mar09_entirereport.pdf (accessed April 1, 2013).

———. 2010. *Report to the Congress: Aligning incentives in Medicare*. http://www.medpac.gov/documents/jun10_entirereport.pdf (accessed March 28, 2013).

———. 2012. *Hospice services payment system*. http://www.medpac.gov/documents/MedPAC_Payment_Basics_12_hospice.pdf (accessed April 1, 2013).

Meier, D. 2012. *Learning from Amy Berman: Barriers to palliative care and how to overcome them*. http://healthaffairs.org/blog/2012/04/30/learning-from-amy-berman-barriers-to-palliative-care-and-how-we-might-overcome-them/ (accessed August 8, 2013).

Meropol, N. J., D. Schrag, T. J. Smith, T. M. Mulvey, R. M. Langdon, Jr., D. Blum, P. A. Ubel, and L. E. Schnipper. 2009. American Society of Clinical Oncology guidance statement: The cost of cancer care. *Journal of Clinical Oncology* 27(23):3868-3874.

Meyer, H. 2011. Changing the conversation in California about care near the end of life. *Health Affairs (Millwood)* 30(3):390-393.

Milne, D., M. Jefford, P. Schofield, and S. Aranda. 2013. Appropriate, timely referral to palliative care services: a name change will not help. *Journal of Clinical Oncology* 31(16):2055.

Moore, P. M., S. R. Mercado, M. G. Artigues, and T. A. Lawrie. 2013. Communication skills training for healthcare professionals working with people who have cancer. *Cochrane Database of Systematic Reviews* 3:CD003751.

Morden, N. E., C. H. Chang, J. O. Jacobson, E. M. Berke, J. P. Bynum, K. M. Murray, and D. C. Goodman. 2012. End-of-life care for Medicare beneficiaries with cancer is highly intensive overall and varies widely. *Health Affairs (Millwood)* 31(4):786-796.

Moriates, C., N. T. Shah, and V. M. Arora. 2013. First, do no (financial) harm. *Journal of the American Medical Association* (epub ahead of print).

NAEP (National Assessment of Educational Progress). 2010. *The nation's report card: Grade 12 reading and mathematics 2009 national and pilot state results*. Washington, DC: U.S. Department of Education.

NCCS (National Coalition for Cancer Survivorship). 2012a. *Cancer is a crisis*. http://www.canceradvocacy.org/resources/remaining-hopeful/cancer-is-a-crisis (accessed September 24, 2012).

————. 2012b. *NCCS applauds establishment of cancer treatment planning and care coordina-tion reimbursement codes.* http://www.canceradvocacy.org/news/nccs-applauds-establishment-treatment-care-reimbursement-codes.html (accessed September 24, 2012).

————. 2012c. *Cancer survivor toolbox.* http://www.canceradvocacy.org/toolbox (accessed January 4, 2013).

————. 2013. *Support the PACT Act.* http://www.canceradvocacy.org/pact-act (accessed August 1, 2013).

NCI (National Cancer Institute). 2012. *Breast cancer risk in American women.* http://www.cancer.gov/cancertopics/factsheet/detection/probability-breast-cancer (accessed April 24, 2013).

————. 2013a. *Cancer Education and Career Development Program (R25T).* http://www.cancer.gov/researchandfunding/cancertraining/outsidenci/R25T (accessed May 2, 2013).

————. 2013b. *NCI dictionary of cancer terms.* http://www.cancer.gov/dictionary (accessed July 19, 2013).

NCSL (National Conference of State Legislatures). 2013. *State and federal actions related to transparency and disclosure of health charges and provider payments.* http://www.ncsl.org/issues-research/health/transparency-and-disclosure-health-costs.aspx#State_Efforts (accessed April 30, 2013).

Neumann, P. J., J. A. Palmer, E. Nadler, C. Fang, and P. Ubel. 2010. Cancer therapy costs influence treatment: A national survey of oncologists. *Health Affairs (Millwood)* 29(1):196-202.

NHPCO (National Hospice and Palliative Care Organization). 2012. *NHPCO facts and figures: Hospice care in America.* http://www.nhpco.org/sites/default/files/public/Statistics_Research/2012_Facts_Figures.pdf (accessed April 30, 2013).

————. 2013. *Advance care planning.* http://www.nhpco.org/advance-care-planning (accessed April 1, 2013).

NQF (National Quality Forum). 2006. *A national framework and preferred practices for palliative and hospice care quality.* http://www.qualityforum.org/Publications/2006/12/A_National_Framework_and_Preferred_Practices_for_Palliative_and_Hospice_Care_Quality.aspx (accessed May 22, 2013).

NRC (National Research Council). 2012. *Improving adult literacy instruction: Options for practice and research.* Washington, DC: The National Academies Press.

OHRI (Ottawa Hospital Research Institute). 2013. *A to Z inventory of decision aids.* http://decisionaid.ohri.ca/AZinvent.php (accessed March 29, 2013).

Oncotalk. 2002. *Learning module 2: Giving bad news.* http://depts.washington.edu/oncotalk/learn/modules.html (accessed May 15, 2013).

Orlander, J. D., B. G. Fincke, D. Hermanns, and G. A. Johnson. 2002. Medical residents' first clearly remembered experiences of giving bad news. *Journal of General Internal Medicine* 17(11):825-831.

Oshima Lee, E., and E. J. Emanuel. 2013. Shared decision making to improve care and reduce costs. *New England Journal of Medicine* 368(1):6-8.

Osta, B. E., J. L. Palmer, T. Paraskevopoulos, B. L. Pei, L. E. Roberts, V. A. Poulter, R. Chacko, and E. Bruera. 2008. Interval between first palliative care consult and death in patients diagnosed with advanced cancer at a comprehensive cancer center. *Journal of Palliative Medicine* 11(1):51-57.

Parry, C., E. E. Kent, L. P. Forsythe, C. M. Alfano, and J. H. Rowland. 2013. Can't see the forest for the care plan: A call to revisit the context of care planning. *Journal of Clinical Oncology* 31(21):2651-2653.

Partin, M. R., D. Nelson, A. B. Flood, G. Friedemann-Sanchez, and T. J. Wilt. 2006. Who uses decision aids? Subgroup analyses from a randomized controlled effectiveness trial of two prostate cancer screening decision support interventions. *Health Expectations* 9(3):285-295.

Patient Advocate Foundation. 2012. *Resources*. http://www.patientadvocate.org/resources.
php (accessed January 4, 2013).

PCORI (Patient-Centered Outcomes Research Institute). 2012. *National priorities for research and research agenda*. http://www.pcori.org/assets/PCORI-National-Priorities-and-Research-Agenda-2012-05-21-FINAL.pdf (accessed May 2, 2013).

———. 2013a. *Development and pilot of three patient decision aids for implanted defibrillators.* http://www.pcori.org/pilot-projects/development-and-pilot-of-three-patient-decision-aids-for-implanted-defibrillators (accessed May 2, 2013).

———. 2013b. *Patient-centered outcomes research*. http://www.pcori.org/research-we-support/pcor (accessed March 29, 2013).

Peppercorn, J. M., T. J. Smith, P. R. Helft, D. J. Debono, S. R. Berry, D. S. Wollins, D. M. Hayes, J. H. Von Roenn, and L. E. Schnipper. 2011. American Society of Clinical Oncology statement: Toward individualized care for patients with advanced cancer. *Journal of Clinical Oncology* 29(6):755-760.

Peters, E., J. Hibbard, P. Slovic, and N. Dieckmann. 2007. Numeracy skill and the communication, comprehension, and use of risk-benefit information. *Health Affairs (Millwood)* 26(3):741-748.

Picker Institute. 2013. *Principles of patient-centered care*. http://pickerinstitute.org/about/picker-principles (accessed July 17, 2013).

Porter-O'Grady, T., and K. Malloch. 2007. *Quantum leadership: A resource for healthcare innovation, second edition*. Sudbury, MA: Jones and Bartlett Publishers.

Quill, T. E., and A. P. Abernethy. 2013. Generalist plus specialist palliative care—creating a more sustainable model. *New England Journal of Medicine* 368(13):1183-1174.

Quill, T. E., and P. Townsend. 1991. Bad news: Delivery, dialogue, and dilemmas. *Archives of Internal Medicine* 151(3):463-468.

Quinn, E. M., M. A. Corrigan, S. M. McHugh, D. Murphy, J. O'Mullane, A. D. Hill, and H. P. Redmond. 2012. Breast cancer information on the internet: Analysis of accessibility and accuracy. *Breast* 21(4):514-517.

Ramsey, S., and V. Shankaran. 2012. Managing the financial impact of cancer treatment: The role of clinical practice guidelines. *Journal of the National Comprehensive Cancer Network* 10(8):1037-1042.

Ramsey, S. D., D. Blough, A. Kirchhoff, K. Kreizenbeck, C. R. Fedorenko, K. S. Snell, P. Newcomb, W. Hollingworth, and K. Overstreet. 2013. Washington state cancer patients found to be at greater risk for bankruptcy than people without a cancer diagnosis. *Health Affairs (Millwood)* 10.1377/hlthaff.2012.1263. (epub ahead of print).

Ratzan, S. C., and R. M. Parker. 2001. Introduction. In *National Library of Medicine Current Bibliographies in Medicine: Health Literacy. NLM Pub. No. CBM 2000-1*, edited by C. R. Selden, M. Zorn, S. C. Ratzan, and R. M. Parker. Bethesda, MD: National Institutes of Health.

Rau, J. 2013. *Medicare lags in project to expand hospice*. http://www.kaiserhealthnews.org/Stories/2013/May/09/Medicare-delays-experiment-on-hospice-and-curative-care.aspx (accessed May 14, 2013).

Reinhardt, U. E. 2011. The many different prices paid to providers and the flawed theory of cost shifting: Is it time for a more rational all-payer system? *Health Affairs (Millwood)* 30(11):2125-2133.

Rose, J. H., E. E. O'Toole, N. V. Dawson, R. Lawrence, D. Gurley, C. Thomas, M. B. Hamel, and H. J. Cohen. 2004. Perspectives, preferences, care practices, and outcomes among older and middle-aged patients with late-stage cancer. *Journal of Clinical Oncology* 22(24):4907-4917.

Roseman, D., J. Osborne-Stafsnes, C. Helwig, S. Boslaugh, and K. Slate-Miller. 2013. Early lessons from four "Aligning Forces for Quality" communities bolster the case for patient-centered care. *Health Affairs (Millwood)* 32(2):232-241.

Rosenthal, J. A., X. Lu, and P. Cram. 2013. Availability of consumer prices from U.S. hospitals for a common surgical procedure. *Journal of the American Medical Association Internal Medicine* 173(6):427-432.

Schwartz, M. D., H. B. Valdimarsdottir, T. A. DeMarco, B. N. Peshkin, W. Lawrence, J. Rispoli, K. Brown, C. Isaacs, S. O'Neill, R. Shelby, S. C. Grumet, M. M. McGovern, S. Garnett, H. Bremer, S. Leaman, K. O'Mara, S. Kelleher, and K. Komaridis. 2009. Randomized trial of a decision aid for BRCA1/BRCA2 mutation carriers: impact on measures of decision making and satisfaction. *Health Psychology* 28(1):11-19.

Sepucha, K. R., J. F. J. Fowler, and J. A. G. Mulley. 2004. Policy support for patient-centered care: The need for measurable improvements in decision quality. *Health Affairs (Millwood)* Suppl Variation:VAR54-62.

Shah, A., J. J. Paly, J. A. Efstathiou, and J. E. Bekelman. 2013. Physician evaluation of internet health information on proton therapy for prostate cancer. *International Journal of Radiation Oncology, Biology, Physics* 85(4):e173-e177.

Shankaran, V., S. Jolly, D. Blough, and S. D. Ramsey. 2012. Risk factors for financial hardship in patients receiving adjuvant chemotherapy for colon cancer: A population-based exploratory analysis. *Journal of Clinical Oncology* 30(14):1608-1614.

Shepperd, S., B. Wee, and S. E. Strauss. 2011. Hospital at home: home-based end of life care. *Cochrane Database of Systematic Reviews* 7:CD009231.

Sheridan, S. L., R. P. Harris, and S. H. Woolf. 2004. Shared decision making about screening and chemoprevention: A suggested approach from the U. S. Preventive Services Task Force. *American Journal of Preventive Medicine* 26(1):56-66.

Siegel, K., D. G. Karus, V. H. Raveis, G. H. Christ, and F. P. Mesagno. 1996. Depressive distress among the spouses of terminally ill cancer patients. *Cancer Practice* 4(1):25-30.

Silveira, M. J., S. Y. H. Kim, and K. M. Langa. 2010. Advance directives and outcomes of surrogate decision making before death. *New England Journal of Medicine* 362(13): 1211-1218.

Siminoff, L. A., N. H. Gordon, P. Silverman, T. Budd, and P. M. Ravdin. 2006. A decision aid to assist in adjuvant therapy choices for breast cancer. *Psycho-Oncology* 15(11):1001-1013.

Smith, T. J. 2003. Tell it like it is. *Journal of Clinical Oncology* 21(9 Suppl):12s-16s.

Smith, T. J., and B. E. Hillner. 2010. Concrete options and ideas for increasing value in oncology care:The view from one trench. *Oncologist* (15 Suppl 1):65-72.

———. 2011. Bending the cost curve in cancer care. *New England Journal of Medicine* 364(21): 2060-2065.

Smith, T. J., and D. L. Longo. 2012. Talking with patients about dying. *New England Journal of Medicine* 367(17):1651-1652.

Smith, T. J., L. A. Dow, E. Virago, J. Khatcheressian, L. J. Lyckholm, and R. Matsuyama. 2010. Giving honest information to patients with advanced cancer maintains hope. *Oncology (Williston Park)* 24(6):521-525.

Smith, T. J., L. A. Dow, E. A. Virago, J. Khatcheressian, R. Matsuyama, and L. J. Lyckholm. 2011. A pilot trial of decision aids to give truthful prognostic and treatment information to chemotherapy patients with advanced cancer. *Journal of Supportive Oncology* 9(2):79-86.

Smith, T. J., S. Temin, E. R. Alesi, A. P. Abernethy, T. A. Balboni, E. M. Basch, B. R. Ferrell, M. Loscalzo, D. E. Meier, J. A. Paice, J. M. Peppercorn, M. Somerfield, E. Stovall, and J. H. Von Roenn. 2012. American Society of Clinical Oncology provisional clinical opinion: The integration of palliative care into standard oncology care. *Journal of Clinical Oncology* 30(8):880-887.

Sommers, R., S. D. Goold, E. A. McGlynn, S. D. Pearson, and M. Danis. 2013. Focus groups highlight that many patients object to clinicians' focusing on costs. *Health Affairs (Millwood)* 32(2):338-346.

Spinks, T., H. W. Albright, T. W. Feeley, R. Walters, T. W. Burke, T. Aloia, E. Bruera, A. Buzdar, L. Foxhall, D. Hui, B. Summers, A. Rodriguez, R. Dubois, and K. I. Shine. 2012. Ensuring quality cancer care: A follow-up review of the Institute of Medicine's 10 recommendations for improving the quality of cancer care in America. *Cancer* 118(10):2571-2582.

Stacey, D., R. Samant, and C. Bennett. 2008. Decision making in oncology: A review of patient decision aids to support patient participation. *CA: A Cancer Journal of Clinicians* 58(5):293-304.

Stacey, D., C. L. Bennett, M. J. Barry, N. F. Col, K. B. Eden, M. Holmes-Rovner, H. Llewellyn-Thomas, A. Lyddiatt, F. Légaré, and R. Thomson. 2011. Decision aids to help people who are facing health treatment or screening decisions. *Cochrane Database of Systematic Reviews*(10):CD001431.

Stump, T. K., N. Eghan, B. L. Egleston, O. Hamilton, M. Pirollo, J. S. Schwartz, K. Armstron, J. R. Beck, N. J. Meropol, and Y.-N. Wong. 2013. Cost concerns of patients with cancer. *Journal of Oncology Practice* (epub ahead of print).

Surbone, A. 2010. Cultural competence in oncology: Where do we stand? *Annals of Oncology* 21(1):3-5.

Tai-Seale, M., C. Wilson, S. Tapper, P. Cheng, S. Lai, F. Wu, and J. Newman. 2012. CC1-03: Documentations of advanced health care directives in the electronic health record: Where are they? *Clinical Medicine & Research* 10(3):167.

Tamman, M. 2013. *U.S. federal judge lifts ban on public access to Medicare data.* http://www.reuters.com/article/2013/05/31/medicare-lawsuit-idUSL2N0EC25U20130531 (accessed July 31, 2013).

Temel, J. S., J. A. Greer, A. Muzikansky, E. R. Gallagher, S. Admane, V. A. Jackson, C. M. Dahlin, C. D. Blinderman, J. Jacobsen, W. F. Pirl, J. A. Billings, and T. J. Lynch. 2010. Early palliative care for patients with metastatic non-small-cell lung cancer. *New England Journal of Medicine* 363(8):733-742.

Temel, J. S., J. A. Greer, S. Admane, E. R. Gallagher, V. A. Jackson, T. J. Lynch, I. T. Lennes, C. M. Dahlin, and W. F. Pirl. 2011. Longitudinal perceptions of prognosis and goals of therapy in patients with metastatic non-small-cell lung cancer: Results of a randomized study of early palliative care. *Journal of Clinical Oncology* 29(17):2319-2326.

Teno, J. M., B. R. Clarridge, V. Casey, L. C. Welch, T. Wetle, R. Shield, and V. Mor. 2004. Family perspectives on end-of-life care at the last place of care. *Journal of the American Medical Association* 291(1):88-93.

The, A.-M., T. Hak, G. Koeter, and G. van Der Wal. 2000. Collusion in doctor-patient communication about imminent death: An ethnographic study. *BMJ* 321(7273):1376-1381.

Tilburt, J. C., M. K. Wynia; R. D. Sheeler, B. Thorsteinsdottir, K. M. James, J. S. Egginton, M. Liebow, S. Hurst, M. Danis, and S. D. Goold. 2013. *Journal of the American Medical Association* 310(4):380-388.

Tinetti, M. E. 2012. The retreat from advanced care planning. *Journal of the American Medical Association* 307(9):915-916.

UCSF Carol Franc Buck Breast Cancer Center. 2012. *Decision services.* http://www.decisionservices.ucsf.edu (accessed January 4, 2013).

Uitterhoeve, R. J., J. M. Bensing, R. P. Grol, P. H. Demulder, and T. van Achterberg. 2010. The effect of communication skills training on patient outcomes in cancer care: A systematic review of the literature. *European Journal of Cancer Care* 19(4):442-457.

Veroff, D., A. Marr, and D. E. Wennberg. 2013. Enhanced support for shared decision making reduced costs of care for patients with preference-sensitive conditions. *Health Affairs (Millwood)* 32(2):285-293.

Villas Boas, P. J., R. S. Spagnuolo, A. Kamegasawa, L. G. Braz, A. Polachini do Valle, E. C. Jorge, H. H. Yoo, A. J. Cataneo, I. Correa, F. B. Fukushima, P. do Nascimento, N. S. Modolo, M. S. Teixeira, E. I. de Oliveira Vidal, S. R. Daher, and R. El Dib. 2012. Systematic reviews showed insufficient evidence for clinical practice in 2004: What about in 2011? The next appeal for the evidence-based medicine age. *Journal of Evaluating Clininical Practice* 19(4):633-637.

Volandes, A. E., M. K. Paasche-Orlow, S. L. Mitchell, A. El-Jawahri, A. D. Davis, M. J. Barry, K. L. Hartshorn, V. A. Jackson, M. R. Gillick, E. S. Walker-Corkery, Y. Chang, L. López, M. Kemeny, L. Bulone, E. Mann, S. Misra, M. Peachey, E. D. Abbo, A. F. Eichler, A. S. Epstein, A. Noy, T. T. Levin, and J. S. Temel. 2013. Randomized controlled trial of a video decision support tool for cardiopulmonary resuscitation decision making in advanced cancer. *Journal of Clinical Oncology* 31(3):380-386.

Wagner, E. H., E. J. Aiello Bowles, S. M. Greene, L. Tuzzio, C. J. Wiese, B. Kirlin, and S. B. Clauser. 2010. The quality of cancer patient experience: perspectives of patients, family members, providers and experts. *Quality and Safety in Health Care* 19(6):484-489.

Weeks, J. C., P. J. Catalano, A. Cronin, M. D. Finkelman, J. W. Mack, N. L. Keating, and D. Schrag. 2012. Patients' expectations about effects of chemotherapy for advanced cancer. *New England Journal of Medicine* (17):1616-1625.

Wentlandt, K., M. K. Krzyzanowska, N. Swami, G. M. Rodin, L. W. Le, and C. Zimmermann. 2012. Referral practices of oncologists to specialized palliative care. *Journal of Clinical Oncology* 30(35):4380-4386.

Wilson, C. J., J. Newman, S. Tapper, S. Lai, P. H. Cheng, F. M. Wu, and M. Tai-Seale. 2013. Multiple locations of advance care planning documentation in an electronic health record: Are they easy to find? *Journal of Palliative Medicine* 16(9):1089-1094.

Wilson, K., and S. Schettle. 2013. A grassroots initiative for end-of-life planning. *Health Affairs (Millwood)* 34(4):823-824.

Wittenberg-Lyles, E., J. Goldsmith, B. Ferrell, and S. L. Ragan. 2013. *Communication in palliative nursing*. New York: Oxford University Press.

Wright, A. A., A. Ray, B. Zhang, J. W. Mack, S. L. Mitchell, M. E. Nilsson, E. T. Trice, S. D. Block, P. K. Maciejewski, and H. G. Prigerson. 2008. Medical care and emotional distress associated with advanced cancer patients' end-of-life discussions with their physicians. *Journal of Clinical Oncology* (May 20 Suppl):abstr 6505.

Wright, A. A., N. L. Keating, T. A. Balboni, U. A. Matulonis, S. D. Block, and H. G. Prigerson. 2010. Place of death: Correlations with quality of life of patients with cancer and predictors of bereaved caregivers' mental health. *Journal of Clinical Oncology* 28(29):4457-4464.

Yung, V. Y., A. M. Walling, L. Min, N. S. Wenger, and D. A. Ganz. 2010. Documentation of advance care planning for community-dwelling elders. *Journal of Palliative Medicine* 13(7):861-867.

Zabora, J., K. BrintzenhofeSzoc, B. Curbow, C. Hooker, and S. Piantadosi. 2001. The prevalence of psychological distress by cancer site. *Psychooncology* 10(1):19-28.

Zafar, S. Y., J. M. Peppercorn, D. Schrag, D. H. Taylor, A. M. Goetzinger, X. Zhong, and A. P. Abernethy. 2013. The financial toxicity of cancer treatment: A pilot study assessing out-of-pocket expenses and the insured cancer patient's experience. *Oncologist* 18(4):381-390.

Zikmund-Fisher, B. J., M. P. Couper, E. Singer, P. A. Ubel, S. Ziniel, F. J. Fowler, Jr., C. A. Levin, and A. Fagerlin. 2010. Deficits and variations in patients' experience with making 9 common medical decisions: The DECISIONS survey. *Medical Decision Making* 30(5 Suppl):85S-95S.

4

The Workforce Caring for
Patients with Cancer

A diverse team of professionals provides cancer care, reflecting the complexity of the disease, its treatments, and survivorship care (C-Change, 2013). The cancer care team includes those with specialized training in oncology, such as oncologists and oncology nurses, other specialists and primary care clinicians, as well as family caregivers and direct care workers. Patients, at the center of the committee's conceptual framework, are encircled by the cancer care workforce (see Figure S-2), depicting the idea that high-quality cancer care depends on the workforce providing competent, trusted interprofessional care that is aligned with the patients' needs, values, and preferences. To achieve this standard, the workforce must include adequate numbers of health care clinicians with training in oncology. The members of interprofessional cancer care teams must be coordinated with each other and with the patients' other care teams (e.g., primary care/geriatrics care teams or other specialty care teams). Additionally, the workforce must have the skills necessary to implement the committee's conceptual framework for a high-quality cancer care system. The focus on the workforce caring for patients with cancer is consistent with the Institute of Medicine's (IOM's) 1999 report on the quality of cancer care, which recognized the importance of cancer care being delivered by coordinated, experienced professionals (IOM and NRC, 1999).

Current practice falls far short of this standard. Workforce shortages among many of the professionals involved in providing cancer care are projected to worsen in the near future, and the educational system lacks the capacity to quickly train new members of the workforce (IOM, 2009b).

Care is often uncoordinated among the various clinicians and care teams, leaving patients to navigate a fragmented cancer care delivery system. Caregivers are also expected to assume a significant amount of medical tasks without any training or support (Reinhard and Levine, 2012).

At the same time, shifting demographics are placing new demands on this delivery system, with the incidence of cancer increasing due to the aging population and cancer survivors living longer (see Chapter 2). Medical advances, such as new chemotherapy regimens that involve less toxic, but more frequent administration, are increasing the volume of cancer care (IOM, 2009b). In addition, the Patient Protection and Affordable Care Act (ACA)[1] is expected to expand health insurance coverage to an estimated 25 million previously uninsured persons, many of whom are likely to require cancer care at some point during their lifetimes (CBO, 2013). A number of studies show that the quality of care is detrimentally impacted by workforce shortages (AHRQ, 2004; Aiken et al., 2010; Blegen et al., 2011; Needleman et al., 2011). Patients can experience delays in diagnosis and treatment, longer wait times to see a clinician, less frequent interaction with clinical and supportive services, delays in the evaluation and management of symptoms, worsening health disparities, and decreased clinical trial enrollment.

This chapter assesses the capacity and competence of the workforce to meet the growing need for high-quality cancer care. The first section provides a review of the cancer care team members, including estimates of workforce supply and demand. The next section focuses on strategies for ensuring the quantity and quality of the clinicians on cancer care teams, including the recruitment and retention of clinicians, the importance of team-based cancer care, training the workforce, and telemedicine. The chapter concludes with a discussion of the role of family caregivers and direct care workers in providing cancer care. The committee relied heavily on the IOM's previous research on the health care workforce to derive the evidence base for this chapter, including the National Cancer Policy Forum's workshop summary on *Ensuring Quality Cancer Care Through the Oncology Workforce* (2009b) and recent consensus studies addressing the geriatric, nursing, and mental health workforces (IOM, 2008b, 2011a, 2012c). The committee identifies two recommendations to strengthen the workforce that cares for patients with cancer.

---

[1] Patient Protection and Affordable Care Act, Public Law 111-148, 111th Congress (March 23, 2010).

DEFINING THE WORKFORCE CARING
FOR PATIENTS WITH CANCER

High-quality cancer care is provided by a diverse team of professionals. This portion of the chapter reviews many of the clinicians who comprise the cancer care team: physicians, nurses, advanced practice registered nurses, physician assistants, palliative care specialists, clinicians providing psychosocial support, spiritual workers, rehabilitation clinicians, pharmacists, and, for care at the end-of-life, hospice clinicians. Each section describes the general role of the profession in cancer care and the projected workforce supply and demand. Many other professionals are also involved in cancer care teams, such as laboratory personnel, public health workers, and cancer registrars. Annex 4-1 provides a detailed list of professionals involved in cancer care, their general roles on the cancer care team, and an overview of available information about the workforce.

In general, data suggest that the growth in the absolute number of older adults is likely to result in a greater total volume of patients with cancer and a greater need for services than our current workforce can provide. As noted in previous IOM reports, however, it can be challenging to accurately translate data on illness prevalence into estimates of workforce supply and demand (IOM, 2005, 2008b, 2012c). Data on health care professions are not routinely or systematically collected across the multiple disciplines involved in cancer care, giving an incomplete picture of the current workforce. Several provisions of the ACA may improve available information on the workforce, including the National Center for Health Workforce Analysis and National Health Care Workforce Commission, but it is unclear whether funding will continue for these activities (see Annex 2-1). In addition, many factors can lead to forecasting errors, such as changes in utilization patterns of medical technologies, changes in the organization of care, and changes in patient demands.

Physicians

Several recent studies estimate that the physician workforce lacks the capacity to meet the future demand for health care services. The Association of American Medical Colleges (AAMC) estimated that the United States will have a shortage of 90,000 physicians in the next 10 years due to the aging and growing population (AAMC, 2011b). Sargen and colleagues (2011) projected further into the future, calculating a current physician shortage of around 8 percent, which could rise to more than 20 percent by 2025 if the rate of medical residents being trained does not increase. The escalating amount of time physicians are devoting to documentation, compliance, and other indirect patient care services could further increase demand for physician services by an additional 10 to 15 percent during the same time period.

A major driver of the physician shortage is the aging workforce. Currently, 40 percent of practicing physicians are older than 55 and roughly one-third of physicians are expected to retire over the next 10 years (AAMC, 2011b, 2013). These physicians are being replaced by a younger generation of physicians who more often prefer to work part time or in specialties that have less demanding on-call responsibilities (Hauer et al., 2008). A study by Staiger and colleagues found that the mean hours worked by physicians decreased by more than 7 percent between 1996 and 2008, with the largest decrease in hours worked among physicians younger than 45 years (Staiger et al., 2010).

The distribution of physicians across urban and rural areas may also contribute to the physician shortage. For example, only 11 percent of the 300,000 primary care physicians practicing in the United States are located in rural areas (UnitedHealth, 2011). Specialists are also more concentrated in urban areas than in rural areas. Thus, patients in rural areas have less access to medical services, including oncology, and often have to drive long distances to receive health care services.

The medical education system is unlikely to keep pace with the rising demand for physician services. Although medical school enrollment has increased by 30 percent over the previous 5 years (AHR, 2012b), the federal government has not substantially increased the number of residency slots that it supports to train newly graduated medical students. This is problematic because Medicare is the largest payer of Graduate Medical Education (GME) (Health Affairs, 2012). The Balanced Budget Act of 1997 froze the number of resident slots and fellowships funded by Medicare without regard to whether the number of physicians generated would meet future demands for health care services (AAMC, 2011b). Recent proposals to reduce the federal debt have included further cuts to Medicare's GME support. An ongoing IOM consensus study is examining this issue in more detail and will be proposing solutions to GME's governance and financing (IOM, 2012b).

These general trends in the physician workforce have a substantial impact on the physicians and specialists who provide care for cancer patients, such as oncologists, primary care physicians, and geriatricians. These clinicians are the focus of the remainder of this section.

Physicians Providing Cancer Care

There are numerous types of physicians who provide cancer care, including surgical oncologists who operate, radiation oncologists who treat with radiation, and medical oncologists who provide systemic treatments. There are also a limited number of geriatric oncologists who primarily conduct academic research on caring for older adults with cancer (Bennett et al., 2010). Additionally, many cancer patients are treated by other types of physicians, such as urologists for prostate cancer, pulmonologists for early-stage lung cancer, dermatologists for early-stage melanoma, and gastroenterologists for early-stage colon cancer. This section focuses on medical oncologists because they are the primary physicians involved in cancer care, and their workforce has been studied extensively by the American Society of Clinical Oncology (ASCO). Less information is available about other physician workforces who provide cancer care. The American Society for Radiation Oncology, however, is currently conducting a survey of the radiation oncology workforce in order to assess the profession's supply, education, and employment situation (ASTRO, 2012b).

In order to become board certified in medical oncology, physicians must complete a 3-year residency program in internal medicine followed by an oncology fellowship (at least 2 clinical years of training, often with additional time for research). Few medical oncology fellowship programs currently have plans to increase the number of training slots, which limits the size of the workforce (AAMC, 2007; Erikson et al., 2007). Training new medical oncologists is expensive and there is little financial support available from the government to expand these programs.

In addition, merely increasing the size of existing oncology fellowship programs would not solve the workforce problem. The size of the oncology workforce is constrained by the pipeline of residents. Medical oncologists must first complete a residency in internal medicine, but the number of students undergoing training in internal medicine has increased only marginally in recent years. There is also a growing number of subspecialties available to internal medicine interns (Salsberg et al., 2008), and medical oncology fellowship programs must compete against interventional subspecialties, such as cardiology and pulmonology, for this limited supply of internal medicine residents. Moreover, many medical students are opting for specialties that do not require a residency in internal medicine, such as dermatology, orthopedic surgery, or radiology, as well as radiation oncology and surgical oncology.

A study commissioned by ASCO predicts that the demand for medical oncologists will increase dramatically between now and 2020 due to a 48 percent increase in cancer incidence and an 81 percent increase in people living with or surviving cancer (AAMC, 2007; Erikson et al., 2007). During this same time period, the supply of oncologists is predicted to increase only 14 percent. The study found that more than half of currently practicing medical oncologists are age 50 or older and will reach retirement age by 2020. Medical oncologists younger than 45 are also working fewer hours on average than those ages 45 to 64, exacerbating the problem of an aging workforce. Based on these trends, the study concluded that there will be a shortage of 2,500 to 4,080 medical oncologists by 2020. It is likely that the other professionals involved in providing cancer care will also face similar imbalances between the workforce supply and demand.

Primary Care Physicians

Primary care physicians are generalists who provide comprehensive and continuous care to patients regardless of the diagnosis, the organ system involved, or the origin of the medical problem (biological, behavioral, or social) (AAFP, 2012). Box 4-1 describes the diverse roles that primary care clinicians play in caring for patients with cancer.

In 2007, there were more than 200,000 general internal medicine and family medicine physicians in the United States, the principal primary care medical specialties (AAMC, 2008). This number has been increasing steadily over the past several years because more medical students have been matching into primary care residencies (AAMC, 2011a). However, a number of factors may limit the long-term supply of primary care physicians.

In a survey of fourth-year medical students, only 2 percent of the respondents planned a career in internal medicine without specialization (Hauer et al., 2008). The respondents identified a number of concerns about careers in general internal medicine, including inadequate administrative and technical support to deal with the paperwork demands, the complexity of caring for older adults and chronically ill patients, and preferences for work schedules that provide fewer demands on time and more opportunities for personal satisfaction outside of work. A major deterrent to becoming a primary care physician is also the more than $135,000 median annual income gap between primary care physicians and subspecialists, a difference of $3.5 million in expected income over a lifetime (RGC, 2010). These factors have likely contributed to approximately 20 percent of primary care physicians departing from general internal medicine within a decade of becoming certified to practice, with many leaving to work in another medical field (Lipner et al., 2006).

It may be possible to offset the need for additional primary care physicians by diverting some patients to nonphysician professionals, such as advanced practice registered nurses and physician assistants (discussed below in the sections on advanced practice registered nurses and physician assistants), and using patient-clinician electronic communication (see discussion in Chapter 6) (Green et al., 2012; Kuo et al., 2013).

BOX 4-1
The Roles of Primary Care Clinicians in
Caring for Patients with Cancer

Primary care clinicians fulfill a diverse set of roles in cancer care. They are often the first clinicians that patients see when they have signs or symptoms of cancer and are the most likely to screen their patients for cancer. Thus, they are usually the ones diagnosing cancer and providing patients with referrals to oncologists or other specialists for treatment.

During active cancer treatment, primary care clinicians provide patients with ongoing health promotion, disease prevention, health maintenance, counseling, education, and diagnosis and treatment of other acute and chronic illnesses. This is especially important in older adults with cancer who tend to require treatment for other chronic conditions, such as high-blood pressure and diabetes (Unroe and Cohen, 2012).

It is important for the cancer care team to effectively coordinate with a patient's primary care clinicians during the acute cancer treatment phase. Primary care clinicians often have known their patients longer than the cancer care team and are more likely to be familiar with their patients' needs, values, and preferences. It is also important that primary care clinicians be informed about their patients' cancer treatments. They often provide continuous treatment for their patients' concurrent illnesses and conditions, which may need to be adjusted or monitored differently during cancer treatment, as well as survivorship care and cancer surveillance after their acute cancer treatment is complete. Primary care clinicians can also play a role during active treatment in establishing advance directives and coordinating with family caregivers and direct care workers (IOM, 2011b; Klabunde et al., 2009).

Cohen (2009) has described the ideal relationship between the primary care team and the cancer team as "shared care," where both care teams are involved in a patient's care during the entire continuum of the disease, but have a bigger or smaller role at a given time depending on the needs of the patient and the disease status. In a survey by Del Giudice and colleagues, primary care clinicians reported that they are interested in being involved in their patients' cancer care, especially if they have a long-term relationship with the particular patient, but often feel they lack the preparation and knowledge to do so effectively (Del Giudice et al., 2009). A more recent survey by Potosky and colleagues (2011) found that primary care clinicians differ significantly from oncologists in their knowledge, attitudes, and practices related to follow-up care for breast and colon cancer. Cancer care plans which summarize a patient's needs, treatment information, and follow-up care, are tools to aid primary care clinicians in coordinating with the cancer care team and providing complementary health care services to their patients (see discussion on care plans in Chapter 3) (IOM, 2005, 2011b).

Geriatricians

Geriatricians are primary care physicians trained to meet the unique health care needs of older adults. Currently, the number of geriatricians does not adequately meet the health care needs of the older adult population, and the situation is growing worse (IOM, 2008b). There are over 9,000 certified geriatricians (ABIM, 2012). In 2011, there was 1 geriatrician for every 2,620 Americans 75 years or older. By 2030 that ratio is expected to drop to 1 geriatrician for every 3,798 Americans 75 years or older. Many geriatric fellowship slots are not being filled due to lack of interest. For academic year 2009-2010, only 56 percent (273 out of 489) of allopathic geriatric training slots were filled and only 2 out of 46 osteopathic geriatric medicine fellowship slots were filled (AGS, 2012).

The recent IOM report *Retooling for an Aging America: Building the Health Care Workforce* (2008b) made a series of recommendations intended to improve and grow the geriatric workforce by enhancing geriatric competence, increasing recruitment and retention of geriatric specialists, and redesigning models of care to meet the rising needs of older adults. The committee believes that these recommendations are important to improving the quality of cancer care in this country and efforts should be made to implement them.

Nurses

The American Nurses Association defines nursing as "the protection, promotion, and optimization of health and abilities, prevention of illness and injury, alleviation of suffering through the diagnosis and treatment of human response, and advocacy in the care of individuals, families, communities, and populations" (ANA, 2012). Nursing is a multilevel profession, and includes (1) licensed practical nurses who are trained through 12- to 18-month programs in vocational/technical schools or community colleges; (2) registered nurses (RNs), who must complete a 4-year bachelor's degree program, a 2-year associate degree program, or a 3-year diploma program and pass a national licensure examination; and (3) advanced practice registered nurses (APRNs), who have master's or doctorate's degrees in nursing and work with more independence. There are currently more than 3 million nurses in the United States and they make up the largest segment of the health care workforce (IOM, 2011a).

A number of analyses suggest that the existing nursing workforce is insufficient to meet the rising demand for services. The Bureau of Labor Statistics has predicted that nursing will be one of the fastest-growing professions in the United States and that the country will need over 1 million new nurses by 2020 to fill new jobs and replace vacancies resulting from retiring nurses (BLS, 2012a). Juraschek and colleagues (2012) forecasted the RN job shortage in all 50 states between 2009 and 2030 and assigned letter grades based on the projected RN job shortage ratio. The number of states receiving a grade of "D" or "F" for their RN job shortage ratio is projected to increase from 5 in 2009 to 30 by 2030. This translates into a deficit of almost 1 million RNs by 2030.

Buerhaus and colleagues published several studies showing that people who have turned to nursing in response to the recent economic downturn have eliminated the current nursing shortage (Buerhaus et al., 2009; Staiger et al., 2012). Older nurses are delaying retirement or returning to the workforce and part-time nurses are becoming full-time employees in response to their own and their spouses' employment insecurity. In addition, the number of RNs has grown faster than predicted (Auerbach et al., 2011). Between 2002 and 2009, the number of full-time RNs between the ages of 23 and 26 increased by 62 percent. Nonetheless, Buerhaus and colleagues cautioned that these trends may not continue and that a number of factors suggest there will be nursing shortages in the future (Buerhaus et al., 2009; Staiger et al., 2012).

The workforce is rapidly aging, with an increasing number of baby boomers nearing retirement. There has also been a decline in RN earnings relative to other career options. Nurses express more dissatisfaction with their jobs than do people in other professions, and the changing demographics in the United States have led to an older and less healthy population, which discourages younger generations from entering nursing (AHR, 2012a). In a survey of the current RN workforce conducted by AMN Healthcare, almost one-third of the nurses reported planning to make career changes in the next 1 to 3 years (AMN Healthcare, 2012). Only 56 percent of respondents said that if they were starting out today they would choose nursing as their career.

The shortage of nursing faculty is compounding the shortage of nurses. A recent IOM study recommended that the nursing workforce increase the number of nurses with a baccalaureate degree from 50 percent to 80 percent of the workforce and double the number of nurses with a doctorate by 2020 (IOM, 2011a). However, nursing schools lack the capacity to train this workforce. A 2007 survey by the American Association of Colleges of Nursing (AACN) found that 85 percent of nursing schools have faculty vacancies or need more faculty members but lack the budget to pay their salaries (AACN, 2012b). In 2011, more than 75,000 qualified nursing applicants were not accepted into a nursing program due primarily to a shortage of faculty and resource constraints (AACN, 2012a).

One of the major factors contributing to the faculty shortage is the requirement for faculty to hold Ph.D.s (Berlin and Sechrist, 2002). In 2007, enrollment in nursing Ph.D. programs was up less than 1 percent from previous years despite the demand for nurses with this qualification (AACN, 2008). A major deterrent to nurses becoming faculty is the fact that advanced practice registered nurses earn significantly higher salaries if they work in clinical positions than if they work in academic positions. The aging workforce is also a factor. Nursing faculty tend to retire earlier than other medical professions, with an average retirement age of 62.5 years (Berlin and Sechrist, 2002). The average age of doctorate-level faculty in nursing is currently 60.5 years for professors (AACN, 2011).

This nursing shortage means that there is likely to be an insufficient number of nurses knowledgeable in oncology and able to meet the needs of the growing number of patients with cancer and cancer survivors. General nursing programs cover a limited amount of information about oncology, and the number of nursing schools with a specialty in oncology has been drastically reduced in recent years (Ferrell et al., 2003; IOM, 2005). Out of the more than 1 million registered nurses with a certification in a clinical specialty, only 1.2 percent are certified in oncology (HRSA, 2010).

Advanced Practice Registered Nurses

APRNs are nurses who have completed graduate-level education and have national certification and licensure from a state board. Nurses meeting this requirement include certified registered nurse anesthetists, certified nurse-midwives, clinical nurse specialists, certified nurse practitioners, and individuals who hold a doctorate of nursing practice (DNP). APRNs are credentialed to practice in a specific patient population (e.g., family/individual across lifespan, adult-gerontology, neonatal, pediatrics, women's health/gender, or psychiatric–mental health), and their credentials allow them to work independently or in collaboration with a physician (NCBSN, 2010, 2012).

In most states, APRNs can diagnose disease, order tests, refer patients to specialists, and prescribe medication without physician oversight (Christian et al., 2007). As a result, they often serve as patients' primary care clinicians and develop long-term relationships with their patients. (See Box 4-1 for a description of the role of primary care clinicians in cancer care.) The inclusion of APRNs on care teams has been shown to improve the quality of care that health care delivery organizations provide to patients, especially when they are involved in patients' transitions between care settings (Naylor and Keating, 2008; Naylor et al., 1994, 1999, 2004, 2005, 2009, 2011).

APRNs wishing to become certified in oncology can go through one of the Oncology Nursing Certification Corporation's three advanced oncology nursing certification programs: (1) Advanced Oncology Certified Nurse Practitioner, (2) Advanced Oncology Certified Clinical Nurse Specialist, or (3) Advanced Oncology Certified Nurse (ONCC, 2012). In 2008, there were approximately 250,000 APRNs and 2.6 percent were certified in oncology (HRSA, 2010). The DNP was launched in 2008, and as of April 2013, there were 217 DNP programs with 97 additional programs in the planning stages (AACN, 2013). DNPs play an important role in collaborative cancer care teams, specifically because of their training as agents of system change and their focus on quality as clinical leaders (Bajorin and Hanley, 2011).

Physician Assistants

Physician assistants (PAs) are medically trained and licensed professionals who practice medicine as part of a care team. They perform duties under the supervision of a physician, including providing physical examinations, diagnosing and treating illnesses, ordering and interpreting lab tests, providing patient education, and establishing and managing care plans. They have prescription privileges in all 50 states and the District of Columbia (AAPA, 2012b).

The American Academy of Physician Assistants projected that the number of PAs will increase from 75,000 in 2008 to between 137,000 and 173,000 certified in 2020 (AAPA, 2012a). They are the second-fastest-growing profession behind nurses. PAs receive a generalist education and then must pass a national certification examination, which includes content on the diagnosis and treatment of all of the major cancers for each organ system. There is also one postgraduate PA residency program in oncology (Coniglio et al., 2011). However, the majority of PAs who work in oncology receive on-the-job training though mentorship with their cancer care team (Ross et al., 2010), and they are playing an increasingly important role on collaborative cancer care teams (Coniglio, 2013; Coniglio et al., 2011).

Palliative and Hospice Care Clinicians

Palliative care and hospice care are essential components of high-quality cancer care (see discussion in Chapter 3). Palliative care is specialized medical care that provides patients with pain and symptom management, counseling on goals of treatment, coordination of care services, support when ending anti-cancer therapy, and end-of-life care. It can be provided at any point along the continuum of cancer care, often in conjunction with anti-cancer therapy. Hospice care is a form of palliative care and is focused on maintaining the quality of life for patients with advanced cancers. In order to provide these services, the cancer care team should include clinicians with training in palliative and hospice medicine.

Integrating palliative care and hospice care into standard cancer practice, however, is likely to strain the palliative and hospice workforce due to the increased utilization of these clinicians.

Currently, there are 4,400 physicians specializing in palliative and hospice medicine. A study sponsored by the American Academy of Hospice and Palliative Medicine estimated that this equates to a shortage of around 3,000 to 7,000 full-time physicians, or 6,000 to 18,000 part-time physicians (Lupu, 2010). It is unlikely that the education system will be able to quickly train new physicians in this field because there are only 234 palliative and hospice medicine fellowship positions. Similarly, the number of nurses with this expertise may be insufficient to meet increased demand. There are currently 17,000 certified hospice and palliative nurses (NBCHPN, 2013a). Nurses with this certification must hold a registered nursing license, have 2 years of relevant experience, and recertify every 4 years (NBCHPN, 2013b).

Cancer care teams are exploring new models of integrating palliative care and hospice care into their practices. For example, U.S. Oncology embeds a palliative care clinician directly within its oncology practices (Alesi et al., 2011). Other oncology practices refer patients with advanced cancer to a palliative care specialist soon after their diagnoses (Yoong et al., 2013). Many academic cancer centers, such as MD Anderson and Memorial Sloan-Kettering, have internal pain management programs to which cancer care teams can refer patients (MDACC, 2013; MSKCC, 2013).

Quill and Abernethy (2013) proposed creating a palliative care model that differentiates between primary palliative care (skills that all clinicians should have) and specialist palliative care (skills for managing more complex and difficult cases). For this model, the physicians and nurses providing cancer care would meet most of their patients' palliative care needs but refer patients to a palliative care clinician for complex and refractory problems. They would refer all patients to hospice clinicians for end-of-life care.

Clinicians Providing Psychosocial Support and Spiritual Workers

A recent IOM report concluded that attending to patients' psychosocial needs is an integral part of high-quality cancer care (IOM, 2008a). It is also a key consideration in developing patients' care plans across the cancer care continuum (see Chapter 3). A wide range of clinicians can provide psychosocial support, including social workers, psychologists, psychiatrists, and chaplains. Because it is important that the provision of psychosocial support be coordinated with a patient's biomedical health care (IOM, 2008a), clinicians providing psychosocial support and spiritual workers should be included on the cancer care team.

Social workers are one of the main professions providing psychosocial support to cancer patients. They assist "individuals, groups, or communities to restore or enhance their capacity for social functioning, and work to create societal conditions that support communities in need" (NASW, 2013b). They help patients manage the stress of a cancer diagnosis, decide on a care plan, and adapt to daily life with this disease (Lauria et al., 2001). For older adults with cancer, they often assist with advance care planning, loss and grief, independent living, and lifestyle adjustments, among many other issues related to the aging process. They can also provide emotional support for individuals serving as family caregivers (NASW, 2013c).

To practice, social workers must obtain a bachelor's, master's, or doctoral degree and be licensed to practice in the state where they work (BLS, 2013f). Master's-level social workers may specialize in health care by meeting specific continuing education and supervised work requirements (NASW, 2013a) and can further specialize in oncology or gerontology, although many social workers practice in health care settings without obtaining these certifications. Of the estimated 650,500 social workers in the United States (BLS, 2013f), 13 percent of licensed social workers specialize in health care (NASW, 2006). There are 1,000 oncology social workers and 428[2] certified oncology social workers (AOSW, 2013; Blum et al., 2006). In a survey from 2006, 78 percent of licensed social workers reported working with older adults; however, only 9 percent identified aging as their primary field of practice (NASW, 2006). Because the social work workforce is significantly older than the U.S. civilian labor force, these numbers may decline (NASW, 2006).

Psychologists also provide psychosocial services to cancer patients, typically using psychotherapy and behavior modification interventions (APA, 2013b; BLS, 2013e). Psychologists can teach cancer patients strategies for controlling their stress, grief, fear, and depression stemming from their disease. For example, some people lose sleep, stop exercising, eat unhealthily, or turn to alcohol and drugs following a diagnosis with cancer. Psychologists can help these patients develop better coping strategies, such as relaxation exercises, meditation, self-hypnosis, imagery, and techniques to relieve nausea or other side effects of treatment. They can also help patients to communicate more effectively with the other members of the cancer care team and help them to decide on an appropriate care plan. In addition, psychologists can play an important role in helping the families of cancer patients cope with their own stress, as well as work through sexual and relationship challenges (APA, 2013a; Clay, 2010).

To practice, psychologists must obtain licensure in the state where

---

[2] Personal communication, G. Vaitones, Board of Oncology Social Work Certification, March 1, 2013.

they work (BLS, 2013e; IOM, 2008a). Licensing laws vary by state; however, most states require a doctoral degree, a 1-year internship, several years of work experience, and passage of the Examination for Professional Practice in Psychology (BLS, 2013e). Psychologists may become board certified in over 10 specialty areas, including clinical psychology, counseling psychology, school psychology, child psychology, clinical health psychology, family psychology, and rehabilitation psychology (APA, 2013c; BLS, 2013e; IOM, 2008a). However, board certification is not a requirement for practice and has not been obtained by the majority of psychologists (IOM, 2008a).

Due to the increasing number of cancer survivors and older adults, the demand for psychologists is expected to grow, as is the number of professionals in the field (BLS, 2013e; IOM, 2008a). There were an estimated 174,000 psychologists in 2010, with 154,300 practicing clinical, counseling, or school psychology. By 2020, projections suggest there will be roughly 211,600 psychologists, with 188,000 practicing clinical, counseling, or school psychology (BLS, 2013e).

Psychiatrists also provide psychosocial support for cancer patients. According to the American Psychiatric Association, "a psychiatrist is a medical doctor who specializes in the diagnosis, treatment and prevention of mental illnesses, including substance use disorders" (American Psychiatric Association, 2013, p. 1). The main difference between psychiatrists and other clinicians providing psychosocial support is that psychiatrists are medically qualified to treat both the mental and the physical aspects of psychological disorders; thus, they can prescribe medication and other medical treatments (American Psychiatric Association, 2013). In cancer care, they often prescribe drugs to treat patients' psychiatric disorders stemming from their diagnosis, including anxiety and depression. They can also provide cancer patients with psychotherapy, which can help patients to cope with their disease and reduce distress (Arehart-Treichel, 2012; Barraclough, 1997). To practice, psychiatrists must complete a medical degree, at least 4 years of residency training, and pass written and oral examinations (American Psychiatric Association, 2013). There were roughly 24,210 psychiatrists practicing in the United States in 2012 (BLS, 2012b).

In addition, chaplains are an important group of professionals involved in meeting the psychosocial needs of cancer patients. Although accrediting groups often require hospitals to meet their patients' spiritual needs, the role of chaplains on the cancer care team is often less prominent and less recognized than it should be. In one study, close to 90 percent of cancer patients receiving palliative radiation therapy reported that their spiritual needs were an important component of their psychological health. More than 90 percent of cancer patients, however, said that the cancer care team did not ask them about those needs (Balboni et al., 2013). Patients whose spiritual needs are supported by the cancer care team, compared to patients whose spirital needs are not, have better quality of life, better quality of care near the end of life, with less aggressive end-of-life care (intubation, ventilation, resuscitation), and use hospice care three to five times more frequently (Balboni et al., 2010). Patients whose spiritual needs are not supported by the cancer care team are more likely to receive hospice care for less than 1 week, more likely to die in an intensive care unit, and generally have higher end-of-life care costs (Balboni et al., 2010). Because chaplains are not reimbursed, however, it is difficult to expand chaplaincy care services. The new models of payment discussed in Chapter 8 may help address this obstacle.

Rehabilitation Clinicians

Cancer and its treatment can lead to changes in individuals' physical, cognitive, and emotional well-being. Rehabilitation clinicians, including physical therapists and occupational therapists, are trained to address these changes and help individuals with cancer maximize their quality of life. Physical therapists are experts in movement and function. They help individuals maintain and restore strength, stamina, flexibility, gross motor function, and mobility (Stubblefield, 2011). Occupational therapists are experts in modifying "activities and environments to allow individuals to do the things they want and need to do to maintain quality of life" (Longpré and Newman, 2011, p. 1). They assist individuals in tasks related to self-care, orthotic fabrication and fitting, home safety, and cognitive function (Stubblefield, 2011).

Rehabilitation clinicians do not currently play a prominent enough role in cancer care (Alfano et al., 2012). Most cancer patients have limited access to comprehensive rehabilitation services due to limited reimbursement and the dependence on referral for these services (Alfano et al., 2012). The importance of including rehabilitation clinicians as members of the cancer care team, however, is increasingly being recognized in the cancer community (Alfano et al., 2012; Stubblefield, 2011; Stubblefield et al., 2012). Rehabilitation clinicians can be involved in patients' care across the cancer care continuum (Stubblefield, 2011; Stubblefield et al., 2012). There are around 200,000 physical therapists and 100,000 occupational therapists in the United States (BLS, 2013b,d) and both workforces are rapidly increasing. To practice, individuals must obtain a graduate-level degree and state licensure (BLS, 2013b,d).

Pharmacists

Pharmacists are an integral part of the cancer care team. They are typically responsible for filling prescriptions, checking for potential drug-drug and drug-disease interactions for patients using multiple medications, instructing patients on how and when to take their medication, and working with clinicians and insurance companies to ensure that patients are receiving the medication they need. To practice, pharmacists must be licensed by the state where they work, which usually requires a Pharm.D. degree and passing two licensing exams (the first tests pharmacists' skills and knowledge and the second tests pharmacists' understanding of the state licensing laws). Pharmacists may obtain an advanced pharmacy position, often in clinical settings. This requires completion of a 1 to 2-year residency program.

There were approximately 274,900 pharmacists practicing in the United States in 2010. This number is expected to increase by 25 percent by 2020, to approximately 344,600 pharmacists (BLS, 2013c).

ENSURING THE QUANTITY AND QUALITY OF THE WORKFORCE

The current workforce crisis has created an opportunity for reforming the cancer care delivery system. This portion of the chapter reviews the main strategies for ensuring that the workforce caring for patients with cancer has sufficient numbers of professionals to meet the demand for cancer care; that the team of professionals providing care is functional and well-coordinated; and that the workforce is prepared with the knowledge, skills, and experiences necessary to provide high-quality cancer care.

Recruitment and Retention of Professionals Who Provide Cancer Care

A key aspect of ensuring that there are sufficient numbers of professionals to care for patients with cancer is attracting individuals into oncology careers and retaining individuals once they choose a career in oncology. Many professionals who provide cancer care experience tremendous career satisfaction from administering care and developing relationships with their patients (Grunfeld et al., 2005; Shanafelt et al., 2006). However, there are numerous challenges to improving the recruitment and retention of professionals in cancer care, and many groups are developing strategies to overcome these challenges.

Job dissatisfaction and job-related stress are major deterrents to recruiting professionals to provide cancer care. Careers in oncology require individuals to deal with death and grieving regularly. Oncology professionals are particularly vulnerable to stress and career burnout due to the limited number of successful treatment options for many cancers and the difficult conversations about end-of-life decisions (IOM, 2009a; Losses, 2006). More general systemic pressures may also lead to dissatisfaction with oncology jobs and high rates of job-related stress, such as a heavy clinical workload, seeing high numbers of patients, short patient visits, the increasing levels of documentation required for reimbursement, and unpredictable work schedules that are driven by patient needs (Shanafelt et al., 2006). These problems are magnified during periods of workforce shortages (AAHC, 2008).

Surveys of medical oncologists confirm that professionals providing care to cancer patients experience significant career burnout, defined as emotional exhaustion and the lack of motivation to continue working in a given field (Allegra et al., 2005; Grunfeld et al., 2005; Kash et al., 2000; Ramirez et al., 1995, 1996; Shanafelt et al., 2005; Whippen and Canellos, 1991). In addition, many professionals who work in oncology report that their professional responsibilities regularly interfere with their family and personal lives, and lead to feelings of guilt and personal dissatisfaction (Allegra et al., 2005; Geurts et al., 1999; Grunfeld et al., 2005; Linzer et al., 2001; Warde et al., 1999). Similar levels of job dissatisfaction and stress are reported among other professionals involved in cancer care. For example, a 2001 survey of nurses found that hospital nurses were three to four times more likely than the average U.S. worker to be unhappy with their job and almost one-quarter of U.S. nurses reported that they were planning on leaving their jobs in the next year (Aiken et al., 2001).

Student debt also impedes the recruitment of physician-level professionals who provide cancer care. Medical school tuition has increased over the last two decades by 165 percent in private medical schools and by 312 percent in public medical schools (Jolly, 2005). In a survey conducted for the AAMC, students who appeared to be academically qualified for medical school were asked why they had not applied. All of the respondents listed cost as a major factor, with African American, Hispanic, and Native American students identifying cost as the top deterrent (Jolly, 2005). At the same time, reimbursement rates for medical care have declined and the threat of malpractice liability has increased (AAHC, 2008). When these factors are weighed against the number of training years required to become an oncologist or any of the other physician-specialists who provide cancer care, many potential recruits may choose alternate professions.

The recruitment of racial and ethnic minorities is particularly challenging. A previous IOM report recognized that increasing the proportion of populations underrepresented in medicine is an important mechanism for addressing disparities in care (IOM, 2003a). However, the clinical workforce is not currently representative of the general population. For example, 75 percent of the physician workforce is White and just over 12 percent is composed of African Americans, American Indians/Alaska Natives, and Hispanics (AAMC, 2010). Similarly small proportions of minorities are represented in the nursing and social work workforces (HRSA, 2010; NASW, 2006).

The health care community has implemented several strategies to improve the recruitment of oncology and other health professionals, including national campaigns, early exposure to health professionals, and loan forgiveness and scholarship programs. For example, the Johnson & Johnson Campaign for Nursing's Future was a national campaign that emphasized the positive aspects of nursing. An evaluation of this program showed that the campaign successfully improved nursing students' attitudes about their decisions to become nurses (Donelan et al., 2005).

Many academic cancer centers have created opportunities for students to gain early exposure to careers in oncology, such as providing speakers to schools and hosting high school and college students as interns (IOM, 2009b). In a survey of nurses, 65 percent of respondents reported that they were motivated to go into nursing due to information and advice from practicing nurses (Buerhaus et al., 2005).

There are also several examples of loan forgiveness and scholarship programs in oncology. ASCO's Loan Repayment Program will pay off up to $70,000 in loans for oncologists who commit to providing cancer care in medically underserved regions of the United States for 2 years (ASCO, 2009). The National Cancer Institute's (NCI's) Cure Program is similarly designed to draw underserved minority students into oncology professions by providing promising high school through junior investigator–level individuals with funding opportunities (NCI, 2012a). The National Institutes of Health also has a loan-forgiveness program that will provide payment for up to $35,000 in loans each year for clinical researchers who work to meet critical health needs, including cancer care needs (NIH, 2013).

Retaining professionals with training in cancer care is equally important to recruiting professionals who provide cancer care. The average turnover rate for health care professionals changing their place of employment is around 15 to 20 percent, depending on the region of the country (Jenkins and Fina, 2008; Kosel and Olivo, 2002). The average turnover rate for nurse practitioners and PAs is more than 12 percent; for nurses, 14 percent; and for physicians, around 6 percent (AACN, 2012b; AMGA, 2012).

The first few years are the most important for retention. A study by PricewaterhouseCoopers found that the average annual nursing turnover rate in hospitals was 8 percent, but average annual turnover rate for first-year nurses was 27 percent (PricewaterhouseCoopers, 2007). Factors that influence the retention of health care workers include salary, benefits, work culture, potential for promotion, and flexible work schedules (IOM, 2009b).

Duke University Hospital is an example of an organization that has instituted extensive programs and policies to retain its health professionals. The hospital offers training programs and educational-assistance programs; orientation, coaching, and mentoring programs for new employees and emerging leaders; and flexible work arrangements. The hospital's professional development institute allows employees who work part time to be paid for full-time work while they go to school; as a result, the annual turnover rate is 12 percent overall and only around 5 percent for first-year hires, significantly below the average for academic hospitals (IOM, 2009b).

Some health policy experts, however, are concerned that retention efforts like the program at Duke University may be unsustainable and too expensive (May et al., 2006). Thus, additional strategies for retaining professionals who provide cancer care may be needed.

Team-Based Cancer Care

Team-based care is an essential component of high-quality, patient-centered cancer care. It can be defined as "the provision of health services to individuals, families, and/or their communities by at least two health clinicians who work collaboratively with patients and their caregivers—to the extent preferred by each patient—to accomplish shared goals within and across settings to achieve coordinated, high quality care" (Mitchell et al., 2012, p. 5). A white paper published by the IOM recently identified a core set of principles common to high-functioning health care teams (see Box 4-2).

Several literature reviews have found that team-based care can improve health care quality and outcomes (Boult et al., 2009; IOM, 2011c; Naylor et al., 2010). Team-based care can also lead to better care coordination among clinicians by establishing standard practices for transmitting information, communicating, and providing follow-up care (NQF, 2010). Health information technology can be a tool for facilitating the coordination of care between team members and across care settings (see discussion in Chapter 6).

A clinician's ability to work well in interdisciplinary teams is particularly important in cancer care because, as discussed throughout this chapter, cancer is a complex disease that requires the coordination of multiple professionals to treat and alleviate the symptoms of the disease. It is unlikely that merely increasing the number of oncology professionals will adequately address oncology workforce needs. A number of innovative strategies for organizing the cancer care team and delivering care

---

BOX 4-2
Principles of Team-Based Health Care

Shared goals: The team—including the patient and, when appropriate, family members or other support persons—works to establish shared goals that reflect patient and family priorities, and can be clearly articulated, understood, and supported by all team members.

Clear roles: There are clear expectations for each team member's functions, responsibilities, and accountabilities, which optimize the team's efficiency and often make it possible for the team to take advantage of division of labor, thereby accomplishing more than the sum of its parts.

Mutual trust: Team members earn each other's trust, creating strong norms of reciprocity and greater opportunities for shared achievement.

Effective communication: The team prioritizes and continuously refines its communication skills. It has consistent channels for candid and complete communication, which are accessed and used by all team members across all settings.

Measurable processes and outcomes: The team agrees on and implements reliable and timely feedback on successes and failures in both the functioning of the team and achievement of the team's goals. These are used to track and improve performance immediately and over time.

SOURCE: Mitchell et al., 2012.

---

have been proposed that rely more heavily on team-based care compared to traditional oncology practice, such as collaborative practice arrangements and in survivorship care (see Box 4-3), as well as oncology patient-centered medical homes and accountable care organizations (see discussion in Chapter 8).

In a high-quality cancer care system, all of the professionals involved in a patient's care should act as a single, coordinated care team. In practice, a patient's care team will usually be composed of a number of smaller care teams that work in coordination, and an individual with cancer will be treated by a cancer care team and a primary care or geriatrics care team (see Box 4-1), as well as other specialty care teams (e.g., clinicians addressing a patient's comorbidities) (see Figure 4-1). **The committee identified as a goal that all of the members of the cancer care team coordinate with each other and with primary/geriatrics and specialist care teams to implement patients' care plans and deliver comprehensive, efficient, and patient-centered care (Recommendation 3).** The cancer care team should include all of the clinicians involved in implementing a patient's care plan, including the clinicians focusing on cancer treatment and those providing psychosocial support and pain management (see Figure 4-2).

There are a number of obstacles to team-based care. A recent IOM report concluded that the "coordination and integration of patient services currently are poor" (IOM, 2012a, p. 24). The sheer number of individuals involved in patients' care make coordination challenging. For example, patients with Medicare see an average of seven physicians, including five specialists, split among four different practices per year (Pham et al., 2007). The typical primary care physician coordinates with 229 other physicians in 117 different practices in a single year for his or her Medicare patients (Pham et al., 2009). A national survey in 2011 found that around one-quarter of patients reported that their clinicians failed to share important information about test results or medical history with other clinicians involved in their care (Stremikis et al., 2011). Establishing effective care teams requires time and effort, and there are few incentives for health care clinicians to make this investment. Health care organizations often lack the experience and expertise to form clinical teams, and the "siloed" nature of the professionals involved in care creates cultural barriers. Additionally, the health care infrastructure and reimbursement system are not set up to support team-based care (IPEC, 2011b; Mitchell et al., 2012).

Regulatory and policy barriers prevent many of the professionals on cancer care teams from practicing to the full extent of their education and training. The IOM recognized this problem in *Crossing the Quality Chasm: A New Health System for the 21st Century* (2001), noting that achieving high-quality care will mean modifying the regulation of health professionals, such as scope-of-practice acts and other workforce regulations. More recently, in *Future of Nursing: Leading Change, Advancing Health* (2011), the IOM found that the regulations defining scope-of-practice limitations for nurses often limit nurses in the types of tasks they are allowed to perform, for reasons unrelated to their ability, education, or training. The report recommended a number of steps to remove scope-of-practice barriers for nurses, including changing Medicare reimbursement policy to cover nursing services and encouraging state legislatures to reform scope-of-practice regulations to conform to model laws (IOM, 2011a).

Policy makers, however, have made limited progress in implementing these recommendations (Iglehart, 2013). Similar changes in federal and state laws will be necessary to enable all members of the cancer care team to be fully functioning, valuable team members. The reimbursement system must also create incentives for engaging all members of the cancer care team to the full extent of their abilities (IOM, 2012a). **Thus, the committee recommends that federal and state legislative and regulatory bodies eliminate reimbursement and scope-of-practice barriers**

BOX 4-3
Examples of Team-Based Cancer Care

Collaborative Practice Arrangements

Collaborative practice arrangements address the anticipated shortfall of oncologists by expanding the roles of physician assistants and nurse practitioners, also called nonphysician practitioners. The American Society of Clinical Oncology (ASCO) has taken the lead in pursuing this strategy. In 2005, ASCO commissioned the American Association of Medical Colleges to conduct a national survey of oncology practices and their use of nonphysician practitioners (n=226) (AAMC, 2007). Half of the practices reported working with nonphysician practitioners, and more than two-thirds of these practices reported that using nonphysician practitioners benefited their practice by improving patient care, efficiency, and physician satisfaction. In response to this positive feedback, ASCO initiated a pilot program to assess how oncologists can work most efficiently with nonphysician practitioners (Towle et al., 2011). The pilot was conducted in 33 oncology practices that varied in terms of practice size, structure, and geography. These practices submitted data to ASCO on staffing information, volume of patient visits, and expenses, and also completed physician, nonphysician practitioners, and patient surveys. The results of the pilot indicated that patients were aware when an nonphysician practitioner provided their clinical care, and were almost universally satisfied with this arrangement. Both the physicians and nonphysician practitioners were also highly satisfied with their collaborative practice models. Nonphysician practitioners were most productive in sites where they worked with all of the physicians in the practice, as opposed to sites where they worked exclusively with one or more physicians in the practice.

Survivorship Care

Another model of team-based care in oncology is treating patients who no longer require active cancer treatment (e.g., chemotherapy, radiation) in settings outside of an oncologist's office. The vast majority of visits to an oncologist's office are currently for the provision of survivorship care (AAMC, 2007). However, there are a number of other potential sites of care for meeting patients' survivorship needs.

to team-based care. This could have the added benefit of improving job satisfaction among professionals involved in cancer care as well as the recruitment and retention of oncology professionals.

The new models of payment discussed in Chapter 8, such as bundled payments, accountable care organizations, and oncology patient-centered medical homes, may remove many of the reimbursement barriers to team-based care. These models reward clinicians for providing high-quality of care at lower costs, unlike traditional fee-for-service models that incentivize the volume of services provided and reimburse certain clinicians at

Primary care clinicians often play a significant role in their patients' surveillance and ongoing survivorship care (Grunfeld et al., 2006; McCabe et al., 2013). In an analysis of Medicare claims data, Earle and Neville (2004) concluded that there is a lack of clarity around the roles of the primary care clinician and oncologist in survivorship care. Approximately 50 percent of cancer survivors in their study saw an oncologist for survivorship care and 8 percent of those saw only an oncologist; 38 percent of survivors saw only a primary care physician; and 46 percent saw both an oncologist and a primary care physician. The patients who saw only a primary care physician were more likely to receive preventive health interventions, but were less likely to receive ongoing cancer surveillance. In contrast, the patients who only saw an oncologist were unlikely to receive preventive care, but did receive follow-up cancer care. Thus, the type of doctor that the patients visited had a significant impact on the type of care that they received. More recently, Snyder and colleagues also found that there is a need to clarify the role of primary care clinicians and oncologists in survivorship care. In their review of the SEER-Medicare database, adults with a history of cancer were most likely to receive appropriate survivorship care and preventive care if they saw both an oncologist and a primary care clinician (Snyder et al., 2008, 2009, 2011).

In order to more effectively transition from acute cancer care to primary care, oncologists and primary care clinicians need to be better coordinated and the role of the primary care clinician in cancer survivorship care needs to be clearly delineated. Care should be tailored to the individual patient based on the type of cancer, treatment intensity, and risk of cancer-related complications. Nurse practitioners can help ease this transition (Oeffinger and McCabe, 2006). At the University of Pennsylvania, for example, the same nurse practitioners meet with patients throughout their cancer treatment and for the duration of a survivorship program. One of the goals of the survivorship program is to develop a treatment summary and care plan that can be used to inform the primary care clinician about the patients' cancer follow-up needs (Penn Medicine, 2012).

An alternative model of survivorship care relies on nurse practitioners to provide survivorship care. At Memorial-Sloan Kettering Cancer Center, nurse practitioners administer examinations and preventive care, evaluate and manage long-term or late effects of cancer and its treatment, provide cancer screening, and coordinate with each patient's primary care team through disease-specific survivorship clinics (MSKCC, 2012).

a higher rate than others. Thus, new models of payment may reduce the disincentive for physicians to work together with other clinicians. In addition, several other components of the committee's conceptual framework will facilitate team-based care. These include care plans, which facilitate coordinated care by summarizing all relevant information into a single location that can be shared among members of the cancer care team, the primary care/geriatrics care team, and other clinicians involved in a patient's care (see Chapter 3). Shared electronic health records also may

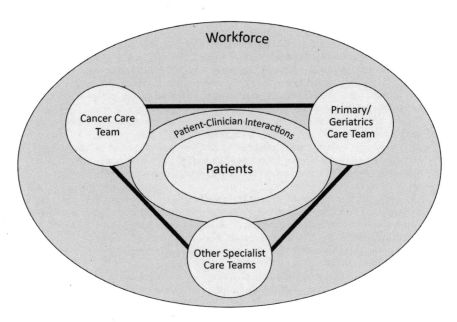

FIGURE 4-1 An illustration of a coordinated workforce.

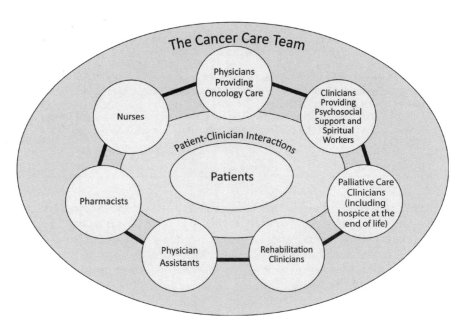

FIGURE 4-2 An illustration of a coordinated cancer care team.

make it easier for clinicians to communicate, share information, and provide coordinated care (see Chapter 6).

Interprofessional Education

Interprofessional education is designed to teach health professionals how to engage in teamwork and improve individuals' abilities to work in interdisciplinary environments. It occurs "when students from two or more professions learn about, from, and with each other to enable effective collaboration and improve health outcomes" (WHO, 2010, p. 7). The Pew Health Professions Commission identified working with interdisciplinary teams as one of the key competencies for all health professionals in the 21st century (PHPC, 1998). Six professional organizations formed the Interprofessional Education Collaboration to develop and endorse competencies in interdisciplinary care, including the American Association of Colleges of Osteopathic Medicine, AAMC, AACN, the American Association of Colleges of Pharmacy, the American Dental Education Association, and the Association of Schools of Public Health (IPEC, 2011a). Interprofessional education is also consistent with the vision statement included in a previous IOM report on health professional education, which stated that "all health professionals should be educated to deliver patient-centered care as members of an interdisciplinary team, emphasizing evidence-based practice, quality improvement approaches, and informatics" (IOM, 2003b, p. 45).

The majority of health professional education is currently conducted in silos where professional students are isolated from each other based on the professional degree they are pursuing. However, a growing number of universities are undertaking efforts to develop successful interprofessional education programs (see Box 4-4 for several examples) (IOM, 2013; NHPF, 2011). Some universities are even establishing interprofessional education programs that involve the collaboration of multiple institutions. For example, Hunter College, which offers coursework in nursing, public health, and social work, has partnered with Weill Cornell College of Medicine to offer a full range of interprofessional classes (JMF, 2013; Thibault and Schoenbaum, 2013).

As the delivery of cancer care becomes more team based, academic institutions and professional societies should develop interprofessional education programs to train the workforce in team-based cancer care and promote coordination with primary/geriatrics and specialist care teams. These programs could be provided by academic institutions or by oncology, geriatric, and primary care/internal medicine professional societies, and should target both current and future workforces.

Additional research is needed to identify the most effective methods

---

BOX 4-4
Examples of Interprofessional Educational Programs

Rush University Medical Center's Geriatric Integrated Team Training Program

Rush University Medical Center's Geriatric Integrated Team Training Program provides interprofessional training in the care of older adults for students from 12 different disciplines, including medicine, nursing, social work, and pharmacy. In this program, interprofessional classes meet weekly for 3 hours and students are placed in clinical settings that offer interprofessional practice opportunities. The program has received positive alumni feedback regarding job placements and subsequent team performance.

University of Colorado's Interprofessional Educational Program

The University of Colorado's interprofessional educational program consists of two major components: (1) the Realizing Educational Advancement for Collaborative Health (REACH) program and (2) the Frontier Center Project. In the REACH program, all health professional students participate in a longitudinal curriculum that integrates preclinical and clinical training, and helps students develop competencies in teamwork, communication, collaborative interprofessional practice, quality, and safety. Hoping to "forge a new link between dentistry and medicine for better patient care," the Frontier Center Project provides educational and clinical activities to students from a variety of disciplines. Its activities are designed to focus on oral health and preventive practices in primary care.

---

of aligning interprofessional education programs with health care delivering organizations to advance team-based cancer care (Thibault and Schoenbaum, 2013). Fortunately, the Health Resources and Services Administration's Coordinating Center for Interprofessional Education and Collaborative Practice is currently providing financial support for efforts to develop successful interprofessional educational programs (HRSA, 2013). A number of private foundations have also pledged additional resources to this coordinating center (Thibault and Schoenbaum, 2013).

It is possible that the predicted workforce shortages may persist and create an obstacle to high-quality cancer care, even in an environment of interprofessional, team-based cancer care. The National Workforce Commission is charged with collecting health workforce data to predict future workforce needs. **The committee recommends that Congress fund this Commission, and that the Commission take into account the aging population, the increasing incidence of cancer, and the complexity of cancer care in this planning.**

University of Minnesota's 1Health Program

The University of Minnesota's 1Health Program is an interprofessional program that gives students an opportunity to learn from and interact with their counterparts from other health disciplines. This program consists of three phases: (1) orientation, (2) necessary skills, and (3) expertise in practice. Over the course of these three phases, students from a variety of disciplines meet in six moderated, face-to-face interprofessional groups, participate in workshops geared toward developing the skills necessary for interprofessional collaboration, and engage with community-based partners while applying the concepts of interprofessional collaboration. While this program is still evolving, it has already received positive feedback from alumni.

University of Washington's Center for Health Science Interprofessional Education, Research, and Practice

The University of Washington's Center for Health Science Interprofessional Education, Research, and Practice provides educational opportunities for students to develop interprofessional skills and for faculty to be leaders and facilitators of interprofessional education. The goal is to integrate interprofessional educational content into existing core health sciences curriculum, expand student access to opportunities to become involved in collaborative practice, and build facilities that encourage formal and informal interprofessional interactions.

SOURCES: RUMC, 2012; UMN, 2013; University of Colorado, 2013a,b; UW, 2012, 2013.

Training the Workforce That Cares for Patients with Cancer

Training the workforce that cares for patients with cancer to ensure appropriate skills, knowledge, and experiences is a key component of ensuring the quality of cancer care. Professionals trained in oncology and nononcology professionals who often provide care to patients with cancer need distinct sets of skills. **The committee identified as a goal that all individuals caring for patients with cancer have appropriate core competencies (Recommendation 4). To achieve this, professional organizations that represent clinicians who care for patients with cancer should define cancer core competencies for their memberships.** In addition, professionals caring for patients with cancer should be able to respond to the changing demographics in the United States. The committee strongly endorses the IOM's previous recommendation that the "maintenance of certification for health care professionals should include demonstration of competence in the care of older adults as a criterion" (IOM, 2008b, p. 9).

Competencies for the Members of the Cancer Care Team

Cancer care delivery organizations should require that members of the cancer care team have the necessary competencies to deliver high-quality cancer care, as demonstrated through training, certification, or credentials. These competencies should include all of the components of the committee's conceptual framework for high-quality cancer care, such as

- Providing patient-centered communication in order to support all patients and caregivers in making informed medical decisions that are consistent with their needs, values, and preferences, and documenting these decisions in each patient's care plan; this includes communicating about advance care planning and end-of-life decisions (see Chapter 3)
- Working in interprofessional care teams and coordinating with other care teams (see discussion above in the section on team-based cancer care)
- Demonstrating knowledge about established and evolving clinical and health services research (see Chapter 5)
- Participating in a learning health care system for cancer and using advancements in information technology to improve cancer care delivery and health outcomes (see Chapter 6)
- Investigating and evaluating care practices, translating knowledge gained from research into the delivery of patient care, and improving patient care practices (see Chapter 7)
- Understanding how the larger health care system influences the accessibility and affordability of cancer care (see Chapter 8)

Core Competencies for Nononcology Clinicians

Primary care clinicians and other medical and surgical specialists—such as urologists, pulmonologists, dermatologists, and gynecologists, who have not spent years training in oncology—provide much of the cancer care in the United States. Facilitating the development of core competencies among these professionals can improve their basic skills and knowledge about cancer that are essential for delivering high-quality cancer care. For example, C-Change has started a Cancer Core Competency Initiative to develop a web-based toolkit that other organizations can use to create programs in cancer core competencies (C-Change, 2012). The tools can be applied to a wide variety of disciplines, including medicine, nursing, social work, and public health, and can be used to educate individuals with varying levels of experience and expertise. Several pilot programs have demonstrated measurable improvement in participants' knowledge, skills, and attitudes after using C-Change's toolkit (Cox et al., 2012; Smith et al., 2009).

The potential of these programs to improve the health care workforce's knowledge of basic cancer care is enormous. For example, there are only 21,000 oncology-certified nurses. However, there are close to 3 million RNs in this country, many of whom work with cancer patients and cancer survivors. If a larger proportion of these 3 million nurses had basic knowledge about cancer care, the health care system would be better equipped to meet the needs of people at risk of or living with cancer (C-Change, 2012). It would also be beneficial if other specialists understood, for example, the effects of chemotherapy on cardiac, pulmonary, and endocrine systems, and the interactions of treatment for cancer with many noncancer care treatments. **Thus, the committee recommends that organizations responsible for accreditation, certification, and training of nononcology clinicians promote the development of relevant core competencies across the cancer care continuum.**

Training in core competencies can take place during academic training, continuing education programs, or work-site training programs. The relevant professional organizations representing primary care clinicians and other medical specialists who work in oncology should define the cancer core competencies for these workforces. In order to ensure that members of the cancer care team have core competencies in other relevant fields, professional organizations representing nononcology clinicians should reciprocate by sharing tools and information about their specialties with the cancer care community.

Telemedicine in Cancer Care

Telemedicine or telehealth is "the use of electronic information and communications technologies to provide and support health care when distance separates participants" (IOM, 1996, p. 1). Increasing the use of telemedicine in cancer care may help to address the projected workforce shortages and ensure that patients with cancer have access to clinicians with the necessary expertise. Telemedicine's potential to improve access to high-quality care is especially great for patients living in rural, vulnerable, or underserved communities (IOM, 2012d).

There are a number of ongoing initiatives that are exploring the potential of telemedicine to improve the quality of care. The Centers for Medicare & Medicaid Services (CMS) Innovation Center has awarded several grants for innovative telehealth programs targeted at Medicare- and Medicaid-eligible populations (CMS, 2013). For example, the University of New Mexico received a grant for its Extension for Community Healthcare Outcomes (ECHO) program, which is using telemedicine to educate clinicians and bring expertise to rural communities (UNM, 2013). The Veterans Health Administration has also invested significant resources in adopting telehealth strategies. It currently operates the world's largest telehealth program and serves more than 50,000 veterans (VHA, 2012).

There have been a number of clinical trials, pilot programs, and other initiatives that utilize telehealth to improve care for patients with cancer. Examples include programs in the areas of managing patient risk, addressing treatment-related dermatologic toxicities, managing pain and depression, monitoring long-term side effects of treatment, providing genetic counseling, and treating patients in rural areas (Gibelli et al., 2008; Gordon, 2012; Hitt et al., 2013; Kroenke et al., 2010; MacDonald et al., 2010; Pruthi et al., 2013; Zilliacus et al., 2011). Telemedicine is also being applied in radiology and pathology, where images can easily be captured digitally and read by clinicians at off-site locations (IOM, 2012d). As discussed in Chapter 8, the committee recommends that CMS and other payers evaluate new models of care delivery and payment for cancer care, which could include telemedicine.

There are a number of obstacles to the widespread use of telemedicine, however, that will need to be addressed in order for it to reach its full potential. One of the major obstacles is reimbursement policies. Medicare and Medicaid both place restrictions on telehealth coverage based on the patient populations, clinicians, sites of care, and services.[3] For example, Medicare Part B only reimburses patients living in rural areas for telehealth services.[4] In addition, few states have laws requiring private health insurance plans to cover telehealth services. As a result, there is great variability in what services are reimbursable (NCSL, 2013).

Professional licensure is another obstacle to telemedicine. As mentioned above, many clinicians are required to be licensed by the state where they practice. This limits the ability of telehealth programs to cross state lines. Similarly, many state medical boards require in-person consultations before initiating telemedicine services, further limiting the potential geographic reach of telemedicine programs (IOM, 2012d).

CAREGIVERS

Caregivers, including family caregivers and direct care workers, are critical members of the cancer care team. The IOM has defined family caregivers (also called informal caregivers) as "relatives, friends, or neigh-

---

[3] Medicare, Medicaid, and SCHIP Benefits Improvement and Protection Act of 2000, Public Law 554, 106th Cong., 2nd sess. (December 21, 2000).
[4] Social Security Act § 1834(m); 42 U.S.C. § 1395m(m)(4)(C).

bors who provide assistance related to an underlying physical or mental disability, but who are unpaid for those services" (IOM, 2008b, p. 247). Direct care workers are the primary clinicians of paid hands-on care, and they include nurse aides, home health aides, and personal and home care aides (IOM, 2008b). Both family caregivers and direct care workers are particularly important in cancer care because of the debilitating effect of the disease; the side effects associated with many of the common cancer treatments; the complexity of the medical decisions; and the ongoing need for medical treatment, home care, and surveillance. The fragmented nature of the current cancer care delivery system, which requires individuals to take the lead in coordinating their own care, furthers the importance of caregivers.

Family Caregivers

In *Retooling for an Aging America: Building the Health Care Workforce*, family caregivers were characterized as "the backbone for much of the care that is received by older adults in the United States" (IOM, 2008b, p. 241). Between 2008 and 2009, approximately 65.7 million people served as unpaid family caregivers, and on average, they spent approximately 20 hours each week providing care (NAC and AARP, 2009). Live-in caregivers often provide more intensive care and can spend around 40 hours per week providing care, equal to time spent in a full-time job (NAC and AARP, 2009). The overall burden of care is considered high for 32 percent of caregivers, moderate for 19 percent of caregivers, and relatively low for 46 percent of caregivers (NAC and AARP, 2009). Many individuals providing family caregiving serve in this role for an extended period of time, with the average length of time being 4.6 years. Thirty-one percent of family caregivers have provided care for 5 years or more (NAC and AARP, 2009).

The demographic trends of family caregivers are similar to the trends in the general population. Family caregivers and their care recipients are now older than their counterparts were 5 years ago. The average age of individuals caring for adults has increased from 46.4 to 49.2 years of age. The average age of a person receiving help from a caregiver has also increased from 66.5 to 69.3 years over the past 5 years. The majority of caregivers are female (NAC and AARP, 2009).

Distance caregiving, or providing care remotely, is an increasingly common alternative to the more familiar caregiving models where the care recipient and caregiver(s) live nearby or in the same household.

Approximately 5 to 7 million Americans act as distant caregivers,[5] a statistic expected to double by 2022 (Benefield and Beck, 2007). Examples of common support provided by distance caregivers include ensuring the coordination of care, maintenance of independence, and socialization.

Serving as a family caregiver can be a rewarding experience. Although few studies have examined the benefits of caregiving for the care provider, existing research suggests that the experience of caring for an individual with cancer leads to personal growth, an improved sense of self-worth, a deepening of the relationship with the cancer patient, the discovery of personal strength and mastery, and a greater appreciation for life and family (NCI, 2012b; Sanjo et al., 2009). Caregivers are more likely to report a positive experience if they receive psychological support, the care team validates the care they are providing, and health care professionals assist in solving any problems that arise with the care recipient (Haley, 2003; Kim et al., 2007).

Caregiving, however, can also have a negative impact on the quality of life, health, and well-being of the care provider (Girgis et al., 2013). Family caregivers are required to balance the competing demands of providing care and meeting all of their other obligations. There are serious financial repercussions of serving as a caregiver, which may include the burden of insurance deductibles, copayments, and uncovered services (e.g., transportation, home care) (NCI, 2012b). There is also the cost of taking the time to provide the needed care, such as helping with transportation for medical appointments, waiting with the patient for appointments, preparing for surgery and medical procedures, visiting the hospital, and addressing insurance issues (Glajchen, 2009; NCI, 2012b). This can lead to missed work, reduced wages, and disruptions in family and friendships.

Many caregivers experience social isolation due to the lack of time they spend on their usual activities and relationships. Caregivers are also prone to neglecting their own health by not getting enough sleep or exercise (NCI, 2012b). In addition, caregivers are likely to experience distress from witnessing someone close to them suffer, with some studies suggesting that caregivers may experience the same level of distress as patients (Hodges et al., 2005; Weitzner et al., 1999).

Direct Care Workers

Direct care work is the fastest-growing job in the United States due to the aging population's need for in-home care. In 2008, there were approximately 3 million individuals serving as direct care workers in

---

[5] Distant caregivers are defined as individuals who live at least an hour from the care recipient.

the United States (Hess and Henrici, 2013). The size of this workforce is expected to increase by 70 percent between 2010 and 2020 (BLS, 2013a). The workforce is predominantly female and includes many individuals who are racial or ethnic minorities. A study from the Institute for Women's Policy Research estimated that immigrants make up approximately 28 percent of the workforce, with around 20 percent being undocumented (Hess and Henrici, 2013). There are no formal education requirements for most of these workers and most training takes place on the job (BLS, 2013a).

Serving as a direct care worker is a physically and emotionally demanding job that is poorly rewarded. Direct care workers have higher than average work-related injuries due to overexertion during the care of patients (BLS, 2013a; Burnham and Theodore, 2012). At the same time, the average hourly salary is only $9.70, or approximately $20,000 per year (BLS, 2013a). Many individuals work part time and do not get benefits (Burnham and Theodore, 2012). More than 40 percent rely on public assistance programs, such as Medicaid or food stamps (Kurtz, 2013).

A primary reason for the low salaries is that many direct care workers are exempt from federal minimum wage and overtime laws, due to a provision in the Fair Labor Standards Act of 1974. In 2011, the Department of Labor issued a Notice of Proposed Rulemaking to amend this law; however, the health care industry has blocked any changes (DOL, 2012). A survey by the National Domestic Workers Alliance found that almost one-quarter of direct care workers are still paid wages less than those required by state minimum wage laws (Burnham and Theodore, 2012).

Integration with the Cancer Care Team

Caregivers may provide assistance at any point in the continuum of cancer care, starting with diagnosis, treatment, palliative care, survivorship, through the end-of-life phases of cancer care. They may assist with various patient responsibilities, such as taking medication, managing symptoms, ensuring adherence to care plans, running errands, paying bills, providing emotional support, coordinating care, monitoring use of medical devices, and communicating with clinicians. They may also assist with activities of daily living including bathing, dressing, feeding, and toileting. In addition, many of the tasks these individuals provide require physical activity, such as lifting, positioning, and transferring the care recipient.

To successfully provide care, these individuals may have to rely on an expansive set of everyday skills (e.g., planning, interpreting, decision making, problem solving, time management, accessing resources). They must also learn new skills (e.g., negotiating with the health care system and providing hands-on direct care). Medical skills that many caregivers learn include administering intravenous infusions and injections, providing wound care, using feeding tubes, running mechanical ventilators, and gaining knowledge of specialty pharmacies and medications (Given, 2011; Reinhard and Levine, 2012).

It is equally important that the cancer care team communicate as effectively with a patient's caregivers as with the patient. In *Crossing the Quality Chasm*, the IOM committee recognized that clinicians should "focus on accommodating family and friends on whom patients may rely, involving them as appropriate in decision making, supporting them as caregivers, making them welcome and comfortable in the care delivery setting, and recognizing their needs and contributions" (IOM, 2001, p. 50).

The cancer care team often does not know the best methods for better involving caregivers, but it should make an effort to incorporate caregivers in decision-making processes. Family caregivers and direct care workers often have different informational needs and ways of communicating (e.g., technological sophistication) compared to the patient, and there are sometimes conflicting values and preferences between patients and family caregivers (IOM, 2011c). Any incongruence between the patient and family caregiver will need to be addressed by the care team to ensure the quality of care and an ongoing beneficial caregiving relationship. Ultimately, it is the patient's values, preferences, and needs that should dictate the care plan (Gillick, 2013).

A lack of available training and support makes the task of integrating caregivers with the cancer care team challenging. Caregivers are regularly asked to perform a number of tasks for which they may feel unprepared. For example, a survey by Reinhard and Levine (2012) found that almost half of family caregivers report performing medical/nursing tasks but the majority reported that they had received little or no training (Reinhard and Levine, 2012). Similarly, many direct care workers have no more than a high school education and report that they could benefit from further training (Menne et al., 2007; Montgomery et al., 2005; Smith and Baughman, 2007). Instructions on how to perform basic care tasks, as well as education and informational resources, could improve patient care and reduce the stress and burden placed on caregivers.

There are a few programs that support research, training, and pilot programs to increase knowledge and test approaches to assist caregivers (HJWF, 2013; RCIC, 2013; VA, 2013). The IOM committee on *Retooling for an Aging America* recognized a growing need in this area and recommended further education and training for both direct care workers and family caregivers (IOM, 2008b). More recently, Naylor (2012) recommended prioritizing research on the best methods of training family caregivers and direct care workers to be integrated members of care teams. **The committee echoes these findings and recommends that HHS and other funders support demonstration projects to train family caregivers and direct care workers in relevant core competencies related to caring for cancer patients.**

Specific areas in cancer care where additional information could be helpful are the disease trajectory, the anticipated course of treatment, and the management of pain, weakness, and fatigue (Wong et al., 2002). Caregivers' informational and training needs change depending on the point in the cancer care continuum. Periods when trainings should be administered include at diagnosis, during hospitalization, at the start of new treatments, at recurrence, and during end-of-life care (McCorkle and Pasacreta, 2001).

SUMMARY AND RECOMMENDATIONS

A diverse team of professionals provides cancer care, reflecting the complexity of the disease, its treatments, and survivorship care. These teams include professionals with specialized training in oncology, such as medical, surgical, and radiation oncologists and oncology nurses, as well as other specialists and primary care clinicians. In addition, family caregivers (e.g., relatives, friends, and neighbors) and direct care workers (e.g., nurse aides, home health aides, and personal and home care aides) provide a great deal of care to cancer patients. Patients, at the center of the committee's conceptual framework, are encircled by the workforce (see Figure S-2), depicting the idea that high-quality cancer care depends on the workforce providing competent, trusted interprofessional care that is aligned with patients' needs, values, and preferences. To achieve this standard, the workforce must include adequate numbers of health clinicians with training in oncology. New models of interprofessional, team-based care are an effective mechanism of responding to the existing workforce shortages and demographic changes, as well as in promoting coordinated and patient-centered care.

Recommendation 3: An Adequately Staffed, Trained, and Coordinated Workforce

Goal: Members of the cancer care team should coordinate with each other and with primary/geriatrics and specialist care teams to implement patients' care plans and deliver comprehensive, efficient, and patient-centered care.

To accomplish this:

- Federal and state legislative and regulatory bodies should eliminate reimbursement and scope-of-practice barriers to team-based care.
- Academic institutions and professional societies should develop interprofessional education programs to train the workforce in team-based cancer care and promote coordination with primary/geriatrics and specialist care teams.
- Congress should fund the National Workforce Commission, which should take into account the aging population, the increasing incidence of cancer, and the complexity of cancer care, when planning for national workforce needs.

The workforce must also have the distinct set of skills necessary to implement the committee's conceptual framework for a high-quality cancer care delivery system. The recent IOM report *Retooling for an Aging America: Building the Health Care Workforce* recommended enhancing the geriatric competency of the general health care workforce. The committee endorses this recommendation as it is especially important to cancer care, where the majority of patients are older adults. Currently, many clinicians also lack essential cancer core competencies.

Recommendation 4: An Adequately Staffed, Trained, and Coordinated Workforce

Goal: All individuals caring for cancer patients should have appropriate core competencies.

To accomplish this:

- Professional organizations that represent clinicians who care for patients with cancer should define cancer core competencies for their memberships.
- Cancer care delivery organizations should require that the members of the cancer care team have the necessary competencies to deliver high-quality cancer care, as demonstrated through training, certification, or credentials.
- Organizations responsible for accreditation, certification, and training of nononcology clinicians should promote the development of relevant core competencies across the cancer care continuum.

- **The U.S. Department of Health and Human Services and other funders should fund demonstration projects to train family caregivers and direct care workers in relevant core competencies related to caring for cancer patients.**

REFERENCES

AACN (American Association of Colleges of Nursing). 2008. *Enrollment growth in U.S. Nursing colleges and universities hits an 8-year low according to new data released by AACN.* http://www.apps.aacn.nche.edu/Media/NewsReleases/2008/EnrlGrowth.html (accessed January 9, 2009).

———. 2010. *Shortage of faculty and resource constraints hinder growth in U.S. nursing schools according to the latest AACN data.* http://www.aacn.nche.edu/news/articles/2010/faculty-shortage (accessed June 18, 2013).

———. 2011. *2011 annual report: Shaping the future of nursing education.* http://www.aacn.nche.edu/aacn-publications/annual-reports/AR2011.pdf (accessed June 18, 2013).

———. 2012a. *New AACN data show an enrollment surge in baccalaureate and graduate programs amid calls for more highly educated nurses.* http://www.aacn.nche.edu/news/articles/2012/enrollment-data (accessed September 10, 2012).

———. 2012b. *Nursing shortage fact sheet.* http://www.aacn.nche.edu/media-relations/fact-sheets/nursing-shortage (accessed September 20, 2012).

———. 2013. *DNP fact sheet.* http://www.aacn.nche.edu/media-relations/fact-sheets/dnp (accessed April 18, 2013).

AAFP (American Academy of Family Physicians). 2012. *Primary care.* http://www.aafp.org/online/en/home/policy/policies/p/primarycare.html#Parsys0004 (accessed September 7, 2012).

AAHC (Association of Academic Health Centers). 2008. *Out of order, out of time: The state of the nation's health workforce.* http://www.aahcdc.org/policy/AAHC_OutofTime_4WEB.pdf (accessed September 19, 2012).

AAMC (Association of American Medical Colleges). 2007. *Forecasting the supply of and demand for oncologists: A report to the American Society of Clinical Oncology from the AAMC Center for Workforce Studies.* http://www.asco.org/ASCO/Downloads/Cancer%20Research/Oncology%20Workforce%20Report%20FINAL.pdf (accessed January 14, 2009).

———. 2008. *2008 physician specialty data.* https://www.aamc.org/download/47352/data/specialtydata.pdf (accessed September 7, 2012).

———. 2010. *Diversity in the physician workforce: Facts & figures 2010.* https://members.aamc.org/eweb/DynamicPage.aspx?Action=Add&ObjectKeyFrom=1A83491A-9853-4C87-86A4-F7D95601C2E2&WebCode=PubDetailAdd&DoNotSave=yes&ParentObject=CentralizedOrderEntry&ParentDataObject=Invoice+Detail&ivd_formkey=69202792-63d7-4ba2-bf4e-a0da41270555&ivd_prc_prd_key=A6A4AF05-91F1-47EC-9842-F60CB45F2356 (accessed March 21, 2013).

———. 2011a. *For second year, more U.S. Medical school seniors match to primary care residencies.* https://www.aamc.org/newsroom/newsreleases/2011/180410/110317.html (accessed September 7, 2012).

———. 2011b. *Physician shortages factsheet.* https://www.aamc.org/download/150584/data/physician_shortages_factsheet.pdf (accessed September 6, 2012).

———. 2013. Policies targeted toward aging physicians may keep doctors working longer, smarter. https://www.aamc.org/newsroom/reporter/april2013/334334/aging-physicians.html (accessed June 18, 2013).

AAPA (American Academy of Physician Assistants). 2012a. *Quick facts.* http://www.aapa.
    org/the_pa_profession/quick_facts/resources/item.aspx?id=3840 (accessed Septem-
    ber 10, 2012).
————. 2012b. *What is a PA?* http://www.aapa.org/the_pa_profession/what_is_a_pa.aspx
    (accessed September 10, 2012).
ABIM (American Board of Internal Medicine). 2012. *Candidates certified—all candidates.* http://
    www.abim.org/pdf/data-candidates-certified/all-candidates.pdf (accessed October 22,
    2012).
ACCP (American College of Chest Physicians). 2012. *ACCP: The global leader in clinical chest
    medicine.* http://www.chestnet.org/accp/accp-global-leader-clinical-chest-medicine
    (accessed October 22, 2012).
ACG (American College of Gastroenterology). 2012. *Membership.* http://gi.org/membership
    (accessed October 22, 2012).
ACOG (American Congress of Obstetricians and Gynecologists). 2011. *ACOG workforce fact
    sheet.* http://www.acog.org/~/media/Departments/Government%20Relations%20and
    %20Outreach/WF2011CO.pdf?dmc=1&ts=20120918T1601427427 (accessed September
    18, 2012).
ACR (American College of Radiology). 2012. *About us.* http://www.acr.org/About-Us (ac-
    cessed September 18, 2012).
ACS/HPRI (American College of Surgeons/Health Policy Research Institute). 2010. *The
    surgical workforce in the United States: Profile and recent trends.* http://www.acshpri.org/
    documents/ACSHPRI_Surgical_Workforce_in_US_apr2010.pdf (accessed October 22,
    2012).
AGA (American Gastroenterological Association). 2012. *About AGA.* http://www.gastro.
    org/about-aga (accessed October 22, 2012).
AGS (American Geriatrics Society). 2012. *Frequently asked questions about geriatrics.* http://
    www.americangeriatrics.org/advocacy_public_policy/gwps/gwps_faqs (accessed Oc-
    tober 18, 2013).
AHR (Alliance for Health Reform). 2012a. *Health care workforce: Nurses.* http://www.allhealth.
    org/publications/Cost_of_health_care/Nursing_Toolkit_FINAL_8-27-12_111.pdf (ac-
    cessed September 10, 2012).
————. 2012b. *A toolkit: The physician workforce.* http://allhealth.org/publications/
    Physician_Workforce_Shortage_110.pdf (accessed September 6, 2012).
AHRQ (Agency for Healthcare Research and Quality). 2004. *Hospital nurse staffing and quality
    of care.* http://www.ahrq.gov/research/findings/factsheets/services/nursestaffing/
    index.html (accessed May 9, 2013).
Aiken, L. H., S. P. Clarke, D. M. Sloane, J. A. Sochalski, R. Busse, H. Clarke, P. Giovannetti,
    J. Hunt, A. M. Rafferty, and J. Shamian. 2001. Nurses' reports on hospital care in five
    countries. *Health Affairs (Millwood)* 20(3):43-53.
Aiken, L. H., D. M. Sloane, J. P. Cimiotti, S. P. Clarke, L. Flynn, J. A. Seago, J. Spetz, and
    H. L. Smith. 2010. Implications of the California nurse staffing mandate for other states.
    Health Service Research 45(4):904-921.
Alesi, E. R., D. Fletcher, C. Muir, R. Beveridge, and T. J. Smith. 2011. Palliative care and
    oncology partnerships in real practice. *Oncology* 25(13):1287-1290, 1287-1290, 1292-1293.
Alfano, C. M., P. A. Ganz, J. H. Rowland, and E. E. Hahn. 2012. Cancer survivorship and
    cancer rehabilitation: Revitalizing the link. *Journal of Clinical Oncology* 30(9):904-906.
Allegra, C. J., R. Hall, and G. Yothers. 2005. Prevalence of burnout in the U.S. oncology com-
    munity: Results of a 2003 survey. *Journal of Oncology Practice* 1(4):140-147.
American Psychiatric Association. 2013. *About APA & psychiatry.* http://www.psychiatry.
    org/about-apa--psychiatry (accessed July 31, 2013).

AMGA (American Medical Group Association). 2012. *Survey reveals physician shortage challenges medical groups and increases demand for advanced practitioners.* http://www.amga.org/AboutAMGA/News/article_news.asp?k=569 (accessed September 20, 2012).

AMN Healthcare. 2012. *2012 survey of registered nurses: Job satisfaction and career patterns and trajectories.* http://www.amnhealthcare.com/uploadedFiles/MainSite/Content/Healthcare_Industry_Insights/Industry_Research/AMN%202012%20RN%20Survey.pdf (accessed June 18, 2013).

ANA (American Nurses Association). 2012. *What is nursing?* http://www.nursingworld.org/EspeciallyForYou/What-is-Nursing (accessed September 7, 2012).

AOSW (Association of Oncology Social Work). 2013. *About us.* http://www.aosw.org/html/about.php (accessed February 28, 2013).

APA (American Psychological Association). 2013a. Breast cancer. http://www.apa.org/health-reform/breast-cancer.html (accessed August 16, 2013).

———. 2013b. *Public description of clinical psychology.* http://www.apa.org/ed/graduate/specialize/clinical.aspx (accessed July 31, 2013).

———. 2013c. *Recognized specialties and proficiencies in professional psychology.* http://www.apa.org/ed/graduate/specialize/recognized.aspx (accessed July 31, 2013).

Arehart-Treichel, J. 2012. *Cancer patients have much to gain from psychiatric treatment.* http://psychnews.psychiatryonline.org/newsarticle.aspx?articleid=1032923 (accessed August 16, 2013).

ASCO (American Society of Clinical Oncology). 2009. ASCO announces new program designed to increase workforce diversity and reduce cancer care disparities. *Journal of Oncology Practice* 5(6):315-317.

ASCP (American Society for Clinical Pathology). 2004. *The medical laboratory personnel shortage.* http://www.ascp.org/pdf/MedicalLaboratoryPersonnelShortage.aspx (accessed January 13, 2009).

ASH (American Society of Hematology). 2011. *About ASH.* http://www.hematology.org/About-ASH (accessed November 9, 2012).

ASHP (American Society of Health-System Pharmacists). 2007. *ASHP pharmacy staffing survey results.* http://www.ashp.org/DocLibrary/Policy/WorkFrorce/PPM_2007StaffSurvey.pdf (accessed January 15, 2009).

———. 2008. *Confronting the public health workforce crisis.* http://www.asph.org/document.cfm?page=1038 (accessed January 14, 2009).

ASTRO (American Society for Radiation Oncology). 2012a. *About ASTRO.* https://www.astro.org/About-ASTRO/Index.aspx (accessed September 18, 2012).

———. 2012b. *ASTRO's 2012 workforce survey.* https://www.astro.org/Research/Initiatives/ASTRO-Workforce-Survey.aspx (accessed October 24, 2012).

Auerbach, D. I., P. I. Buerhaus, and D. O. Staiger. 2011. Registered nurse supply grows faster than projected amid surge in new entrants ages 23–26. *Health Affairs (Millwood)* 30(12):2286-2292.

Bajorin, D. F., and A. Hanley. 2011. The study of collaborative practice arrangements: Where do we go from here? *Journal of Clinical Oncology* 29(27):3599-3600.

Balboni, M. J., A. Sullivan, A. Amobi, A. C. Phelps, D. P. Gorman, A. Zollfrank, J. R. Peteet, H. G. Prigerson, T. J. Vanderweele, and T. A. Balboni. 2013. Why is spiritual care infrequent at the end of life? Spiritual care perceptions among patients, nurses, and physicians and the role of training. *Journal of Clinical Oncology* 31(4):461-467.

Balboni, T. A., M. E. Paulk, M. J. Balboni, A. C. Phelps, E. T. Loggers, A. A. Wright, S. D. Block, E. F. Lewis, J. R. Peteet, and H. G. Prigerson. 2010. Provision of spiritual care to patients with advanced cancer: Associations with medical care and quality of life near death. *Journal of Clinical Oncology* 28(3):445-452.

Balboni, T., M. Balboni, M. E. Paulk, A. Phelps, A. Wright, J. Peteet, S. Block, C. Lathan, T. Vanderweele, and H. Prigerson. 2011. Support of cancer patients' spiritual needs and associations with medical care costs at the end of life. *Cancer* 117(23):5383-5391.

Barraclough, J. E. 1997. Psycho-oncology and the role of the psychiatrist in cancer patient care. *International Journal of Psychiatry in Clinical Practice* 1:189-195.

Benefield, L. E., and C. Beck. 2007. Reducing the distance in distance-caregiving by technology innovation. *Clinical Interventions in Aging* 2(2):267-272.

Bennett, J. M., W. J. Hall, D. Sahasrabudhe, and L. Balducci. 2010. Enhancing geriatric oncology training to care for elders: A clinical initiative with long term follow-up. *Journal of Geriatric Oncology* 1(1):4-12.

Berlin, L. E., and K. R. Sechrist. 2002. The shortage of doctorally prepared nursing faculty: A dire situation. *Nursing Outlook* 50(2):50-56.

Blegen, M. A., C. J. Goode, J. Spetz, T. Vaughn, and S. H. Park. 2011. Nurse staffing effects on patient outcomes: Safety-net and non-safety-net hospitals. *Medical Care* 49(4):406-414.

BLS (Bureau of Labor Statistics). 2012a. *Economic and employment projections.* http://www.bls.gov/news.release/ecopro.toc.htm (accessed September 10, 2012).

———. 2012b. *Occupational employment and wages, May 2012. 29-1066 Psychiatrists.* http://www.bls.gov/oes/current/oes291066.htm#nat (accessed July 31, 2013).

———. 2013a. *Occupational outlook handbook, 2012-13 edition, home health and personal care aides.* http://www.bls.gov/ooh/healthcare/home-health-and-personal-care-aides.htm (accessed March 21, 2013).

———. 2013b. *Occupational outlook handbook, 2012-13 edition, occupational therapists.* http://www.bls.gov/ooh/healthcare/occupational-therapists.htm (accessed April 29, 2013).

———. 2013c. *Occupational outlook handbook, 2012-13 edition, pharmacists.* http://www.bls.gov/ooh/Healthcare/Pharmacists.htm#tab-1 (accessed July 31, 2013).

———. 2013d. *Occupational outlook handbook, 2012-13 edition, physical therapists.* http://www.bls.gov/ooh/healthcare/physical-therapists.htm (accessed April 29, 2013).

———. 2013e. *Occupational outlook handbook, 2012-13 edition, psychologists.* http://www.bls.gov/ooh/Life-Physical-and-Social-Science/Psychologists.htm (accessed July 31, 2013).

———. 2013f. *Occupational outlook handbook, 2012-13 edition, social workers.* http://www.bls.gov/ooh/Community-and-Social-Service/Social-workers.htm (accessed February 28, 2013).

Blum, D., E. Clark, P. Jacobsen, J. Holland, M. J. Monahan, and P. D. Duquette. 2006. Building community-based short-term psychosocial counseling capacity for cancer patients and their families: The individual cancer assistance network (ICAN) model. *Social Work in Health Care* 43(4):71-83.

Boult, C., A. F. Green, L. B. Boult, J. T. Pacala, C. Snyder, and B. Leff. 2009. Successful models of comprehensive care for older adults with chronic conditions: Evidence for the Institute of Medicine's "Retooling for an aging America" report. *Journal of the American Geriatrics Society* 57(12):2328-2337.

Buerhaus, P., K. Donelan, L. Norman, and R. Dittus. 2005. Nursing students' perceptions of a career in nursing and impact of a national campaign designed to attract people into the nursing profession. *Journal of Professional Nursing* 21(2):75-83.

Buerhaus, P. I., D. I. Auerbach, and D. O. Staiger. 2009. The recent surge in nurse employment: Causes and implications. *Health Affairs (Millwood)* 28(4):w657-w668.

Burnham, L., and N. Theodore. 2012. *Home economics: The invisible and unregulated world of domestic work.* http://www.domesticworkers.org/pdfs/HomeEconomicsEnglish.pdf (accessed March 21, 2013).

CBO (Congressional Budget Office). 2013. *CBO's Estimate of the net budgetary impact of the Affordable Care Act's health insurance coverage provisions has not changed much over time.* http://www.cbo.gov/publication/44176 (accessed September 5, 2012).

C-Change. 2012. *Project overview.* http://www.cancercorecompetency.org/index.php?page=project-overview (accessed September 21, 2012).

———. 2013. *A national strategy to strengthen the cancer workforce: Position statement and call to action.* http://c-changetogether.org/Websites/cchange/images/Documents/C-CHANGE_WORKFORKCE_POSITION_STATEMENT-_February_2012v1.pdf (accessed March 19, 2013).

Christian, S., C. Dower, and E. O'Neil. 2007. *Chart overview of nurse practitioner scopes of practice in the united states.* http://www.health.state.mn.us/healthreform/workforce/npcomparison.pdf (accessed October 24, 2012).

Clay, R. A. 2010. Psychologists' new interventions are helping families cope with what can be a devastating diagnosis. *Monitor on Psychology* 41(7):69.

CMS (Centers for Medicare & Medicaid Services). 2013. *The CMS innovation center.* http://innovation.cms.gov (accessed May 1, 2013).

Cohen, H. J. 2009. A model for the shared care of elderly patients with cancer. *Journal of the American Geriatrics Society* 57(Suppl 2):S300-S302.

Coniglio, D. 2013. Collaborative practice models and team-based care in oncology. *Journal of Oncology Practice* 9(2):1-2.

Coniglio, D., T. Pickard, and S. Wei. 2011. Commentary: Physician assistant perspective on the results of the ASCO study of collaborative practice arrangements. *Journal of Oncology Practice* 7(6):283-284.

Cox, K. A., A. P. Smith, and M. Lichtveld. 2012. A competency-based approach to expanding the cancer care workforce part III: Improving cancer pain and palliative care competency. *Journal of Cancer Education* 27(3):507-514.

CWS (Center for Workforce Studies). 2006. *Assuring the sufficiency of a frontline workforce: A national study of licensed social workers.* http://workforce.socialworkers.org/studies/health/health.pdf (accessed September 18, 2012).

Del Giudice, M. E., E. Grunfeld, B. J. Harvey, E. Piliotis, and S. Verma. 2009. Primary care physicians' views of routine follow-up care of cancer survivors. *Journal of Clinical Oncology* 27(20):3338-3345.

DOL (Department of Labor). 2012. *Notice of proposed rulemaking to amend the companionship and live-in worker regulations.* http://www.dol.gov/whd/flsa/companionNPRM.htm (accessed March 21, 2013).

Donelan, K., P. I. Buerhaus, B. T. Ulrich, L. Norman, and R. Dittus. 2005. Awareness and perceptions of the Johnson & Johnson Campaign for Nursing's Future: Views from nursing students, MSs, and CNOs. *Nursing Economics* 23(4):214-221.

Earle, C. C., and B. A. Neville. 2004. Under use of necessary care among cancer survivors. *Cancer* 101(8):1712-1719.

Erikson, C., E. Salsberg, G. Forte, S. Bruinooge, and M. Goldstein. 2007. Future supply and demand for oncologists: Challenges to assuring access to oncology services. *Journal of Oncology Practice* 3(2):79-86.

Ferrell, B. R., R. Virani, S. Smith, and G. Juarez. 2003. The role of oncology nursing to ensure quality care for cancer survivors: A report commissioned by the National Cancer Policy Board and Institute of Medicine. *Oncology Nursing Forum* 30(1):E1-E11.

Geurts, S., C. Rutte, and M. Peeters. 1999. Antecedents and consequences of work-home interference among medical residents. *Social Science & Medicine* 48(9):1135-1148.

Gibelli, G., B. Gibelli, and F. Nani. 2008. Thyroid cancer: Possible role of telemedicine. *Acta Otorhinolaryngol Italica* 28(6):281-286.

Gillick, M. R. 2013. The critical role of caregivers in achieving patient-centered care. *Journal of the American Medical Association* 310(6):575-576.

Girgis, A., S. Lambert, C. Johnson, A. Waller, and D. Currow. 2013. Physical, psychosocial, relationship, and economic burden of caring for people with cancer: A review. *Journal of Oncology Practice* 9(4):197-202.

Given, B. 2011. The challenge of quality care for family caregivers in adult cancer care. Paper read at Improving Quality of Life and Quality of Care for Oncology Family Caregivers, July 13, Anaheim, CA.

Glajchen, M. 2009. Role of family caregivers in cancer pain management. In *Cancer pain: Assessment and management*, edited by E.D. Bruera and R. K. Portenoy. New York: Cambridge University Press. Pp. 597-607.

Gordon, J. 2012. Dermatologic assessment from a distance: The use of teledermatology in an outpatient chemotherapy infusion center. *Clinical Journal of Oncology Nursing* 16(4):418-420.

Green, L. V., S. Savin, Y. Lu. 2012. Primary care physician shortages could be eliminated through use of teams, nonphysicians, and electronic communication. *Health Affairs (Millwood)* 32(1):11-19.

Grunfeld, E., L. Zitzelsberger, M. Coristine, T. J. Whelan, F. Aspelund, and W. K. Evans. 2005. Job stress and job satisfaction of cancer care workers. *Psychooncology* 14(1):61-69.

Grunfeld, E., M. N. Levine, J. A. Julian, D. Coyle, B. Szechtman, D. Mirsky, S. Verma, S. Dent, C. Sawka, K. I. Pritchard, D. Ginsburg, M. Wood, and T. Whelan. 2006. Randomized trial of long-term follow-up for early-stage breast cancer: A comparison of family physician versus specialist care. *Journal of Clinical Oncology* 24(6): 848-855.

Haley, W. E. 2003. Family caregivers of elderly patients with cancer: Understanding and minimizing the burden of care. *Journal of Supportive Oncology* 1(4 Suppl 2):25-29.

Hauer, K. E., S. J. Durning, W. N. Kernan, M. J. Fagan, M. Mintz, P. S. O'Sullivan, M. Battistone, T. DeFer, M. Elnicki, H. Harrell, S. Reddy, C. K. Boscardin, and M. D. Schwartz. 2008. Factors associated with medical students' career choices regarding internal medicine. *Journal of the American Medical Association* 300(10):21154-21164.

Health Affairs. 2012. Health policy briefs: Graduate Medical Education (Updated). http://www.healthaffairs.org/healthpolicybriefs/brief.php?brief_id=75 (accessed June 18, 2013).

Hess, C., and J. M. Henrici. 2013. *Increasing pathways to legal status for immigrant in-home care workers.* Washington, DC: Institute for Women's Policy Research.

Hillborne, L. 2008. The other big workforce shortage. As laboratory technology wanes as a career choice, a staffing crisis grows. *Modern Healthcare* 38(22):23.

Hitt, W. C., G. Low, T. M. Bird, and R. Ott. 2013. Telemedical cervical cancer screening to bridge medicaid service care gap for rural women. *Telemedicine Journal and E-Health* 19(5):403-408.

HJWF (Harry and Jeanette Weinberg Foundation). 2013. *Family and informal caregiver support program.* http://www.hjweinbergfoundation.org/ficsp (accessed May 2, 2013).

Hodges, L. J., G. M. Humphris, and G. Macfarlane. 2005. A meta-analytic investigation of the relationship between the psychological distress of cancer patients and their careers. *Social Science & Medicine* 60(1):1-12.

HRSA (Health Resources and Services Administration). 2010. *The registered nurse population: Findings from the 2008 national sample survey of registered nurses.* http://bhpr.hrsa.gov/healthworkforce/rnsurveys/rnsurveyfinal.pdf (accessed September 10, 2012).

———. 2012. *Occupational outlook handbook.* http://www.bls.gov/ooh/healthcare/occupational-therapists.htm (accessed October 22, 2012).

———. 2013. *Coordinating Center for Interprofessional Education and Collaborative Practice.* http://www.hrsa.gov/grants/apply/assistance/interprofessional (accessed May 2, 2013).

HWS (Health Workforces Solutions). 2007. *Closing the health workforce gap in California: The education imperative.* San Francisco, CA: Health Workforce Solutions.

Iglehart, J. K. 2013. Expanding the role of advanced practiced nurse practitioners: Risks and rewards. *New England Journal of Medicine* 368(20): 1935-1941.

IOM (Institute of Medicine). 1996. *Telemedicine: A guide to assessing telecommunications for health care.* Washington, DC: National Academy Press.

———. 2001. *Crossing the quality chasm: A new health system for the 21st century.* Washington, DC: National Academy Press.

———. 2003a. *Unequal treatment: Confronting racial and ethnic disparities in health care.* Washington, DC: The National Academies Press.

———. 2003b. *Health professions education: A bridge to quality.* Washington, DC: The National Academies Press.

———. 2005. *From cancer patient to cancer survivor: Lost in transition.* Washington, DC: The National Academies Press.

———. 2008a. *Cancer care for the whole patient: Meeting psychosocial health needs.* Washington, DC: The National Academies Press.

———. 2008b. *Retooling for an aging america: Building the health care workforce.* Washington, DC: The National Academies Press.

———. 2009a. *Assessing and improving value in cancer care: Workshop summary.* Washington, DC: The National Academies Press.

———. 2009b. *Ensuring quality cancer care through the oncology workforce: Sustaining care in the 21st century: Workshop summary.* Washington, DC: The National Academies Press.

———. 2011a. *Future of nursing: Leading change, advancing health.* Washington, DC: The National Academies Press.

———. 2011b. *Patient-centered cancer treatment planning: Improving the quality of oncology care: Workshop summary.* Washington, DC: The National Academies Press.

———. 2012a. *Best care at lower cost: The path to continously learning health care in America.* Washington, DC: The National Academies Press.

———. 2012b. *Governance and financing of graduate medical education.* http://www.iom.edu/Activities/Workforce/GMEGovFinance.aspx (accessed September 7, 2012).

———. 2012c. *The mental health and substance use workforce for older adults.* Washington, DC: The National Academies Press.

———. 2012d. *The role of telehealth in an evolving health care environment.* Washington, DC: The National Academies Press.

———. 2013. *Interprofessional education for collaboration: Learning how to improve health from interprofessional models across the continuum of education to practice: Workshop summary.* Washington, DC: The National Academies Press.

IOM and NRC (National Research Council). 1999. *Ensuring quality cancer care.* Washington, DC: National Academy Press.

IPEC (Interprofessional Education Collaborative). 2011a. *Core competencies for interprofessional colaborative practice: Report of an expert panel.* www.asph.org/userfiles/collaborative practice.pdf (accessed July 26, 2013).

———. 2011b. *Team-based competencies: Building a shared foundation for education and clinical practice.* http://macyfoundation.org/docs/macy_pubs/Team-Based_Competencies.pdf (accessed November 5, 2012).

Jenkins, W., and M. C. Fina. 2008. *Realize the benefits.* http://www.hrmreport.com/article/Issue-7/Incentives-AND-Recognition/Realize-the-Benefits (accessed January 21, 2009).

JMF (The Josiah Masy Jr. Foundation). 2013. *Integrating transdisciplinary education at Cornell Hunter.* http://macyfoundation.org/grantees/profile/integrating-transdisciplinary-education-at-cornell-hunter-iteach (accessed July 26, 2013).

Jolly, P. 2005. Medical school tuition and young physicians' indebtedness. *Health Affairs (Millwood)* 24(2):527-535.

Juraschek, S. P., X. Zhang, V. Ranganathan, and V. W. Lin. 2012. United States registered nurse workforce report card and shortage forecast. *American Journal of Medical Quality* 27(3):241-249.

Kash, K. M., J. C. Holland, W. Breitbart, S. Berenson, J. Dougherty, S. Ouellette-Kobasa, and L. Lesko. 2000. Stress and burnout in oncology. *Oncology* 14(11):1621-1633.

KHN (Kaiser Health News). 2011. *Senior boom creates a demand for home health workers.* http://www.kaiserhealthnews.org/stories/2011/august/16/direct-care-workers-in-demand-as-seniors-ranks-grow.aspx (accessed September 18, 2012).

Kim, Y., R. Schulz, and C. S. Carver. 2007. Benefit-finding in the cancer caregiving experience. *Psychosomatic Medicine* 69(3):283-291.

Klabunde, C. N., A. Ambs, N. L. Keating, Y. He, W. R. Doucette, D. Tisnado, S. Clauser, and K. L. Kahn. 2009. The role of primary care physicians in cancer care. *Journal of General Internal Medicine* 24(9):1029-1036.

Kosel, K. C., and T. Olivo. 2002. *The business case for workforce stability.* Irving, TX: Voluntary Hospitals of America.

Kroenke, K., D. Theobald, J. Wu, K. Norton, G. Morrison, J. Carpenter, and W. Tu. 2010. Effect of telecare management on pain and depression in patients with cancer: A randomized trial. *Journal of the American Medical Association* 304(2):163-171.

Kuo, Y., F. L. Loresto, L. R. Rounds, and J. S. Goodwin. 2013. States with the least restrictive regulations experienced the largest increase in patients seen by nurse practitioners. *Health Affairs (Millwood)* 32(7):1236-1243.

Kurtz, A. 2013. *America's fastest growing job pays poorly.* http://money.cnn.com/2013/03/11/news/economy/fastest-growing-job/index.html?hpt=hp_t3 (accessed March 21, 2013).

Lauria, M. M., E. J. Clark, J. F. Hermann, and N. M. Stearns. 2001. *Social work in oncology: Supporting survivors, families, and caregivers.* Atlanta, GA: American Cancer Society.

Linzer, M., M. R. Visser, F. J. Oort, E. M. Smets, J. E. McMurray, and H. C. de Haes. 2001. Predicting and preventing physician burnout: Results from the United States and the Netherlands. *American Journal of Medicine* 111(2):170-175.

Lipner, R. S., W. H. Bylsma, G. K. Arnold, G. S. Fortna, J. Tooker, C. K. Cassel. 2006. Who is maintaining certification in internal medicine—and why? A national survey 10 years after initial certification. *Annals of Internal Medicine* 144(1): 29-36.

Longpré, S., and R. Newman. 2011. *The role of occupational therapy in oncology.* http://www.aota.org/Consumers/Professionals/WhatIsOT/MH/Facts/OT-Role-Oncology.aspx (accessed April 29, 2013).

Losses, G. 2006. Managing stress and burnout in oncology. *Journal of Oncology Practice* 2(3):130-131.

Lupu, D. 2010. Estimate of current hospice and palliative medicine physician workforce shortage. *Journal of Pain and Symptom Management* 40(6):899-911.

MacDonald, D. J., K. R. Blazer, and J. N. Weitzel. 2010. Extending comprehensive cancer center expertise in clinical cancer genetics and genomics to diverse communities: The power of partnership. *Journal of the National Comprehensive Cancer Network* 8(5):615-624.

May, J. H., G. J. Bazzoli, and A. M. Gerland. 2006. Hospitals' responses to nurse staffing shortages. *Health Affairs (Millwood)* 25(4):W316-W323.

McCabe, M. S., S. Bhatia, K. C. Oeffinger, G. H. Reaman, C. Tyne, D. S. Wollins, and M. M. Hudson. 2013. American Society of Clinical Oncology statement: Achieving high-quality cancer survivorship care. *Journal of Clinical Oncology* 31(5):631-640.

McCorkle, R., and J. V. Pasacreta. 2001. Enhancing caregiver outcomes in palliative care. *Cancer Control* 8(1):36-45.

McDonald, K., and J. Sutton. 2009. *Surgical workforce: An emerging crisis.* http://www.facs.org/fellows_info/bulletin/2009/mcdonald0509.pdf (accessed October 20, 2012).

MDACC (MD Anderson Cancer Center). 2013. *Pain Management Center*. http://www.mdanderson.org/patient-and-cancer-information/care-centers-and-clinics/specialty-and-treatment-centers/pain-management/index.html (accessed June 18, 2013).

Menne, H. L., F. K. Ejaz, L. S. Noelker, and J. A. Jones. 2007. Direct care workers' recommendations for training and continuing education. *Gerontolology and Geriatrics Education* 28(2):91-108.

Mitchell, P., M. Wynia, R. Golden, R. McNellis, S. Okun, C. E. Webb, V. Rohrbach, and I. Von Korhorn. 2012. *Core principles and values of effective team-based health care*. Washington, DC: Institute of Medicine.

Montgomery, R. J., L. Holley, J. Deichert, and K. Kosloski. 2005. A profile of home care workers from the 2000 Census: How it changes what we know. *Gerontologist* 45(5):593-600.

MSKCC (Memorial Sloan-Kettering Cancer Center). 2012. *Adult survivorship program*. http://www.mskcc.org/cancer-care/survivorship/adult-survivorship (accessed September 20, 2012).

———. 2013. *Palliative care & pain management*. http://www.mskcc.org/cancer-care/palliative-care (accessed June 18, 2013).

NAC (National Alliance for Caregiving) and AARP. 2009. *Caregiving in the U.S.* http://www.caregiving.org/data/Caregiving_in_the_US_2009_full_report.pdf (accessed September 27, 2012).

NASW (National Association of Social Workers). 2006. *Assuring the sufficiency of a frontline workforce: A national study of licensed social workers*. http://workforce.socialworkers.org/studies/nasw_06_execsummary.pdf (accessed January 14, 2009).

———. 2013a. *The certified social worker in health care*. http://www.socialworkers.org/credentials/specialty/c-swhc.asp (accessed February 28, 2013).

———. 2013b. *Social work profession*. http://www.socialworkers.org/pressroom/features/general/profession.asp (accessed February 28, 2013).

———. 2013c. *The social worker in gerontology*. http://www.socialworkers.org/credentials/specialty/sw-g.asp (accessed February 28, 2013).

Naylor, M. D. 2012. *Next research steps in caregiving*. Bethesda, MD: National Institute of Aging.

Naylor, M. D., and S. K. Keating. 2008. Transitional care: Moving patients from one care setting to another. State of the science: Supporting family caregivers. *American Journal of Nursing* 108(S9):58-63.

Naylor, M., D. Brooten, R. Jones, R. Lavizzo-Mourey, M. Mezey, and M. Pauly. 1994. Comprehensive discharge planning for the hospitalized elderly: A randomized clinical trial. *Annals of Internal Medicine* 120(12):999-1006.

Naylor, M., D. Brooten, R. Campbell, B. Jacobsen, M. Mezey, M. Pauly, and J. Schwartz. 1999. Comprehensive discharge planning and home follow-up of hospitalized elders: A randomized controlled trial. *Journal of the American Medical Association* 281(7):613-620.

Naylor, M. D., D. A. Brooten, R. L. Campbell, G. M. Maislin, K. M. McCauley, and J. S. Schwartz. 2004. Transitional care of older adults hospitalized with heart failure: A randomized clinical trial. *Journal of the American Geriatric Society* 52(5):675-684.

Naylor, M. D., C. Stephens, K. H. Bowles, and M. B. Bixby. 2005. Cognitively impaired older adults: From hospital to home. A pilot study of these patients and their caregivers. *American Journal of Nursing* 105(2):40-49.

Naylor, M. D., P. Feldman, S. Keating, M. J. Koren, E. T. Kurtzman, M. Maccoy, and R. Krakauer. 2009. Translating research into practice: Transitional care for older adults. *Journal of Evaluation in Clinical Practice* 15:1164-1170.

Naylor, M. D., K. D. Coburn, E. T. Kurtzman, J. Prvu Bettger, H. G. Buck, J. Van Cleave, and C. A. Cott. 2010. *Inter-professional team-based primary care for chronically ill adults: State of the science.* Paper presented at ABIM Foundation meeting to Advance Team-Based Care for the Chronically Ill in Ambulatory Settings, Philadelphia, PA, March 24-25.

Naylor, M. D., K. H. Bowles, K. M. McCauley, M. C. Maccoy, G. Maislin, M. V. Pauly, and R. Krakauer. 2011. High-value transitional care: Ttranslation of research into practice. *Journal of Evaluation in Clinical Practice,* doi: 10.1111/j.1365-2753.2011.01659.x.

NBCHPN (National Board for Certification of Hospice and Palliative Nurses). 2013a. *Certification for hospice and palliative registered nurses.* http://www.nbchpn.org/DisplayPage. aspx?Title=RN Overview (accessed March 13, 2013).

———. 2013b. *Welcome!* http://www.nbchpn.org (accessed March 13, 2013).

NCI (National Cancer Institute). 2012a. *Continuing umbrella of research experiences (cure).* http://crchd.cancer.gov/diversity/cure-overview.html (accessed September 19, 2012).

———. 2012b. *Impacts of caregiving on the caregiver's quality of life.* http://www.cancer.gov/ cancertopics/pdq/supportivecare/caregivers/healthprofessional/page5 (accessed September 27, 2012).

NCRA (National Cancer Registrars Association). 2006. *Frontline workers in cancer data management: Workforce analysis study of the cancer registry field.* http://www.ncra-usa.org/files/ public/execsum0506.pdf (accessed January 15, 2009).

NCSBN (National Council of State Boards of Nursing). 2010. *APM consensus model frequently asked questions.* https://www.ncsbn.org/APRN_Consensus_Model_FAQs_ August_19_2010.pdf (accessed October 24, 2012).

———. 2012. *APM consensus model legislation.* https://www.ncsbn.org/aprn.htm (accessed October 24, 2012).

NCSL (National Conference of State Legislatures). 2013. *State coverage for telehealth services.* http://www.ncsl.org/issues-research/health/state-coverage-for-telehealth-services. aspx (accessed May 1, 2013).

Needleman, J., P. Buerhaus, V. S. Pankratz, C. L. Leibson, S. R. Stevens, and M. Harris. 2011. Nurse staffing and inpatient hospital mortality. *New England Journal of Medicine* 364(11):1037-1045.

NIH (National Institutes of Health). 2013. *Loan repayment programs.* http://www.lrp.nih. gov/index.aspx (accessed June 18, 2013).

NQF (National Quality Forum). 2010. *Preferred practices and performance measures for measuring and reporting care coordination.* http://www.qualityforum.org/Publications/2010/10/ Preferred_Practices_and_Performance_Measures_for_Measuring_and_Reporting_Care_ Coordination.aspx (accessed November 5, 2012).

Oeffinger, K. C., and M. S. McCabe. 2006. Models for delivering survivorship care. *Journal of Clinical Oncology* 24(32):5117-5124.

ONCC (Oncology Nursing Certification Corporation). 2012. *Advanced practice.* http://www. oncc.org/Advanced (accessed September 7, 2012).

Passiment, E. 2006. Update on the laboratory workforce-shortage crisis. *Medical Laboratory Observer.* http://www.mlo-online.com/articles/0306/0306washreport.pdf (accessed January 13, 2008).

Penn Medicine. 2012. *Livestrong Cancer Survivorship Clinic.* http://www.penncancer.org/ patients/centers-programs-services/livestrong-cancer-survivorship-center (accessed September 20, 2012).

Pham, H. H., D. Schrag, A. S. O'Malley, B. Wu, and P. B. Bach. 2007. Care patterns in medicare and their implications for pay for performance. *New England Journal of Medicine* 356(11):1130-1139.

Pham, H. H., A. S. O'Malley, P. B. Bach, C. Saiontz-Martinez, and D. Schrag. 2009. Primary care physicians' links to other physicians through medicare patients: The scope of care coordination. *Annals of Internal Medicine* 150(4):236-242.

PHPC (Pew Health Professions Commission). 1998. *Recreating health professional practice for a new century.* http://futurehealth.ucsf.edu/Content/29/1998-12_Recreating_Health_Professional_Practice_for_a_New_Century_The_Fourth_Report_of_the_Pew_Health_Professions_Commission.pdf (accessed September 21, 2012).

Potosky, A. L., P. K. Han, J. Rowland, C. N. Klabunde, T. Smith, N. Aziz, C. Earle, J. Z. Ayanian, P. A. Ganz, and M. Stefanek. 2011. Differences between primary care physicians' and oncologists' knowledge, attitudes and practices regarding the care of cancer survivors. *Journal of General Internal Medicine* 26(12):1403-1410.

PricewaterhouseCoopers. 2007. *What works: Healing the healthcare staffing shortage.* http://www.pwc.com/extweb/pwcpublications.nsf/docid/674d1e79a678a0428525730d006b74a9 (accessed January 15, 2009).

Pruthi, S., K. J. Stange, G. D. Malagrino, Jr., K. S. Chawla, N. F. LaRusso, and J. S. Kaur. 2013. Successful implementation of a telemedicine-based counseling program for high-risk patients with breast cancer. *Mayo Clinic Proceedings* 88(1):68-73.

Quill, T. E., and A. P. Abernethy. 2013. Generalist plus specialist palliative care—creating a more sustainable model. *New England Journal of Medicine* 368(13):1183-1174.

Ramirez, A. J., J. Graham, M. A. Richards, A. Cull, W. M. Gregory, M. S. Leaning, D. C. Snashall, and A. R. Timothy. 1995. Burnout and psychiatric disorder among cancer clinicians. *British Journal of Cancer* 71(6):1263-1269.

Ramirez, A. J., J. Graham, M. A. Richards, A. Cull, and W. M. Gregory. 1996. Mental health of hospital consultants: The effects of stress and satisfaction at work. *Lancet* 347(9003):724-728.

RCIC (Rosalynn Carter Institute for Caregiving). 2013. *Education & training.* http://www.rosalynncarter.org/national_quality_caregiving_network (accessed May 2, 2013).

Reinhard, S. C., and C. Levine. 2012. *Home alone: Family caregivers providing complex chronic care.* http://www.aarp.org/home-family/caregiving/info-10-2012/home-alone-family-caregivers-providing-complex-chronic-care.html (accessed March 29, 2013).

RGC (Robert Graham Center). 2010. *Income disparities shape medical student specialty choice.* http://www.graham-center.org/online/graham/home/publications/onepagers/2010/op67-income-disparities.html (accessed September 7, 2012).

Ross, A. C., M. N. Polansky, P. A. Parker, and J. L. Palmer. 2010. Understanding the role of physician assistants in oncology. *Journal of Oncology Practice* 6(1):26-30.

Routson, J. 2010. *Shortage of oncology nurses could get worse as population ages.* http://www.healthecareers.com/article/shortage-of-oncology-nurses-could-get-worse-as-population-ages/158441 (accessed September 7, 2012).

RUMC (Rush University Medical Center). 2012. *Geriatric integrated team training.* http://www.rush.edu/professionals/training/geriatrics/index.html (accessed September 21, 2012).

Salsberg, E., P. Rockey, K. Rivers, S. Brotherton, and G. Jackson. 2008. U.S. residency training before and after the 1997 Balanced Budget Act. *Journal of the American Medical Association* 300(10):1205-1207.

Sanjo, M., T. Morita, M. Miyashita, M. Shiozaki, K. Sato, K. Hirai, Y. Shima, and Y. Uchitomi. 2009. Caregiving consequences inventory: A measure for evaluating caregiving consequences from the bereaved family member's perspective. *Psychooncology* 18(6):657-666.

Sargen, M., R. Hooker, and R. Coolper. 2011. Gaps in the supply of physicians, advanced practice nurses, and physician assistants. *Journal of the American College of Surgeons* 212(6):991-999.

Shanafelt, T. D., P. Novotny, M. E. Johnson, X. Zhao, D. P. Steensma, M. Q. Lacy, J. Rubin, and J. Sloan. 2005. The well-being and personal wellness promotion strategies of medical oncologists in the North Central Cancer Treatment Group. *Oncology* 68(1):23-32.

Shanafelt, T., H. Chung, H. White, and L. Lyckholm. 2006. Shaping your career to maximize personal satisfaction in the practice of oncology. *Journal of Clinical Oncology* 24(24):4020-4026.

Sheldon, G. F. 2010. The surgeon shortage: Constructive participation during health reform. *Journal of the American College of Surgeons* 210(6):887-894.

Smith, A. P., M. Y. Lichtveld, K. R. Miner, S. L. Tyus, and L. N. Gase. 2009. *A competency-based approach to expanding the cancer care workforce: Proof of concept.* http://c-changetogether. org/Websites/cchange/Images/MedSurg%20Journals/2009/MSJN109_Cancer.pdf (accessed November 5, 2012).

Smith, K., and R. Baughman. 2007. Caring for america's aging population: A profile of the direct-care workforce. *Monthly Labor Review* 130(9):20-26.

Snyder, C. F., C. C. Earle, R. J. Herbert, B. A. Neville, A. L. Blackford, and K. D. Frick. 2008. Trends in follow-up and preventive care for colorectal cancer survivors. *Journal of General Internal Medicine* 23(3):254-259.

Snyder, C. F., K. D. Frick, K. S. Peairs, M. E. Kantsiper, R. J. Herbert, A. L. Blackford, A. C. Wolff, and C. C. Earle. 2009. Comparing care for breast cancer survivors to non-cancer controls: A five-year longitudinal study. *Journal of General Internal Medicine* 24(4):469-474.

Snyder, C. F., K. D. Frick, R. J. Herbert, A. L. Blackford, B. A. Neville, M. A. Carducci, and C. C. Earle. 2011. Preventive care in prostate cancer patients: Following diagnosis and for five-year survivors. *Journal of Cancer Survivorship* 5(3):283-291.

Staiger, D., D. I. Auerbach, and P. I. Buerhaus. 2010. Trends in the work hours of physicians in the United States. *Journal of the American Medical Association* 303(8):747-753.

———. 2012. Registered nurse labor supply and the recession—Are we in a bubble? *New England Journal of Medicine* 366(16):1463-1465.

Stremikis, K., C. Schoen, and A. Fryer. 2011. *A call for change: The 2011 Commonwealth Fund survey of public views of the U.S. health system.* http://www.commonwealthfund.org/~/media/Files/Publications/Issue%20Brief/2011/Apr/1492_Stremikis_public_views_2011_ survey_ib.pdf (accessed May 2, 2013).

Stubblefield, M. D. 2011. Cancer rehabilitation. *Seminars in Oncology* 38(3):386-393.

Stubblefield, M. D., M. L. McNeely, C. M. Alfano, and D. K. Mayer. 2012. A prospective surveillance model for physical rehabilitation of women with breast cancer: Chemotherapy-induced peripheral neuropathy. *Cancer* 118(8 Suppl):2250-2260.

Thibault, G. E., and S. C. Schoenbaum. 2013. *Forging collaboration within academia and between academia and health care delivery organizationsL Importance, successes, and future work.* http://www.iom.edu/forgingcollaboration (accessed July 26, 2013).

Towle, E. L., T. R. Barr, A. Hanley, M. Kosty, S. Williams, and M. A. Goldstein. 2011. Results of the ASCO study of collaborative practice arrangements. *Journal of Oncology Practice* 7(5):278-282.

UMN (University of Minnesota). 2013. *1health.* http://www.ahceducation.umn.edu/1Health (accessed August 2, 2013).

UnitedHealth. 2011. *Modernizing rural health care: Coverage, quality and innovation.* http:// www.unitedhealthgroup.com/hrm/unh_workingpaper6.pdf (accessed September 6, 2012).

University of Colorado. 2013a. *Frontier Center.* http://www.ucdenver.edu/academics/ colleges/dentalmedicine/CommunityService/Pages/Frontier-Center.aspx (accessed August 2, 2013).

————. 2013b. *Interprofessional education for quality and collaborative care*. http://www.ucdenver. edu/academics/degrees/health/REACH/Pages/Default.aspx (accessed August 2, 2013).

UNM (University of New Mexico). 2013. *Project ECHO*. http://echo.unm.edu (accessed July 26, 2013).

Unroe, K. T., and H. J. Cohen. 2012. Chapter 31: Multidisciplinary models of care. In *Cancer and aging handbook: Research and practice*. First ed, edited by K. M. Bellizzi and M. A. Gosney. Hoboken, NJ: John Wiley & Sons, Inc.

UT (Urology Times). 2007. *Is there a urologist in the house? Maybe not for long*. http://urology times.modernmedicine.com/urologytimes/News+Feature/Is-there-a-urologist-in-the-house-Maybe-not-for-lo/ArticleStandard/Article/detail/423954 (accessed September 18, 2012).

UW (University of Washington). 2012. *Interprofessional education at the University of Washington: Vision for a collaborative future. Final report of the Health Sciences Interprofessional Education and Facilities Committee*. http://sph.washington.edu/strategicplan/implementation/IPE_report.pdf (accessed August 2, 2013).

————. 2013. *Center for Health Science Interprofessional Education, Research, and Practice*. http:// collaborate.uw.edu (accessed August 2, 2013).

VA (Department of Veterans Affairs). 2013. *Caregiver services*. http://www.caregiver.va.gov/ support_services.asp (accessed May 2, 2013).

VHA (Veterans Health Administration). 2012. A new era of telehealth expansion. *VHA Telehealth Quarterly*. http://www.telehealth.va.gov/newsletter/2012/021312-Newsletter_Vol11Iss01.pdf (accessed May 1, 2013).

Warde, C. M., K. Moonesinghe, W. Allen, and L. Gelberg. 1999. Marital and parental satisfaction of married physicians with children. *Journal of General Internal Medicine* 14(3):157-165.

Weitzner, M. A., S. C. McMillan, and P. B. Jacobsen. 1999. Family caregiver quality of life: Differences between curative and palliative cancer treatment settings. *Journal of Pain and Symptom Management* 17(6):418-428.

Whippen, D. A., and G. P. Canellos. 1991. Burnout syndrome in the practice of oncology: Results of a random survey of 1,000 oncologists. *Journal of Clinical Oncology* 9(10): 1916-1920.

White, S. 2005. Will there be a pharmacy leadership crisis? An ASHP Foundation scholar-in-residence report. *American Journal of Health-System Pharmacy* 62(8):845-855.

WHO (World Health Organization). 2010. *Framework for action on interprofessional education & collaborative practice*. http://whqlibdoc.who.int/hq/2010/WHO_HRH_HPN_10.3_eng. pdf (accessed September 21, 2012).

Wong, R. K., E. Franssen, E. Szumacher, R. Connolly, M. Evans, B. Page, E. Chow, C. Hayter, T. Harth, L. Andersson, J. Pope, and C. Danjoux. 2002. What do patients living with advanced cancer and their carers want to know? A needs assessment. *Supportive Care in Cancer* 10(5):408-415.

Yoong, J., E. R. Park, J. A. Greer, V. A. Jackson, E. R. Gallagher, W. F. Pirl, A. L. Back, and J. S. Temel. 2013. Early palliative care in advanced lung cancer: A qualitative study. *JAMA Internal Medicine* 173(4):283-290.

Zilliacus, E. M., B. Meiser, E. A. Lobb, P. J. Kelly, K. Barlow-Stewart, J. A. Kirk, A. D. Spigelman, L. J. Warwick, and K. M. Tucker. 2011. Are videoconferenced consultations as effective as face-to-face consultations for hereditary breast and ovarian cancer genetic counseling? *Genetics in Medicine* 13(11):933-941.

ANNEX 4-1 PROFESSIONALS INVOLVED IN CANCER CARE

Health Care Professional	Role in Cancer Care	Overview of Available Information
Physicians		
Physicians (general)	• Principal clinicians of medical care	• Current shortage of ~8% • Shortage will increase to >20% by 2025 if no new residency slots are added
Oncology Physicians		
Geriatric Oncologists	• Diagnose and treat cancer in older adults	• No information available
Hematologists	• Diagnose and treat blood disorders, including cancer	• American Society of Hematology has +14,000 members
Medical Oncologists	• Diagnose and treat cancer	• Shortage of 2,500-4,080 oncologists by 2020 predicted • More than 14,000 medical oncologists and 8,000 hematologists in 2012
Radiation Oncologists	• Treat cancer with radiation therapy	• The American Society for Radiation Oncology has ~10,000 members
Surgical Oncologists	• Specialize in the surgical management of cancer	• The number of general surgical subspecialties, including surgical oncology, grew 20% between 2004 and 2008
Medical and Surgical Specialists		
Gastroenterologists	• Diagnose and treat cancers in the digestive system	• 15,000 in 2012
Gynecologists	• Diagnose, treat, and manage patients with gynecological cancers (e.g., ovarian, cervical)	• 49% of counties in the United States lack an ob-gyn physician • 18% shortage by 2030 and 25% shortage by 2050 • 15,000+ will likely retire in next 10 years

Hospice and Palliative Care Physicians	• Palliative care physicians prevent and relieve the suffering of patients throughout the continuum of cancer care • Experts in hospice care relieve the symptoms of terminally ill patients and provide emotional support	• 4,400 hospice and palliative care physicians • Majority work part time in the palliative care field. • Current shortage of 2,787 to 7,510 full-time employees, which equals 6,000-18,000 individual physicians
Pulmonologists	• Diagnose and treat patients with cancers in the respiratory track	• ~15,000 certified in pulmonary disease in 2012 • American College of Chest Physicians has 18,500 members
Radiologists	• Use imaging and radiation technologies to diagnose and treat cancer	• The American College of Radiology has +35,000 members, including radiation oncologists
Surgeons	• Remove diseased tissue from the body	• The workforce decreased by 16.3% between 1996 and 2006, and is projected to increase by only 3% between 2005 and 2020 • One-third of critical access hospitals lack a surgeon living in the county
Urologists	• Diagnose, treat, and manage patients with urological cancers (e.g., prostate, kidney, bladder)	• Ranks last among all specialties in "production rate" of new physicians • 45% of all urologists are 55 years or older
Primary Care Clinicians		
Geriatricians	• Specialize in the care for older adults	• 9,000+ in 2012
Primary Care Physicians	• Provide comprehensive and continuous care for patients regardless of diagnosis, organ system, or problem origin	• More than 200,000 primary care physicians in 2007 • Only 2% of internal medicine residents planned to go into primary care in 2009
Nurses and Physician Assistants		
Nurses (general)	• Focused on caring for and dealing with individual responses to health problems	• 3 million registered nurses • Shortage of 1 million registered nurses predicted by 2020 • 6.9% nursing school faculty vacancy rate in 2010 • 30% drop-out rate for first-year nurses

continued

Health Care Professional	Role in Cancer Care	Overview of Available Information
Advanced Practice Registered Nurses (APRNs)	• Have master's degrees, doctorates of nursing practice, or Ph.D.s in nursing and work with a high level of independence in the care of patients	• 250,000 APRNs in 2008; 2.6% were certified in oncology
Oncology Nurses	• Provide care to individuals with cancer	• The Oncology Nursing Society has more than 35,000 members • 2.6% of advanced practice nurses are trained in oncology
Physician Assistants	• Provide care under the supervision of a physician • Prescription privileges across the entire United States	• Fastest-growing profession behind nursing • Projected to increase from 75,000 professionals in 2008 to between 137,000-173,000 in 2020
Other Health Professionals		
Cancer Registrars	• Collect and analyze data for national and regional cancer priority research	• 72,800 registrars in 2006 • 800 new registrars will be needed by 2020
Direct care workers (i.e., personal and home care aides)	• Provide long-term care and personal assistance • Help clients bathe, dress, and other daily tasks	• 3.2 million people • Predicted to account for 40% of new health care jobs in 2008-2018
Laboratory personnel	• Collect samples and perform tests to analyze body fluids, tissue, and other substances	• 60% of the health care workforce • By 2015, an additional 81,000 clinical laboratory technologists are needed to replace retiring personnel; 68,000 to fill newly created positions • Aging 78% faster than the general U.S. labor market
Occupational Therapists	• Help patients develop, recover, and improve skills necessary for everyday living that are impaired due to cancer or cancer treatment	• ~100,000 in 2010 • 33% increase between 2010 and 2020

Profession	Role	Workforce Information
Patient Navigators	• Help patients navigate through the various components of the health care system, including physicians' offices, clinics, hospitals, outpatient centers, insurance and payment systems, and patient-support organizations	• No information available • Education and training varies widely
Pharmacists	• Provide chemotherapy, medications for palliative care, and patient education on drug side effects and interactions	• 25% of pharmacists are approaching retirement age • 75% of pharmacy directors and middle managers anticipate retiring from their positions within the next decade • 6.4% vacancy rate in 2007
Physical Therapists	• Promote mobility, functional ability, quality of life, and movement potential	• ~200,000 in 2010 • 39% increase projected between 2010 and 2020
Public Health Workers	• Screening, prevention, and early detection of cancer • Surveillance of cancer incidence, prevalence, and mortality	• 250,000 more workers are needed by 2020 • 50,000 fewer workers in 2000 than in 1980 • 23% of the current workforce was eligible to retire in 2012 • Schools of public health would have to train three times the current number of graduates to replenish the workforce
Social Workers	• Provide patient navigation, psychosocial screening and assessment, and support for cancer-related depression and anxiety	• 650,500 social workers; 1,000 in oncology • 13% of licensed social workers specialize in health care • 29% of licensed social workers are over 55 years • 85% of all health care social workers are likely to practice in metropolitan areas; 2% are likely to practice in rural areas

NOTE: The information presented for each professional varies, depending on what information is available about that workforce.

SOURCES: AACN, 2010; AAMC, 2007, 2008; AAPA, 2012a; ABIM, 2012; ACCP, 2012; ACG, 2012; ACOG, 2011; ACR, 2012; ACS/HPRI, 2010; AGA, 2012; AOSW, 2013; ASCP, 2004; ASH, 2011; ASHP, 2007, 2008; ASTRO, 2012a; BLS, 2013b,f; Blum et al., 2006; Buerhaus et al., 2009; CWS, 2006; Hauer, 2008; Hillborne, 2008; HRSA, 2010, 2012; HWS, 2007; IOM, 2011a; KHN, 2011; Lupu, 2010; McDonald and Sutton, 2009; NASW, 2006; NCRA, 2006; Passiment, 2006; PricewaterhouseCoopers, 2007; Routson, 2010; Sargen et al., 2011; Sheldon, 2010; UT, 2007; White, 2005.

5

The Evidence Base for
High-Quality Cancer Care

"Decisions about the care of individual patients should be based on the conscientious, explicit, and judicious use of current best evidence" (IOM, 2008b, p. 2). The committee's conceptual framework (see Figure S-2) depicts the evidence base as supporting patient-clinician interactions, because a high-quality cancer care delivery system uses results from scientific research, such as clinical trials and comparative effectiveness research (CER), to inform medical decisions. A high-quality cancer care delivery system depends upon clinical research that gathers evidence of the benefits and harms of various treatment options so that patients, in consultation with their clinicians, can make treatment decisions that are consistent with their needs, values, and preferences.

The relative weight that patients place on each consideration related to their diagnosis and treatment tends to vary across different populations. Older adults faced with a cancer diagnosis, for example, may value outcomes different from the ones younger patients value, and may be more apt to choose treatment options that will maintain quality of life for as long as possible rather than focusing solely on increasing the length of survival or disease remission as measured by biomarkers (see discussion in Chapter 2 on the unique needs of older adults with cancer). The recent emphasis on molecularly targeted medicine in clinical cancer research could greatly improve the quality of cancer care by enabling physicians to effectively target therapeutic interventions to the patients for whom they are most suited and to avoid treating patients for whom the interventions will not be effective and may be unsafe (see discussion in Chapter 2 on trends in cancer research and practice changes). The focus on improving the evidence base for cancer is consistent with the Institute of Medicine's (IOM's) 1999 report *Ensuring Quality Cancer Care*, which recommended investing in clinical trials to address questions about cancer care management and health services research to understand care patterns associated with good health outcomes (IOM and NRC, 1999).

A recent IOM report concluded that "despite the accelerating pace of scientific discovery, the current clinical research enterprise does not sufficiently address pressing clinical questions. The result is decisions by both patients and clinicians that are inadequately informed by the evidence" (IOM, 2012a, p. 20). For example, Villas Boas and colleagues (2012) and El Dib and colleagues (2007) found that about half of Cochrane systematic reviews had sufficient evidence to inform clinical practice.

Oftentimes, research participants are not representative of the population that actually contracts the disease; older adults, individuals with comorbidities, members of racial and ethnic minorities, and people who live in rural areas are consistently underrepresented in clinical research (EDICT, 2008). Investigators also often fail to collect data that could be used to draw conclusions about factors that influence the course of the disease and provide information about the patient experience with care (e.g., quality of life, functional and cognitive status, symptoms, socioeconomic status, literacy, numeracy, language, culture, education, transportation, social supports, neighborhood, behavioral health, housing, family capacity, comorbidity, and psychological state) (Ganz, 2012). Although health information technology (IT) has great promise for improving research and clinical knowledge to guide decisions, there need to be advances in health IT infrastructure, computational capabilities, and research methods to fulfill this potential (IOM, 2012a).

The complexity of cancer and the diverse treatment options available exacerbate the challenges of developing an evidence base that will adequately support clinical decision making. There are hundreds of different types of cancer, with multiple stages of disease (e.g., precancer, early-stage disease, metastatic disease). The multiple treatment modalities and combination strategies for cancer treatment necessitate coordinated teams of professionals with multiple skill sets. Additionally, the toxicity of many treatment options often requires patients and clinicians to make difficult decisions that weigh the benefits and harms of alternative treatment approaches. Although cancer care is evolving quickly, with manufacturers marketing new drugs and devices that have the potential to improve current treatment, those innovations come with substantial human and financial costs.

This chapter summarizes how the evidence base for decision making in cancer care is generated and discusses the need to improve the breadth and depth of information collected in clinical cancer research, as well as the potential to improve the use of technology to collect, organize, and analyze data from various sources. The chapter focuses on clinical research with the potential to generate evidence that could directly inform medical decision making; a discussion of basic research is outside the scope of this report. Other topics relevant to delivering evidence-based cancer care are discussed elsewhere in this report. New models of care delivery are discussed in Chapter 8 and performance improvement initiatives are discussed in Chapter 7. This chapter builds on the IOM's previous consensus studies on cancer clinical trials, CER, and a learning health care system (IOM, 2008a,b, 2009a,b, 2010a,b, 2012a,b). The committee identifies two recommendations to improve the evidence base for high-quality cancer care.

HOW THE EVIDENCE BASE FOR CANCER CARE DECISIONS IS GENERATED

Both publicly and privately funded research will be necessary to improve the evidence base for cancer care. For-profit industries generally fund research focused on developing new drugs and devices for treating cancer, while public funders often support research addressing "questions that are important to patients but are less likely to be top priorities of industry" (IOM, 2010b, p. 1). This section addresses trials of new drugs, biologics, and devices, as well as CER.

Trials of New Drugs, Biologics, and Devices

Manufacturers of drugs, biologics, and devices leverage scientific advances to bring new treatments to the market with the potential to improve patient outcomes. The Food and Drug Administration (FDA), the federal agency charged with regulating pharmaceuticals and medical devices, requires manufacturers to submit scientific evidence that establishes the safety and effectiveness of their products prior to making them available to the public (FDA, 2012a,b). The FDA approval or clearance allows the marketing of new drugs, biologics, and devices with the potential to improve outcomes for patients with cancer, although some experts have raised concern that the FDA's medical device approval/clearance processes are less rigorous than for drugs (IOM, 2013; Meropol et al., 2009). An IOM committee reviewing the process by which most medical devices enter the market concluded that the process often fails to adequately ensure safety and effectiveness (IOM, 2011b). The IOM recommended that the FDA design a new medical-device regulatory framework. Nevertheless, clinical trials conducted by manufacturers can provide important information for clinical decision making.

Research conducted by manufacturers tends to be narrowly focused on allowing the manufacturers to market efficacious products that may improve patient care, influence package inserts or labeling claims on their products, or expand market share. As a result, such research often fails to address many additional research questions relevant to clinical care. An IOM report on cancer clinical trials noted that companies often lack incentives to conduct clinical trials that compare the effectiveness of different treatment options already approved for clinical use; combine novel treatments developed by different sponsors; determine optimal duration and dose of drugs in clinical use; or test multimodality treatments, such as radiation therapy, surgery, or devices in combination with drugs (IOM, 2010b).

In addition, manufacturers often conduct their research with highly selective patient populations and through carefully defined and monitored treatment regimens, with the goal of providing safety and efficacy data to the FDA. The data collected by manufacturers may therefore not be generalizable to real-world clinical practice. Certain populations are routinely understudied due to strict eligibility criteria, including older adults and patients with multiple chronic conditions, and outcomes (such as the impact of treatment on physical or cognitive function) that are important to patients and their caregivers are often unmeasured. Manufacturers are also unlikely to study certain types of treatments that do not require regulatory approval, such as surgery and radiation therapy.

Comparative Effectiveness Research

Because of the narrow focus of research conducted for regulatory approval, there are often many remaining practical questions when a drug or device is introduced into the market, which go beyond those typically addressed by regulatory agencies. There has been recent interest in using CER to fill these knowledge gaps (IOM, 2009a, 2011a; Lyman and Levine, 2012; PCORI, 2012a; Ramsey et al., 2013). CER is defined as "the generation and synthesis of evidence that compares the benefits and harms of alternative methods to prevent, diagnose, treat, and monitor a clinical condition or to improve the delivery of care. The purpose of CER is to assist consumers, clinicians, purchasers, and policy makers to make informed decisions that will improve health care at both the individual and population levels" (IOM, 2009a, p. 13). Research that is compatible with the aims of CER has six defining characteristics:

1. The objective is to inform a specific clinical question.
2. It compares at least two alternative interventions, each with the potential to be a "best practice."
3. It addresses and describes patient outcomes at both a population and a subgroup level.
4. It measures outcomes that are important to patients, including harms and benefits.
5. It uses research methods and data sources that are appropriate for the question of interest.
6. It is conducted in settings as close as possible to the settings in which the intervention will be used.

CER can be conducted using multiple research methodologies, including clinical trials as well as observational research and systematic reviews (see Box 5-1). The appropriate methodology depends on the type of question the research is intended to answer.

The American Recovery and Reinvestment Act of 2009[1] appropriated $1.1 billion for CER, and the IOM was charged with identifying an initial set of CER priorities (IOM, 2009a). These priorities included six topics in cancer, including screening technologies for colorectal and breast cancer; management strategies for localized prostate cancer; imaging technologies for diagnosis, staging, and monitoring of all cancers; use of biomarker analysis in risk assessment and treatment strategies for common cancers; and comparing treatment strategies for liver metastases.

The Patient Protection and Affordable Care Act of 2010[2] (ACA) reinforced the importance of CER and created the Patient-Centered Outcomes Research Institute (PCORI), a new institute responsible for establishing and implementing a research agenda that provides "information about the best available evidence to help patients and their health care providers make more informed decisions" (PCORI, 2012a). The institute has a trust fund of $150 million in annual appropriations, plus an annual per-capita charge for each enrollee from insurance plans through 2019 (Clancy and Collins, 2010).

The National Cancer Institute's (NCI's) Clinical Trials Cooperative Group Program is one of the major funders of CER in cancer. Many of the Cooperative Groups' studies have generated data that have informed clinical decision making and set the standard of care in cancer. Their studies regularly compare alternative interventions, describe results at the

---

[1] The American Recovery and Reinvestment Act of 2009, Public Law 111-5, 111th Congress, 1st Sess. (February 17, 2009).

[2] Patient Protection and Affordable Care Act, Public Law 111-148, 111th Congress, 2nd Sess. (March 23, 2010).

BOX 5-1
Types of Comparative Effectiveness Research Studies

Experimental study: A study in which the investigators actively intervene to test a hypothesis.

- **Controlled trials** are experimental studies in which a group receives the intervention of interest while one or more comparison groups receive an active comparator, a placebo, no intervention, or the standard of care, and the outcomes are compared. In **head-to-head** trials, two active treatments are compared.
- In a **randomized controlled trial (RCT),** participants are randomly allocated to the experimental group or the comparison group. **Cluster randomized trials** are RCTs in which participants are randomly assigned to the intervention or comparison in groups (clusters) defined by a common feature, such as the same physician or health plan.

Observational study: A study in which investigators simply observe the course of events.

- In **prospective observational studies,** the exposure of interest is studied using data stored in registries, which can require years to accumulate the needed numbers of patients and outcomes.
- In **cohort studies,** groups with certain characteristics or receiving certain interventions (e.g., premenopausal woman receiving chemotherapy for breast cancer) are monitored over time to observe an outcome of interest (e.g., loss of fertility).
- In **case-control studies,** groups with and without an event or outcome are examined to see whether a past exposure or characteristic is more prevalent in one group than in the other.
- In **cross-sectional studies,** the prevalence of an exposure of interest is associated with a condition (e.g., prevalence of hysterectomy in African American versus white women) and is measured at a specific time or time period.

Systematic review (SR): A scientific investigation that focuses on a specific question and that uses explicit, planned scientific methods to identify, select, assess, and summarize the findings of similar but separate studies. It may or may not include a quantitative synthesis (meta-analysis) of the results from separate studies.

- A **meta-analysis** is an SR that uses statistical methods to combine quantitatively the results of similar studies in an attempt to allow inferences to be made from the sample of studies and applied to the population of interest.

SOURCES: IOM, 2011a. Adapted from Last, 1995.

population and subpopulation levels, and measure benefits and risks that are important to patients. The Cooperative Groups' inclusion of the Community Clinical Oncology Program means that many trials are conducted by community practices, where the majority of cancer patients are treated, representing a more generalizable population. The Cooperative Groups' research regularly addresses interventions not studied in FDA registration trials, such as surgical innovations and in-depth evaluations of imaging and medical devices (Hahn and Schilsky, 2012; Schilsky, 2013).

Despite progress, the NCI convened the IOM to provide advice on improvements and reorganization in the Cooperative Groups' research that could help them reach their full potential and conduct timely, large-scale, and innovative clinical trials needed to improve patient care (IOM, 2010b; NCI, 2012c). The IOM released its recommendations in 2010 and the Cooperative Groups are currently reorganizing within a National Clinical Trials Network (NCTN). Given current financial constraints, the NCI is still grappling with how to prioritize new research and create a balanced portfolio of clinical trials on new cancer treatments, CER, and correlative biomarker research (NCI, 2012b). Thus, there is some uncertainty about the types and focus of research that the NCTN will conduct in the future.

The Agency for Healthcare Research and Quality (AHRQ) Effective Health Care Program is the federal government's major funder of CER. This program includes several initiatives focused on CER: (1) Evidence-Based Practice Centers—which conduct systematic reviews of the literature and are involved in developing the methodology of systemic reviews; (2) Developing Evidence to Inform Decisions about Effectiveness Centers—which are involved in developing new CER evidence; (3) The Centers for Education and Research on Therapeutics—which conduct research and provide education to advance the optimal use of drugs, devices, and biological products; and (4) the John M. Eisenberg Clinical Decisions and Communications Science Center—which translates evidence into lay language (AHRQ, 2013a). AHRQ's Effective Health Care Program has completed more than 50 research summaries, systematic reviews, and reports on cancer, as well as other topics relevant to cancer care (e.g., patient-centeredness, end-of-life issues) (AHRQ, 2013b).

IMPROVING THE BREADTH OF INFORMATION COLLECTED

For clinical research to improve the quality of cancer care, researchers need to study populations that are representative of clinical practice. Participation in a clinical trial can be a valid treatment option for many individuals with cancer, especially for individuals who have exhausted the standard of care options. The ACA acknowledges the importance of participation in clinical trials and requires insurers to cover research participants' routine care costs during approved trials (IOM, 2010b).

Currently, however, only 3 percent of adults with cancer participate in clinical trials (IOM, 2010b). Members of racial and ethnic minorities, individuals with comorbidities, older adults, low-income individuals, and people who live in rural areas are consistently underrepresented in cancer research (EDICT, 2008; IOM, 2010b). And although the majority of cancer patients are treated in community settings, the majority of cancer patients who enroll in clinical trials are treated at academic cancer centers (Cox and McGarry, 2003; IOM, 2010b; Somkin et al., 2005). As cancer treatment moves toward more molecularly targeted therapies, the underrepresentation of certain population segments becomes particularly problematic; this type of research requires large numbers of patients willing to participate in trials.

The committee is particularly concerned about the lack of clinical trial research focused on older adults, given its statement of task. Research shows that not only are older adults often excluded from trials, but when they are included they are not representative of the typical older adult; they are younger and healthier than average (Cerreta et al., 2012; Dhruva and Redberg, 2008; Van Spall et al., 2007). As mentioned in Chapter 2, there are many unique considerations to treating older adults with cancer. Older adults with cancer may have different treatment goals from those of younger patients (e.g., quality of life vs. length of life), often respond differently to treatment than do younger patients, and are more sensitive to toxicity and side effects. They are also more likely to have comorbidities that may influence the effects of treatment on their health.

At the same time, older adults are often some of the first individuals using a newly available drug because the majority of cancer patients are over 65 years. When older adults and individuals with comorbidities are underrepresented in cancer clinical trials, clinicians are forced to extrapolate from clinical trials conducted on younger, healthier adults and apply that information to older adults, hoping that the information will be relevant in the older population. Although federal agencies have mandated the recruitment of women and minorities to oncology trials to address those groups' past exclusion, policies on the inclusion of older adults are less stringent or nonexistent (FDA, 1998; NIH, 2001).[3]

The inclusion of older adults in clinical research is complicated by

---

[3] Under the Food and Drug Administration Modernization Act of 1998 Sec. 115. (b) Women and Minorities. Section 505(b)(1) 21 U.S.C. 355(b)(1) was amended by adding the following: "The Secretary shall, in consultation with the Director of the National Institutes of Health and with representatives of the drug manufacturing industry, review and develop guidance, as appropriate, on the inclusion of women and minorities in clinical trials."

the fact that chronological age is an inadequate method of characterizing individuals. Many individuals qualify as older adults based on their chronologic age, but are functionally much younger, and the opposite can also be true (see discussion in Chapter 2). As a result, even when eligibility criteria are set to match the population with the disease, clinicians and ethics boards often prevent frail individuals from participating in trials (Cerreta et al., 2012). Some researchers have suggested that "clinical trials designed with physiological age in mind would certainly lead to more meaningful results" (Herrera et al., 2010, p. S106).

There are many barriers to older adults' participation in clinical research. Trials often have stringent eligibility criteria with regard to comorbidities, concomitant medications, and medical histories. In an evaluation of older adults participating in NCI-sponsored clinical trials, Lewis and colleagues (2003) found that the majority of trials excluded participation if a person had hematologic, hepatic, renal, or cardiac abnormalities, all of which are common in older adults (see discussion in Chapter 2). Approximately 80 percent of the trials also required participants to be ambulatory and capable of caring for themselves (Lewis et al., 2003). Because many older adults do not drive, transportation and the cost of traveling to the research location can also be challenging.

In addition, the attitudes of both clinicians and patients can impede their participation. A study by Javid and colleagues (2012) found that family-related and personal concerns played a greater role in older adults' decisions not to participate in a clinical trial than in younger cancer patients' decisions. Patients who were older were also less likely than younger patients to believe their participation in a clinical trial would benefit future generations and more likely to believe that participation in a clinical trial would be burdensome.

Clinicians have few incentives to offer patients enrollment in clinical trials, and regularly cite concerns about drug toxicity and the impact of treatment as reasons to not enroll older adults (Javid et al., 2012; Townsley et al., 2005; Trimble et al., 1994). In the Javid study, researchers found that when trials were available, and patients were eligible for enrollment, physicians discussed trial participation with 76 percent of patients under 65 years versus only 58 percent of patients over 65 years. However, several studies have found that older adults are as willing as younger adults to participate in clinical trials when given the opportunity by their clinicians (Kemeny et al., 2003; Kornblith et al., 2002).

The following sections explore the inclusion of older adults and individuals with multiple comorbidities in FDA registration trials and CER.

FDA Registration Trials

Under FDA regulation, manufacturers are required to report clinical trial results by age[4] and to include a "geriatric use" subsection in the label of their product that provides details on how to use the drug or biological product in older adults.[5] The FDA has also issued numerous guidance documents that provide more comprehensive direction to manufacturers about the inclusion of older adults and individuals with comorbidities, but these are not binding legal documents. For example, FDA guidance encourages, but does not require, the routine and thorough evaluation of the effect of drugs in older adults, with the explicit purpose of providing clinicians with sufficient information on how to use drugs properly in this population (FDA, 1989, 2012c).

The guidance states that patients in clinical studies should reflect the population that will receive the drug after it is marketed and notes that it is usually appropriate to include more than 100 geriatric patients in phase 2 and phase 3 trials (FDA, 2012c). It also emphasizes that there is no rationale for excluding patients on the basis of advanced age alone, unless it will make it more difficult to interpret the study results.

The guidance also encourages, but does not require, the inclusion of individuals over 75 years and suggests that exclusion criteria should focus on issues such as the presence of an illness that could make participation in a clinical trial dangerous or impact the individual's ability to provide informed consent. To assist the FDA in determining how many older adults participated in a clinical trial, the guidance makes recommendations on how to report the age of clinical trial participants (e.g., average age, age of the youngest and oldest participants, and the number of participants who fall into specific age categories) (FDA, 1988).

In a report to the Government Accountability Office (GAO), the FDA noted that its medical officers routinely take the representation of older adults into consideration when reviewing drug applications (GAO, 2007). On the other hand, guidance documents have recognized that it can be challenging to include older adults with comorbidities and concomitant treatments in premarketing development studies and that data derived from these populations could be more appropriate for collection in the postmarketing context (FDA, 2012c).

There is substantial evidence that older adults are routinely underrepresented in registration trials for new cancer treatments. Talarico and

---

[4] Investigational New Drug Applications and New Drug Applications, 63 Fed. Reg. 6854, 6862 (Feb 11, 1998) (codified at 21 CFR 314.50(d)(5), (vi)(a); 312.33(a)(2)(2007)).

[5] Specific Requirements on Content and Format of Labeling for Human Prescription Drugs; Addition of "Geriatric Use" Subsection in the labeling, 62 Fed Reg. 45313, 4325 (August 27, 1997).

colleagues (2004) analyzed 28,766 cancer patients from 55 registration trials according to age distribution of 65 years and older, 70 years and older, and 75 years and older. They compared the participation rate of each age group to the corresponding rates in the U.S. cancer population. Individuals age 65 years and older represented 36 percent of the trial participants compared with 60 percent of cancer patients, individuals 70 years and older represented 20 percent of trial participants and 46 percent of cancer patients, and individuals 75 years and older represented 9 percent of trial participants and 31 percent of cancer patients.

In the GAO report mentioned above, the FDA reviewed 36 new drug applications (NDAs) from January 2001 through June 2003. They found that older adults (age 65 years and older) were included in at least one clinical drug trial supporting all 36 of the NDAs reviewed. The sponsors reported the number of older adults included in the clinical trials supporting 28 of the NDAs. In these trials, older adults made up 33 percent of the populations studied (GAO, 2007).

More recently, Scher and Hurria (2012) noted that in the geriatric usage sections of the drug package inserts for 24 drugs approved for cancer treatment between 2007 and June 2010, only 33 percent of the participants were age 65 and older compared with 59 percent of the cancer population that is 65 years and older. Individuals with comorbidities are equally likely to be excluded from registration trials for new cancer treatments because of the complexity of interpreting results when they are participants.

Congress has regularly used market exclusivity to promote public health priorities in the pharmaceutical and biomedical sciences (Kesselheim, 2011). For example, the pediatric patent exclusivity provisions[6] provide manufacturers with an additional 6 months of patent protection for conducting clinical trials of their products in children. The law prevents generic versions of a drug from being marketed during those 6 months. Patent exclusivity applies regardless of the outcome of the trial and is not contingent on a labeling change for pediatric use. The goal of the law is to create an incentive for manufacturers to conduct research in children. This allows the government to subsidize research by providing patent extension, but without directly allocating any resources. The cost of the research is paid for by the manufacturers and passed on to the patients and payers through higher drug prices for the additional 6 months (Kesselheim, 2011).

A recent IOM committee concluded that studies conducted under the pediatric patent exclusivity laws "are yielding important information

---

[6] Included in the FDA Modernization Act of 1997, Section 505A. Renewed in 2002 as part of the Best Pharmaceuticals for Children Act, and again in the Pediatric Research Equity Act of 2007.

BOX 5-2
Knowledge Contributed by Studies Conducted Under
the Best Pharmaceuticals for Children Act (BPCA)
and the Pediatric Research Equity Act (PREA)

Pediatric Studies Support Safety and Efficacy

Insulin glulisine (Apidra), a recombinant, rapid-acting human insulin analog, was approved in 2004 for treatment of type 1 diabetes mellitus in adults, with a requirement for a study with children ages 5 to 17 years (Meyer, 2004). In 2008, on the basis of the findings of one previously submitted pharmacokinetic/pharmacodynamic study and one new safety and efficacy study, the Food and Drug Administration (FDA) approved use of the product by children ages 4 to 17 years, the period of peak onset for this disease (Gabry and Joffe, 2008).

Safe and Effective Dosing in Children Differs from Expectations for Youngest Children

Gabapentin (Neurontin) was first approved in 1993. The FDA requested studies under BPCA in 1999, and the drug was approved in 2000 as adjunctive treatment of partial seizures in children ages 3 years and older (Katz, 2000). Based on staff analyses of pharmacokinetic data, the FDA concluded that children under 5 years of age required higher than anticipated doses (Feeney, 2000). Findings from the study for the 3- to 12-year-old age group also led to a warning on the product's label about adverse neuropsychiatric events, such as concentration problems, hostility, and hyperactivity.

Drug Affects Growth and Development

Pegylated interferon alfa 2b (PegIntron) in combination with ribavirin (Rebetol) was approved in June 2008 for the treatment of chronic hepatitis C virus infection in patients ages 18 years or older, with deferral of PREA-required studies for children ages 3 years or older. In December 2008, after the required studies

---

to guide clinical care for children" (IOM, 2012c, p. 26). This committee summarized knowledge contributed by studies conducted under federal programs designed to increase research in children, including the pediatric patent exclusivity (see Box 5-2).

In addition, the pediatric patent exclusivity has contributed to researchers conducting more than 300 pediatric studies between 1997 and 2002 (Li et al., 2007; Milne, 2002). These studies have led to revised labeling of dosing, safety, efficacy, new pediatric formulations, and extended age limits for many of the studied drugs (Li et al., 2007; Rodriguez et

were submitted, the FDA approved labeling for use by that age group. The clinical review noted that "growth inhibition and hypothyroidism were two notable adverse reactions" and that they were being further evaluated in a 5-year follow-up study (Crewalk, 2008, p. 4). The review also noted that these adverse reactions presented less risk than the risk of untreated hepatitis C. The revised label included warnings about the impact of pediatric use on growth of the child.

Studies Support Different Dosing Calculation

Nevirapine (Viramune), which was first approved in 1996, was approved in 1998 for treatment of HIV infection in children ages 2 months of age to 16 years, with additional information submitted in 2002. The 2002 approval letter specifically required studies to determine dosing for younger groups. The information submitted by the sponsor in 2007 provided for dosing down to age 15 days and also provided data to support calculation of pediatric dosing based on body surface area rather than weight (Belew, 2008).

Risk-Benefit Assessment Does Not Support Pediatric Use

Omalizumab (Xolair) was approved in 2003 for treatment of moderate to severe persistent asthma in individuals 12 years of age or older. Although this approval occurred during a period when pediatric study requirements were not in effect, the FDA encouraged further pediatric studies and noted that pending legislation might require such studies (Risso, 2003). The sponsor submitted studies for the 6-to-11 age group in 2008. After the data were reviewed by FDA staff and considered in a meeting of the joint Pulmonary-Allergy, Pediatric, and Drug Safety and Risk Management Advisory Committee, the product's labeling was revised to include the statement "Considering the risk of anaphylaxis and malignancy seen in Xolair-treated patients ≥12 years old and the modest efficacy of Xolair in the pivotal pediatric study, the risk-benefit assessment does not support the use of Xolair in patients 6 to <12 years of age" (Genentech, 2010; Starke, 2009).

SOURCE: IOM, 2012c.

al., 2008). It is probable that patent exclusivity in cancer would lead to a similar increase in research conducted in older adults and individuals with multiple comorbidities, and to an increase in knowledge about how to treat this population. **Thus, the committee recommends that Congress amend patent law to provide patent extensions of up to 6 months for companies that conduct clinical trials of new cancer treatments in older adults or patients with multiple comorbidities (Recommendation 5).**

The committee is concerned about some of the known limitations of the patent extension program in pediatrics, but believes the need for more data in older adults with cancer and individuals with multiple comorbidities is so great that it justifies modeling this program in drugs used to treat older adults with cancer and individuals with multiple comorbidities. As described in the section on "How the Evidence Base for Cancer Care Decisions Is Generated," FDA registration trials are conducted for the narrow goal of bringing new treatments to the market. Alternative strategies that mandate the inclusion of older adults and patients with multiple comorbidities in FDA registration trials have serious limitations. Such a mandate could make it more challenging to determine the efficacy and safety of a new treatment. This could make drug development more expensive, potentially require larger trials, and delay or prevent new drugs from entering the market.

Some of the main criticisms of the pediatric exclusivity provisions are briefly summarized here. A recent review of the pediatric exclusivity provision noted that it is difficult to measure any improvements in children's health care that have resulted from the program (Kesselheim, 2011). The research conducted for the purpose of achieving a pediatric extension often has serious methodological limitations, including the only rare inclusion of drugs most frequently used by children. Most of the studies are conducted in populations of older pediatric patients (not children under the age of 6 or 2), and often at sites outside of the United States (Boots et al., 2007; Grieve et al., 2005; Pasquali et al., 2010).

The results of the research are often unpublished, and thus, not subject to peer review (Benjamin et al., 2009). When the research is published, it often focuses on findings substantively different from those highlighted in the FDA reviews and labeling changes (Benjamin et al., 2008, 2009).

Additionally, society has borne substantial costs from the delayed entry of less expensive generic versions of a drug onto the market. In a 2001 report to Congress, the FDA estimated the 20-year cost to consumers of the pediatric exclusivity to be $13.9 billion (FDA, 2001). A more recent study estimated the potential impact of the program on the U.S. Medicaid population across three classes of drugs (statins, angiotensin-converting-enzyme inhibitors, and selective serotonin reuptake inhibitors) to be $430 million over 18 months (Nelson et al., 2011). The high cost of patent extension is of particular concern when the higher drug prices are passed on to patients, because this could lead to reduced access and worse medication adherence during the extra 6 months of elevated prices (Kesselheim, 2011).

Due to the high price tag, the program has been criticized for overcompensating manufacturers (Kesselheim, 2011). The median cost of conducting clinical trials under this program was more than $12 million between 2002 and 2004, and the median net economic benefit to manufacturers was more than $134 million (Li et al., 2007). Another study found the ratio of net economic return to cost was 17 to 1 (Baker-Smith et al., 2008). Some of the limitations, however, may be preventable in a geriatric oncology exclusivity program by having stringent requirements on the types of clinical trials that qualify for market exclusivity.

Comparative Effectiveness Research

The need to include older adults and individuals with multiple co-morbidities in CER conducted by the NCI's NCTN and others is as press-ing as the need to study this population in regulatory trials. A systematic review of 345 phase 3 trials conducted by five NCI Cooperative Groups found that 57 percent of trials had no stratification by age and only 12 percent of studies had stratification of age greater than 65 years. Only one of the 345 studies was conducted exclusively in older adults (Kumar et al., 2007).

In another analysis of NCI-sponsored clinical trials between 1997 and 2000, 32 percent of the participants in phase 2 and 3 clinical trials were older adults, compared with 61 percent of individuals with new cancer diagnoses in the United States (Lewis et al., 2003). A study look-ing at SWOG (formerly the Southwest Oncology Group) treatment trials between 1993 and 1996 found that 25 percent of clinical trial participants were 65 years and older versus 63 percent of the overall population with cancer (Hutchins et al., 1999). Researchers' inclusion of individuals with comorbidities in clinical research is equally poor, despite the fact that many patients have comorbidities (Alecxih et al., 2010; Dhruva and Redberg, 2008; Tinetti and Studenski, 2011; Van Spall et al., 2007).

It is unclear if CER supported by other funders does better than the Cooperative Groups at including study populations in clinical research that are representative of the majority population who actually contract the disease being studied. AHRQ has identified older adults and indi-viduals with special health needs (e.g., chronic illness, disabilities, and end-of-life care needs) as priority populations, but no analysis has been conducted to assess whether its research includes representative popula-tions of older adults and individuals with comorbidities (AHRQ, 2011). Similarly, it is too early to determine the impact of PCORI-funded studies on the inclusion of older adults and individuals with comorbidities in research.

Thus, the committee recommends that the NCI, AHRQ, PCORI, and other CER funders require researchers evaluating the role of standard and novel interventions and technologies used in cancer care to include a plan to study a population that mirrors the age distribution and health risk profile of patients with the disease (Recommendation 5). This research should evaluate the efficacy, effectiveness, and toxicity of cancer interventions in these populations.

IMPROVING THE DEPTH OF INFORMATION COLLECTED

Researchers often primarily analyze only very narrow outcomes in clinical trials (e.g., progression-free survival, overall survival, toxicity) (Meropol, 2012). If the goal of clinical research is to improve the quality of cancer care, it is important to produce some of the types of evidence that would be most useful to patients and clinicians when making treatment decisions. For example, patients often want information about the estimated impact of a treatment regimen on their quality of life, functional status, symptoms, and overall experience with the disease, as well as information about other contextual factors (socioeconomic status, literacy, numeracy, language, culture, education, transportation, social supports, neighborhood, behavioral health, housing, functional and cognitive impairment, family capacity).

The PCORI methodology standards direct researchers to measure outcomes that patients "notice and care about;" however, there is currently a lack of consensus about which data are central to reaching this goal (Miriovsky et al., 2012; PCORI, 2012b). Researchers can use certain behavioral and patient data to make new discoveries regarding the benefits and harms of different treatments.

Because of the potential advantages of collecting a broader set of data during clinical trials to improve the quality of cancer care, the committee recommends that the NCI build on ongoing efforts and work with other federal agencies, PCORI, clinical and health services researchers, clinicians, and patients to develop a common set of data elements that captures patient-reported outcomes (PROs), relevant patient characteristics, and health behaviors that researchers should collect in randomized clinical trials and observational studies (Recommendation 6). The NCI could draw heavily on existing standardized formats for collecting data under many of the elements in national health population surveys (e.g., National Health Interview Survey, Behavioral Risk Factor Surveillance System) and in the NIH Toolbox, or develop new standards for use in cancer clinical trials (Ganz, 2012; NIH, 2012).

The committee recognizes that excessive data collection can reduce the overall quality of the data and increase the cost and duration of research, and that the added administrative burden can lead to reluctance by clinicians to participate in clinical research (Abrams et al., 2010; IOM, 2010b). However, the added benefits of collecting a broader set of data points during clinical research outweigh these drawbacks. Each data type that should be included in this broad set is discussed in the following sections: PROs, biomarkers, patient characteristics, behaviors, and cost. The challenge of standardizing data collected in electronic health records is discussed in Chapter 6.

Patient-Reported Outcomes

PROs can be defined as "any report of the status of a patient's health condition that comes directly from the patient, without interpretation of the patient's response by a clinician or anyone else" (FDA, 2009, p. 2). A PRO is measured using a self-report or an interview (if the interviewer records only the patient's response). PROs can include severity of symptoms, quality of life, functional status, adverse events, the stages of a disease, contextual factors, and other outcomes.

Evidence shows that cancer patients are capable and willing to self-report adverse events, and clinicians accept this information in the treatment decision-making process (Trotti et al., 2007). PROs are important because the outcomes that patients' report can be different from those collected by health care clinicians and researchers (Basch et al., 2006; Fromme et al., 2004). PROs provide additional information about treatment side effects and outcomes that are important to patients and can inform health care treatment decisions. They could be used to assess whether the cancer care delivery system is providing care that is concordant with patients' needs, preferences, and goals, as well as to assess the impact of providing a type of care on the quality and cost of care. They also have the potential to improve patient safety in clinical studies by identifying adverse events and outcomes that otherwise would go undetected (Basch et al., 2013).

A study that compared patients and clinicians' reporting across eight symptoms using a validated instrument found that clinicians failed to report about one-half of the symptoms identified by patients as adverse events. Similarly, the patients did not identify approximately one-half of the adverse events reported by the clinicians. The authors concluded that the clinicians' sensitivity and specificity in reporting adverse events of common chemotherapy are limited (Fromme et al., 2004).

The importance of PROs is widely accepted in the regulatory context. The FDA and the European Medicines Agency accept the approval of drugs with labeling claims based on PROs as endpoints of safety and efficacy. In 2006, the FDA issued guidelines on using PRO measures to support labeling claims (FDA, 2006) and published the Final PRO Guidance document in 2009 (FDA, 2009). The guidance states that PRO instruments must be based on an appropriate and clearly defined conceptual framework, which requires patient interviews, focus groups, literature reviews, and expert opinion.

The majority of adverse events that currently appear on medication labels are derived from clinicians' interpretations of a patient's experience in a clinical trial, as opposed to the patient's own report of his or her experience (Trotti et al., 2007). However, as mentioned above, research shows little agreement between the two types of reports, and clinicians often underestimate the severity of patients' symptoms and miss preventable adverse events (Atkinson et al., 2011; Fromm et al., 2009).

An example of a drug that recently had a label change based, in part, on PROs is Incyte Corporation's Jakafi ruxolitinib in treating myelofibrosis. Incyte Corporation measured patients' night sweats, itching, abdominal discomfort, pain under the ribs, early satiety, and bone or muscle pain when using the drug and found that the drug relieved these symptoms (McCallister and Usdin, 2011). However, this type of PRO evaluation and labeling outcome is the exception rather than the rule, and there is a great need for expanding the measurement of PROs in the context of drug development (Basch, 2013).

The NCI supports the use of PROs for identifying adverse events in clinical trials and considers understanding patients' reported experiences with their disease an important goal of research (Clauser et al., 2007). Most adverse events in cancer clinical trials are currently obtained, interpreted, and reported by clinicians using the NCI's Common Terminology Criteria for Adverse Events (CTCAE). However, in October 2008, the NCI issued a contract to develop a PRO version of CTCAE, known as the PRO-CTCAE. This project is not yet complete, but information regarding its development is available on the NCI website. The latest version of the PRO-CTCAE includes 81 symptoms appropriate for patient reporting, and its multiple language translations are being validated (NCI, 2012a). Similarly, NIH has developed the Patient Reported Outcomes Measurement Information System (PROMIS), which is a set of measures that capture patients' physical, mental, and social well-being but is not specific to cancer (NIH, 2013). The measures included in these tools could fulfill part of the committee's recommendation to develop common data elements that should be collected in all phase 3 trials. The NCI should use PROs to gather information from patients, including quality-of-life data, functional status, and adverse events.

Biomarkers, Patient Characteristics, and Behavioral Data

A recent IOM report recognized the growing need for correlative and translational studies that measure the relationship between biomarkers or other patient characteristics collected during clinical trials and health outcomes (IOM, 2010b). This research is important because it is increasingly recognized that patient characteristics and behaviors have an impact on cancer outcomes and will play an important role in personalized cancer treatment (Antoni et al., 2006; Goodwin et al., 2010). Examples of characteristics that impact patient outcomes in cancer include demographics (e.g., age, sex, race/ethnicity, marital status, education); individual genetics (see discussion in Chapter 2); functional status; comorbid conditions; behavioral risk factors (e.g., tobacco use, alcohol use, human immunodeficiency virus and human papillomavirus status, sedentary lifestyle, insomnia); medications and supplements; psychological health status; and physiological health status (e.g., inflammation, coagulation) (Ganz, 2012).

For example, tobacco exposure can influence drug metabolism, response to and toxicity of treatment, and the biological aggressiveness of cancer. Correlative research has led to the observation that individuals with non-small-cell lung cancer who never smoked have a significantly greater likelihood of benefiting from an epidermal growth factor receptor tyrosine kinase inhibitor than do individuals who have smoked (Faehling et al., 2010). However, despite the impact of this observation on clinical practice, most Cooperative Group trials do not collect data on participants' tobacco exposure as part of their clinical trials (Peters et al., 2012). Clinical researchers are also inconsistent in collecting other biomarker, patient characteristics, and behavioral data. The importance of this type of data is particularly salient in older adults with cancer because of the need to identify risk factors for treatment toxicity and to develop more complete geriatric assessment variables (see discussion on geriatric assessments in Chapter 2) (Extermann and Hurria, 2007; Extermann et al., 2012; Hurria et al., 2011).

Cost Data

As noted in Chapter 2, the cost of cancer care is spiraling out of control, yet there has been little effort to regularly collect cost data during clinical trials. Without this type of data, it is challenging to conduct cost-effectiveness analyses. Thus, policy makers cannot make informed decisions about addressing the unsustainable cost of care, and it is difficult for patients to take the cost of care into account in their medical decision-making process (see Chapter 3).

IMPROVING THE USE OF INFORMATION TECHNOLOGY

It is impractical to use a clinical trial to answer all research questions relevant to improving the quality of cancer care. The average cost of a large randomized clinical trial addressing a CER question ranges from $15 to $20 million (Holve and Pittman, 2011). In addition, clinical trials do not address all clinically relevant populations, limiting their generalizability. Clinical trials only cover a limited period of time and thus may not identify long-term side effects. They also often fail to make comparisons relevant to answering questions that are important to patients and clinicians (IOM, 2012a).

Multiple IOM reports have emphasized the need to match research questions with the most appropriate research method (IOM, 2008b, 2011a, 2012a). For example, clinical trials are valuable for answering questions about the efficacy of screening, preventive, and therapeutic interventions, while observational studies can answer questions about potential harms, long-term outcomes, and the use of interventions in real-world scenarios.

In Chapter 6, the committee recommends the development of a learning health care system for cancer, which is an IT system that continually and automatically collects and compiles information from clinical practice, disease registries, clinical trials, and other sources in order to deliver the best, most up-to-date care, personalized for each patient. One of the outcomes of this system would be an enormous clinical data resource that could be used for observational research. The potential for a learning cancer care system to improve research and the generation of new knowledge about cancer care is enormous.

A fully operational learning health care system would allow researchers to use data from electronic health records (EHRs), the SEER-Medicare database, Cooperative Group trials, FDA registration trials, cancer registries, and other sources to conduct systematic reviews and meta-analyses, pooled analyses of patient-level data from many clinical trials, and other types of observational and nonexperimental studies. It would also allow researchers to link patient-level data from multiple sources longitudinally and facilitate the surveillance of long-term side effects and health outcomes from various cancer care plans, as well as capture place of death.

In addition, implementation of a learning health care system would overcome many clinical trial limitations. It would provide researchers with access to data from a large, diverse, population (by gender, geography, ethnicity, age, education, and socioeconomic status), which could lead to the identification of subgroup variations. This would be particularly helpful in studying older adults with cancer because the learning health care system would include data on individuals with multiple comorbidities, concomitant medications, and those who are in the oldest age ranges.

A learning health care system would also benefit cancer research more broadly by providing data on off-label prescribing, which accounts for the majority of cancer treatments, as well as on new technologies and surgical techniques not subject to strict regulatory review (Abernethy et al., 2010;

Etheredge, 2010; IOM, 2010a, 2012a,b). It would also provide information on quality of life and functional status, which would be important to patients' decision making (see discussion in Chapter 3) if this information was regularly collected in clinical trials (see recommendation above on improving the depth of information collected in clinical research) and in EHRs.

The major limitation of this type of research is that data from many of these sources are not collected as systematically as data from clinical trials. As a result, there is the potential for bias and drawing erroneous conclusions. Researchers will need to develop analytic methods to adjust for these data limitations. In addition, this research cannot analyze interventions not already used in clinical practice and thus cannot serve as a substitute for premarket approval of new drugs, biologics, or devices (Armstrong, 2012). Implementation challenges, technical challenges, and ethical oversight challenges to achieving a learning health care system for cancer are discussed in Chapter 6.

SUMMARY AND RECOMMENDATIONS

Because a high-quality cancer care delivery system uses results from scientific research, such as clinical trials and CER, to inform medical decisions, the committee's conceptual framework (see Figure S-2) depicts the evidence base as supporting patient-clinician interactions. The committee envisions clinical research that gathers evidence of the benefits and harms of various treatment options, so that patients, in consultation with their clinicians, can make treatment decisions that are consistent with their needs, values, and preferences.

Currently, many studies are not supported by sufficient evidence. Additionally, research participants are often not representative of the population with the disease, which makes it difficult to generalize the research results to a specific patient. Another limitation of the current evidence base is that it frequently does not capture information about the impact of a treatment regimen on quality of life, functional and cognitive status, symptoms, and overall patient experience with the disease. Given that the majority of cancer patients are over 65 years and have comorbid conditions complicated by other health (e.g., physical and cognitive deficits) and social (e.g., limited or absent social support, low health literacy) risks, the committee is particularly concerned about the lack of clinical research focused on older adults and individuals with multiple chronic diseases.

Recommendation 5: Evidence-Based Cancer Care

Goal: Expand the breadth of data collected on cancer interventions for older adults and individuals with multiple comorbid conditions.

To accomplish this:

- The National Cancer Institute, the Agency for Healthcare Research and Quality, the Patient-Centered Outcomes Research Institute, and other comparative effectiveness research funders should require researchers evaluating the role of standard and novel interventions and technologies used in cancer care to include a plan to study a population that mirrors the age distribution and health risk profile of patients with the disease.
- Congress should amend patent law to provide patent extensions of up to 6 months for companies that conduct clinical trials of new cancer treatments in older adults or patients with multiple comorbidities.

Recommendation 6: Evidence-Based Cancer Care

Goal: Expand the depth of data available for assessing interventions.

To accomplish this:

- The National Cancer Institute should build on ongoing efforts and work with other federal agencies, the Patient-Centered Outcomes Research Institute, clinical and health services researchers, clinicians, and patients to develop a common set of data elements that captures patient-reported outcomes, relevant patient characteristics, and health behaviors that researchers should collect from randomized clinical trials and observational studies.

REFERENCES

Abernethy, A. P., L. M. Etheredge, P. A. Ganz, P. Wallace, R. R. German, C. Neti, P. B. Bach, and S. B. Murphy. 2010. Rapid-learning system for cancer care. *Journal of Clinical Oncology* 28(27):4268-4274.

Abrams, J., R. Erwin, G. Fyfe, and R. L. Schilsky. 2010. Data submission standards and evidence requirements. *Oncologist* 15(5):488-491.

AHRQ (Agency for Healthcare Research and Quality). 2011. *Special emphasis notice: AHRQ announces interest in priority populations research.* http://grants.nih.gov/grants/guide/notice-files/NOT-HS-11-014.html (accessed March 22, 2013).

————. 2013a. *Who is involved in the Effective Health Care Program.* http://www.effective healthcare.ahrq.gov/index.cfm/who-is-involved-in-the-effective-health-care-program1 (accessed July 1, 2013).

————. 2013b. *Search for research summaries, reviews, and reports.* http://www.effective healthcare.ahrq.gov/index.cfm/search-for-guides-reviews-and-reports (accessed July 1, 2013).

Alecxih, L., S. Shen, I. Chan, D. Taylor, and J. Drabek. 2010. *Individuals living in the community with chronic conditions and functional limitations: A closer look.* http://aspe.hhs.gov/daltcp/reports/2010/closerlook.pdf (accessed March 22, 2013).

Antoni, M. H., S. K. Lutgendorf, S. W. Cole, F. S. Dhabhar, S. E. Sephton, P. G. McDonald, M. Stefanek, and A. K. Sood. 2006. The influence of bio-behavioural factors on tumour biology: Pathways and mechanisms. *Nature Reviews. Cancer* 6(3):240-248.

Armstrong, K. 2012. Methods in comparative effectiveness research. *Journal of Clinical Oncology* 30(34):4208-4214.

Atkinson, T. M., Y. Li, C. W. Coffey, L. Sit, M. Shaw, D. Lavene, A. V. Bennett, M. Fruscione, L. Rogak, and J. Hay. 2011. Reliability of adverse symptom event reporting by clinicians. *Quality of Life Research*:1-6.

Baker-Smith, C. M., D. K. Benjamin, Jr., H. G. Grabowski, E. D. Reid, B. Mangum, J. V. Goldsmith, M. D. Murphy, R. Edwards, E. L. Eisenstein, J. Sun, R. M. Califf, and J. S. Li. 2008. The economic returns of pediatric clinical trials of antihypertensive drugs. *American Heart Journal* 156(4):682-688.

Basch, E. 2013. Toward patient-centered drug development in oncology. *New England Journal of Medicine* 369(5):397-400.

Basch, E., A. Iasonos, T. McDonough, A. Barz, A. Culkin, M. G. Kris, H. I. Scher, and D. Schrag. 2006. Patient versus clinician symptom reporting using the National Cancer Institute Common Terminology Criteria for Adverse Events: Results of a questionnaire-based study. *Lancet Oncology* 7(11):903-909.

Basch, E., P. Torda, and K. Adams. 2013. Standards for patient-reported outcome-based performance measures. *Journal of the American Medical Association* 310(2):139-140.

Belew, Y. 2008. *Clinical review for Viramune (nevirapine).* NDA 20636/20933. June 21. Silver Spring, MD: Food and Drug Administration. http://www.fda.gov/downloads/Drugs/DevelopmentApprovalProcess/DevelopmentResources/ucm072777.pdf (accessed March 23, 2012).

Benjamin, D. K., Jr., P. B. Smith, P. Jadhav, J. V. Gobburu, M. D. Murphy, V. Hasselblad, C. Baker-Smith, R. M. Califf, and J. S. Li. 2008. Pediatric antihypertensive trial failures: Analysis of end points and dose range. *Hypertension* 51(4):834-840.

Benjamin, D. K., Jr., P. B. Smith, M. J. Sun, M. D. Murphy, D. Avant, L. Mathis, W. Rodriguez, R. M. Califf, and J. S. Li. 2009. Safety and transparency of pediatric drug trials. *Archives of Pediatric & Adolescent Medicine* 163(12):1080-1086.

Boots, I., R. N. Sukhai, R. H. Klein, R. A. Holl, J. M. Wit, A. F. Cohen, and J. Burggraaf. 2007. Stimulation programs for pediatric drug research: Do children really benefit? *European Journal of Pediatrics* 166(8):849-855.

Cerreta, F., H. G. Eichler, and G. Rasi. 2012. Drug policy for an aging population: The European Medicines Agency's geriatric medicines strategy. *New England Journal of Medicine* 367(21):1972-1974.

Clancy, C., and F. S. Collins. 2010. Patient-Centered Outcomes Research Institute: The intersection of science and health care. *Science Translational Medicine* 2(37):37cm18.

Clauser, S. B., P. A. Ganz, J. Lipscomb, and B. B. Reeve. 2007. Patient-reported outcomes assessment in cancer trials: Evaluating and enhancing the payoff to decision making. *Journal of Clinical Oncology* 25(32):5049-5050.

Cox, K., and J. McGarry. 2003. Why patients don't take part in cancer clinical trials: An overview of the literature. *European Journal of Cancer Care (Engl)* 12(2):114-122.

Crewalk, J.-A. 2008. *Clinical review for PegIntron (peginterferon alfa-2b).* BLA 103949. December 8. Silver Spring, MD: Food and Drug Administration. http://www.fda.gov/downloads/Drugs/DevelopmentApprovalProcess/DevelopmentResources/UCM171341.pdf (accessed March 23, 2012).

Dhruva, S. S., and R. F. Redberg. 2008. Variations between clinical trial participants and Medicare beneficiaries in evidence used for Medicare national coverage decisions. *Archives of Internal Medicine* 168(2):136-140.

EDICT (Eliminating Disparities in Clinical Trials). 2008. *The EDICT project: Policy recommendations to eliminate disparities in clinical trials.* Houston, TX: EDICT Project.

El Dib, R. P., A. N. Atallah, and R. B. Andriolo. 2007. Mapping the Cochrane evidence for decision making in health care. *Journal of Evaluation in Clinical Practice* 13:689-692.

Etheredge, L. M. 2010. Creating a high-performance system for comparative effectiveness research. *Health Affairs (Millwood)* 29(10):1761-1767.

Extermann, M., and A. Hurria. 2007. Comprehensive geriatric assessment for older patients with cancer. *Journal of Clinical Oncology* 25(14):1824-1831.

Extermann, M., I. Boler, R. R. Reich, G. H. Lyman, R. H. Brown, J. DeFelice, R. M. Levine, E. T. Lubiner, P. Reyes, F. J. Schreiber, 3rd, and L. Balducci. 2012. Predicting the risk of chemotherapy toxicity in older patients: The Chemotherapy Risk Assessment Scale for High-age Patients (crash) score. *Cancer* 118(13):3377-3386.

Faehling, M., R. Eckert, S. Kuom, T. Kamp, K. M. Stoiber, and C. Schumann. 2010. Benefit of erlotinib in patients with non-small-cell lung cancer is related to smoking status, gender, skin rash and radiological response but not to histology and treatment line. *Oncology* 78(3-4):249-258.

FDA (Food and Drug Administration). 1988. *Guideline for the format and content of the clinical and statistical sections of an application.* http://www.fda.gov/downloads/Drugs/GuidanceComplianceRegulatoryInformation/Guidances/UCM071665.pdf (accessed November 30, 2012).

———. 1989. *Guidance for industry. Guidelines for the study of drugs likely to be used in the elderly.* http://www.fda.gov/downloads/Drugs/GuidanceComplianceRegulatoryInformation/Guidances/ucm072048.pdf (accessed November 30, 2012).

———. 1998. *FDAMA: Women and minorities guidance requirements.* http://www.fda.gov/downloads/Drugs/GuidanceComplianceRegulatoryInformation/Guidances/ucm080616.pdf (accessed July 1, 2013).

———. 2001. *The pediatric exclusivity provision: January 2001 status report to Congress.* http://www.fda.gov/downloads/drugs/developmentapprovalprocess/developmentresources/ucm049915.pdf (accessed December 3, 2012).

———. 2006. Drug administration: Guidance for industry: Patient-reported outcome measures—use in medical product development to support labeling claims. Food and Drug Administration. *Health Quality of Life Outcomes* 4:79.

———. 2009. *Guidance for industry. Patient-reported outcome measures: Use in medical product development to support labeling claims.* http://www.fda.gov/downloads/Drugs/GuidanceComplianceRegulatoryInformation/Guidances/UCM193282.pdf (accessed December 3, 2012).

———. 2012a. *Device approvals and clearances.* http://www.fda.gov/medicaldevices/productsandmedicalprocedures/deviceapprovalsandclearances/default.htm (accessed November 29, 2012).

———. 2012b. *The FDA's drug review process: Ensuring drugs are safe and effective.* http://www.fda.gov/Drugs/ResourcesForYou/Consumers/ucm143534.htm (accessed November 29, 2012).

————. 2012c. *Guidance for industry. E7 studies in support of special populations: Geriatrics. Questions and answers.* http://www.fda.gov/downloads/Drugs/GuidanceCompliance RegulatoryInformation/Guidances/UCM189544.pdf (accessed November 30, 2012).

Feeney, J. 2000. *Medical review for Neurontin (gabapentin).* NDA 21216. October 6. Silver Spring, MD: Food and Drug Administration. http://www.accessdata.fda.gov/drugsat fda_docs/nda/2000/21- 16.pdf_Neurontin_Medr_P1.pdf (accessed March 23, 2012).

Fromme, E. K., K. M. Eilers, M. Mori, Y. C. Hsieh, and T. M. Beer. 2004. How accurate is clinician reporting of chemotherapy adverse effects? A comparison with patient-reported symptoms from the quality-of-life questionnaire c30. *Journal of Clinical Oncology* 22(17):3485-3490.

Gabry, K. E., and H. V. Joffe. 2008. *Clinical review of Apidra (insulin glulisine).* NDA 21629. October 2. Silver Spring, MD: Food and Drug Administration. http://www.fda.gov/downloads/Drugs/DevelopmentApprovalProcess/DevelopmentResources/ucm072460.pdf (accessed March 23, 2012).

Ganz, P. A. 2012. Host factors, behaviors, and clinical trials: Opportunities and challenges. *Journal of Clinical Oncology* 30(23):2817-2819.

GAO (Government Accountability Office). 2007. *Elderly persons in clinical drug trials.* http://www.gao.gov/assets/100/95182.pdf (accessed December 10, 2012).

Genentech. 2010. *Prescribing information for Xolair (omalizumab).* South San Francisco, CA: Genentech. http://www.gene.com/gene/products/information/pdf/xolair-prescribing. pdf (accessed March 23, 2012).

Goodwin, P. J., J. A. Meyerhardt, and S. D. Hursting. 2010. Host factors and cancer outcome. *Journal of Clinical Oncology* 28(26):4019-4021.

Grieve, J., J. Tordoff, D. Reith, and P. Norris. 2005. Effect of the pediatric exclusivity provision on children's access to medicines. *British Journal of Clinical Pharmacology* 59(6):730-735.

Hahn, O. M., and R. L. Schilsky. 2012. Randomized controlled trials and comparative effectiveness research. *Journal of Clinical Oncology* 30(34):4194-4201.

Herrera, A. P., S. A. Snipes, D. W. King, I. Torres-Vigil, D. S. Goldberg, and A. D. Weinberg. 2010. Disparate inclusion of older adults in clinical trials: Priorities and opportunities for policy and practice change. *American Journal of Public Health* 100 (Suppl 1):S105-S112.

Holve, E., and P. Pittman. 2011. The cost and volume of comparative effectiveness research. In *Learning what works: Infrastructure required for comparative effectiveness research (workshop summary)*, edited by L. Olsen, C. Grossman, and J. M. McGinnis. Washington, DC: The National Academies Press. Pp. 89-96.

Hurria, A., K. Togawa, S. G. Mohile, C. Owusu, H. D. Klepin, C. P. Gross, S. M. Lichtman, A. Gajra, S. Bhatia, V. Katheria, S. Klapper, K. Hansen, R. Ramani, M. Lachs, F. L. Wong, and W. P. Tew. 2011. Predicting chemotherapy toxicity in older adults with cancer: A prospective multicenter study. *Journal of Clinical Oncology* 29(25):3457-3465.

Hutchins, L. F., J. M. Unger, J. J. Crowley, C. A. Coltman, Jr., and K. S. Albain. 1999. Underrepresentation of patients 65 years of age or older in cancer-treatment trials. *New England Journal of Medicine* 341(27):2061-2067.

IOM (Institute of Medicine). 2008a. *Improving the quality of cancer clinical trials: Workshop summary.* Washington, DC: The National Academies Press.

————. 2008b. *Knowing what works in health care: A roadmap for the nation.* Washington, DC: The National Academies Press.

————. 2009a. *Initial national priorities for comparative effectiveness research.* Washington, DC: The National Academies Press.

————. 2009b. *Multi-center phase III clinical trials and NCI cooperative groups: Workshop summary.* Washington, DC: The National Academies Press.

————. 2010a. *A foundation for evidence-driven practice: A rapid learning system for cancer care: Workshop summary.* Washington, DC: The National Academies Press.

———. 2010b. *A national cancer clinical trials system for the 21st century: Reinvigorating the NCI Cooperative Group Program.* Washington, DC: The National Academies Press.

———. 2011a. *Finding what works in health care: Standards for systematic reviews.* Washington, DC: The National Academies Press.

———. 2011b. *Medical devices and the public's health: The FDA 510(k) clearance process at 35 years.* Washington, DC: The National Academies Press.

———. 2012a. *Best care at lower cost: The path to continously learning health care in America.* Washington, DC: The National Academies Press.

———. 2012b. *Informatics needs and challenges in cancer research: Workshop summary.* Washington, DC: The National Academies Press.

———. 2012c. *Safe and effective medicines for children: Pediatric studies conducted under the Best Pharmaceuticals for Children Act and the Pediatric Research Equity Act.* Washington, DC: The National Academies Press.

———. 2013. *Delivering affordable cancer care in the 21st century: Workshop summary.* Washington, DC: The National Academies Press.

IOM and NRC (National Research Council). 1999. *Ensuring quality cancer care.* Washington, DC: National Academy Press.

Javid, S. H., J. M. Unger, J. R. Gralow, C. M. Moinpour, A. J. Wozniak, J. W. Goodwin, P. N. Lara, Jr., P. A. Williams, L. F. Hutchins, C. C. Gotay, and K. S. Albain. 2012. A prospective analysis of the influence of older age on physician and patient decision-making when considering enrollment in breast cancer clinical trials (SWOG S0316). *Oncologist* 17(9):1180-1190.

Katz, R. G. 2000. *Approval letter for Neurontin (gabapentin).* NDA 21216/20235/20882/21129. October 12. Silver Spring, MD: Food and Drug Administration. http://www.accessdata. fda.gov/drugsatfda_docs/nda/2000/21-216.pdf_Neurontin_Approv.pdf (accessed April 3, 2012).

Kemeny, M. M., B. L. Peterson, A. B. Kornblith, H. B. Muss, J. Wheeler, E. Levine, N. Bartlett, G. Fleming, and H. J. Cohen. 2003. Barriers to clinical trial participation by older women with breast cancer. *Journal of Clinical Oncology* 21(12):2268-2275.

Kesselheim, A. S. 2011. An empirical review of major legislation affecting drug development: Past experiences, effects, and unintended consequences. *Milbank Quarterly* 89(3):450-502.

Kornblith, A. B., M. Kemeny, B. L. Peterson, J. Wheeler, J. Crawford, N. Bartlett, G. Fleming, S. Graziano, H. Muss, and H. J. Cohen. 2002. Survey of oncologists' perceptions of barriers to accrual of older patients with breast carcinoma to clinical trials. *Cancer* 95(5):989-996.

Kumar, A., H. P. Soares, L. Balducci, and B. Djulbegovic. 2007. Treatment tolerance and efficacy in geriatric oncology: A systematic review of phase III randomized trials conducted by five National Cancer Institute-sponsored cooperative groups. *Journal of Clinical Oncology* 25(10):1272-1276.

Last, J. M., ed. 1995. *A dictionary of epidemiology.* 3rd ed. New York: Oxford University Press.

Lewis, J. H., M. L. Kilgore, D. P. Goldman, E. L. Trimble, R. Kaplan, M. J. Montello, M. G. Housman, and J. J. Escarce. 2003. Participation of patients 65 years of age or older in cancer clinical trials. *Journal of Clinical Oncology* 21(7):1383-1389.

Li, J. S., E. L. Eisenstein, H. G. Grabowski, E. D. Reid, B. Mangum, K. A. Schulman, J. V. Goldsmith, M. D. Murphy, R. M. Califf, and D. K. Benjamin, Jr. 2007. Economic return of clinical trials performed under the pediatric exclusivity program. *Journal of the American Medical Association* 297(5):480-488.

Lyman, G. H., and M. Levine. 2012. Comparative effectiveness research in oncology: An overview. *Journal of Clinical Oncology* 30(34):4181-4184.

McCallister, E., and S. Usdin. 2011. A PROfessional trial. *BioCentury on Business* 19(49): A1-A4.

Meropol, N. J. 2012. Comparative effectiveness research to inform medical decisions: The need for common language. *Journal of Clinical Oncology* 30:1-2.

Meropol, N. J., D. Schrag, T. J. Smith, T. M. Mulvey, R. M. Langdon, Jr., D. Blum, P. A. Ubel, and L. E. Schnipper. 2009. American Society of Clinical Oncology guidance statement: The cost of cancer care. *Journal of Clinical Oncology* 27(23):3868-3874.

Meyer, R. 2004. *Approval letter for Apidra (insulin glulisine (rDNA origin)).* NDA 21629. April 16. Silver Spring, MD: Food and Drug Administration. http://www.accessdata.fda.gov/drugsatfda_docs/appletter/2004/21629ltr.pdf (accessed April 3, 2012).

Milne, C. P. 2002. Exploring the frontiers of law and science: FDAMA's pediatric studies incentive. *Food Drug Law Journal* 57(3):491-517.

Miriovsky, B. J., L. N. Shulman, and A. P. Abernethy. 2012. Importance of health information technology, electronic health records, and continuously aggregating data to comparative effectiveness research and learning health care. *Journal of Clinical Oncology* 30(34):4243-4248.

NCI (National Cancer Institute). 2012a. *Patient-reported outcomes version of the common terminology criteria for adverse events (pro-ctcae).* http://outcomes.cancer.gov/tools/pro-ctcae_fact_sheet.pdf (accessed March, 2012).

———. 2012b. *Prioritization/scientific quality initiatives.* Place Published. http://transforming trials.cancer.gov/initiatives/ctwg/prioritization (accessed December 6, 2012).

———. 2012c. *Transforming the NCI clinical trial enterprise.* http://transformingtrials.cancer.gov/initiatives/overview (accessed December 6, 2012).

Nelson, R. E., C. McAdam-Marx, M. L. Evans, R. Ward, B. Campbell, D. Brixner, and J. Lafleur. 2011. Patent extension policy for paediatric indications: An evaluation of the impact within three drug classes in a state Medicaid program. *Applied Health Economics and Health Policy* 9(3):171-181.

NIH (National Institutes of Health). 2001. *NIH policy and guidelines on the inclusion of women and minorities as subjects in clinical research.* http://grants.nih.gov/grants/guide/notice-files/NOT-OD-02-001.html (accessed November 30, 2012).

———. 2012. *NIH Toolbox for the Assessment of Neurological and Behavioral Function.* http://www.nihtoolbox.org/Pages/default.aspx (accessed July 3, 2013).

———. 2013. PROMIS® overview. http://www.nihpromis.org/about/overview (accessed July 3, 2013).

Pasquali, S. K., D. S. Burstein, D. K. Benjamin, Jr., P. B. Smith, and J. S. Li. 2010. Globalization of pediatric research: Analysis of clinical trials completed for pediatric exclusivity. *Pediatrics* 126(3):e687-e692.

PCORI (Patient-Centered Outcomes Research Institute). 2012a. *About us.* http://www.pcori.org/about-us/landing (accessed November 29, 2012).

———. 2012b. *PCORI methodology standards.* http://www.pcori.org/assets/PCORI-Methodology-Standards1.pdf (accessed July 1, 2013).

Peters, E. N., E. Torres, B. A. Toll, K. M. Cummings, E. R. Gritz, A. Hyland, R. S. Herbst, J. R. Marshall, and G. W. Warren. 2012. Tobacco assessment in actively accruing National Cancer Institute Cooperative Group Program clinical trials. *Journal of Clinical Oncology* 30(23):2869-2875.

Ramsey, S. D., S. D. Sullivan, S. D. Reed, Y. C. Tina Shih, K. Schaecher, R. Dhanda, D. Patt, K. Pendergrass, M. Walker, J. Malin, L. Schwartzberg, K. Neumann, E. Yu, A. Ravelo, and A. Small. 2013. Oncology comparative effectiveness research: A multistakeholder perspective on principles for conduct and reporting. *Oncologist* 18(6):760-767.

Risso, S. T. 2003. *Approval letter for Xolair (omalizumab)*. BLA 103976/0. June 20. Silver Spring, MD: Food and Drug Administration. http://www.accessdata.fda.gov/drugsatfda_ocs/appletter/2003/omalgen062003L.htm (accessed April 3, 2012).

Rodriguez, W., A. Selen, D. Avant, C. Chaurasia, T. Crescenzi, G. Gieser, J. Di Giacinto, S. M. Huang, P. Lee, L. Mathis, D. Murphy, S. Murphy, R. Roberts, H. C. Sachs, S. Suarez, V. Tandon, and R. S. Uppoor. 2008. Improving pediatric dosing through pediatric initiatives: What we have learned. *Pediatrics* 121(3):530-539.

Scher, K. S., and A. Hurria. 2012. Under-representation of older adults in cancer registration trials: Known problem, little progress. *Journal of Clinical Oncology* 30(17):2036-2038.

Schilsky, R. L. 2013. Publicly funded clinical trials and the future of cancer care. *Oncologist* 18(2):232-238.

Somkin, C. P., A. Altschuler, L. Ackerson, A. M. Geiger, S. M. Greene, J. Mouchawar, J. Holup, L. Fehrenbacher, A. Nelson, A. Glass, J. Polikoff, S. Tishler, C. Schmidt, T. Field, and E. Wagner. 2005. Organizational barriers to physician participation in cancer clinical trials. *American Journal of Managed Care* 11(7):413-421.

Starke, P. 2009. *Clinical review for Xolair (omalizumab)*. BLA 103976/5149. December 4. Silver Spring, MD: Food and Drug Administration. http://www.fda.gov/downloads/Drugs/DevelopmentApprovalProcess/DevelopmentResources/UCM202179.pdf (accessed April 3, 2012).

Talarico, L., G. Chen, and R. Pazdur. 2004. Enrollment of elderly patients in clinical trials for cancer drug registration: A 7-year experience by the U.S. Food and Drug Administration. *Journal of Clinical Oncology* 22(22):4626-4631.

Tinetti, M. E., and S. A. Studenski. 2011. Comparative effectiveness research and patients with multiple chronic conditions. *New England Journal of Medicine* 364(26):2478-2481.

Townsley, C. A., R. Selby, and L. L. Siu. 2005. Systematic review of barriers to the recruitment of older patients with cancer onto clinical trials. *Journal of Clinical Oncology* 23(13):3112-3124.

Trimble, E. L., C. L. Carter, D. Cain, B. Freidlin, R. S. Ungerleider, and M. A. Friedman. 1994. Representation of older patients in cancer treatment trials. *Cancer* 74(7 Suppl):2208-2214.

Trotti, A., A. D. Colevas, A. Setser, and E. Basch. 2007. Patient-reported outcomes and the evolution of adverse event reporting in oncology. *Journal of Clinical Oncology* 25(32):5121-5127.

Van Spall, H. G., A. Toren, A. Kiss, and R. A. Fowler. 2007. Eligibility criteria of randomized controlled trials published in high-impact general medical journals: A systematic sampling review. *Journal of the American Medical Association* 297(11):1233-1240.

Villas Boas, P. J., R. S. Spagnuolo, A. Kamegasawa, L. G. Braz, A. Polachini do Valle, E. C. Jorge, H. H. Yoo, A. J. Cataneo, I. Correa, F. B. Fukushima, P. do Nascimento, N. S. Modolo, M. S. Teixeira, E. I. de Oliveira Vidal, S. R. Daher, and R. El Dib. 2012. Systematic reviews showed insufficient evidence for clinical practice in 2004: What about in 2011? The next appeal for the evidence-based medicine age. *Journal of Evaluating Clinical Practice* 19(4):633-637.

6

A Learning Health Care Information Technology System for Cancer

Information technology (IT) is a key requirement for implementing the components of the committee's conceptual framework for a high-quality cancer care delivery system. Health IT[1] has an important role to play in improving the quality of cancer care delivery, patient health, cancer research, quality measurement, and performance improvement. In the committee's diagram of its conceptual framework (see Figure S-2), IT supports patient-clinician interactions by providing patients and clinicians with the information and tools necessary to make well-informed medical decisions. Health IT plays a critical role in developing the evidence base from research (e.g., clinical trials and comparative effectiveness studies) and capturing data from real-world settings that researchers can then analyze to generate new knowledge. Further, health systems can use health IT to collect and report quality metrics data and to facilitate the implementation of performance improvement initiatives, and it allows payers to identify and reward high-quality care.

The role of health IT has been transformed and greatly expanded since the publication of the Institute of Medicine's (IOM's) 1999 report on the quality of cancer care, which discussed a limited role for health IT in collecting quality metrics data (IOM and NRC, 1999). Several more recent IOM reports have emphasized the potential for health IT to improve the

---

[1] The Institute of Medicine has defined health IT as a broad range of products. "It encompasses a technical system of computers and software that operates in the context of a larger sociotechnical system—a collection of hardware and software working in concert within an organization that includes people, processes, and technology" (IOM, 2011b, p. 2).

quality of care. In *Crossing the Quality Chasm*, the IOM recommended "a renewed national commitment to building an information infrastructure to support health care delivery, consumer health, quality measurement and improvement, public accountability, clinical and health services research, and clinical education" (IOM, 2001, p. 17). In *Best Care at Lower Cost: The Path to Continuously Learning Health Care in America* (hereinafter referred to as the *Best Care* consensus report), the IOM concluded that advances in health IT could improve many features of the health care system, including patient-clinician communication, clinical decision support, capturing the patient experience, population surveillance, planning and evaluation, and the generation of knowledge (IOM, 2012a).

A number of other organizations have also elaborated on the important role of health IT in care delivery and research, citing improvements in patient-centeredness, health outcomes, cost savings, safety, public health monitoring, and the conduct of clinical trials (AHRQ, 2012; Hillestad et al., 2005; Kellermann and Jones, 2013; PCAST, 2010; RAND Health, 2005). The American Society of Clinical Oncology (ASCO) envisions that by 2030 health IT will be the major mechanism for collecting, analyzing, and learning from "big data" in order to drive change in the delivery of care (ASCO, 2013b).

Several national events have pushed the health care sector toward the adoption of health IT. In his 2004 State of the Union Address, President George W. Bush announced the national goal of "wider use of electronic records and other health information technology, to help control costs and reduce dangerous medical errors" (Bush, 2004, p. 344). He followed this announcement with an Executive Order establishing the Office of the National Coordinator for Health Information Technology (ONC), which is charged with overseeing a nationwide effort to create an IT-enabled health care system (ONC, 2013a). The Health Information Technology for Economic and Clinical Health (HITECH) Act of 2009[2] mandated the continuation of ONC and provided billions of dollars in incentives for clinicians and hospitals to adopt electronic health records (EHRs).

Many of the anticipated gains in the quality of care from health IT, however, have been slow to materialize. A National Research Council report found that the "nation faces a health care information technology chasm that is analogous to the quality chasm highlighted by the IOM over the past decade" (NRC, 2009, p. 5). Clinicians' and hospitals' adoption of health IT has been slow, despite the incentives created by the HITECH Act (Kellermann and Jones, 2013), and the EHRs that clinicians use lag behind technological advances in other fields (Mandl and Kohane, 2012).

---

[2] Title XIII of the American Recovery and Reinvestment Act of 2009, Public Law 111:5, 111th Cong., 1st sess. (February. 17, 2009).

Patients have also failed to take full advantage of the benefits of health IT in managing their care (Yamin et al., 2011).

In organizations that have implemented health IT, clinicians have sometimes resisted investing the time and effort necessary to master the use of the technology. Originally designed for billing and coding purposes, health IT systems have not been integrated efficiently into clinical care, do not facilitate the coordination of care, and the need to customize local systems has created a situation where health IT systems cannot communicate with each other (Bitton et al., 2012; Campbell et al., 2009; Cimino, 2013; Kellermann and Jones, 2013; Mandl and Kohane, 2012; McDonnell et al., 2010; Yasnoff et al., 2013). Many of these systems are inflexible and thus are unable to adapt to the changing needs of a modern health care system (NRC, 2009). In addition, the promised cost savings from implementing health IT have not been fully realized (Kellermann and Jones, 2013). These problems are especially challenging in cancer care, which involves a complex disease, multiple clinicians, and complex treatment decisions (see Chapter 1 for further discussion of the unique characteristics of cancer care).

This chapter presents the committee's vision for a learning health care system that uses IT to improve the quality of cancer care. The chapter focuses on components of IT that support a learning health care system. Other topics relevant to the use of IT in improving the quality of cancer care are discussed elsewhere in this report. Patient and clinicians' use of web-based information and decision aids is discussed in Chapter 3 and telemedicine is discussed in Chapter 4; a more general discussion of health IT is outside the scope of this report.

The first section of this chapter provides a description of the committee's vision and outlines how health IT can meet the needs of all of the stakeholders discussed throughout this report, including patients, clinicians, researchers, quality metrics developers, and payers. Subsequent sections describe the challenges to creating a health IT system that meets stakeholders' needs, as well as potential paths to implementation. Much of the evidence base for this chapter is derived from a large body of previous work conducted by the IOM on a learning health care system, including several workshop summaries produced by the Roundtable on Value & Science-Driven Health Care and the National Cancer Policy Forum, as well as the recent *Best Care* consensus report (IOM, 2007, 2011a, 2012a,b). In addition, the committee conducted a literature search, from 1999 to the present, for articles relating to health IT in cancer care.[3] It also solicited

---

[3] The literature search was conducted by Amy McLeod, Administrative Fellow, The University of Texas MD Anderson Cancer Center.

input from several professionals knowledgeable about health IT.[4] The committee's recommendation on health IT addresses the identified gaps.

THE VISION

The committee's vision for health IT in a high-quality cancer care system calls for a learning health care IT system. The concept of a learning health care system gained prominence in 2007 (Eddy, 2007; Etheredge, 2007; Kupersmith et al., 2007; Liang, 2007; Lumpkin, 2007; Neumann, 2007; Pawlson, 2007; Perlin and Kupersmith, 2007; Platt, 2007; Slutsky, 2007; Stewart et al., 2007; Tunis et al., 2007; Wallace, 2007). The IOM subsequently explored the development and application of a learning health care system for improving the quality of care (IOM, 2007, 2010, 2012a,b). A learning health care system can be described as a system that:

> Uses advances in IT to continuously and automatically collect and compile from clinical practice, disease registries, clinical trials, and other sources of information, the evidence needed to deliver the best, most up-to-date care that is personalized for each patient. That evidence is made available as rapidly as possible to users of a [learning health care system], which include patients, physicians, academic institutions, hospitals, insurers, and public health agencies. A [learning health care system] ensures that this data-rich system learns routinely and iteratively by analyzing captured data, generating evidence, and implementing new insights into subsequent care. (IOM, 2010, p. 7 [adapted from Etheredge, 2007])

Thus, a learning health care system uses IT to "learn" by collecting data on care outcomes and cost in a systematic manner, analyzing the captured data both retrospectively and through prospective studies, implementing the knowledge gained from these analyses into clinical practice, evaluating outcomes of the changes in care, and generating new hypotheses to test and implement in clinical care (Abernethy et al., 2010).

There are several distinguishing characteristics of a learning health care system. Foremost, clinical practice and clinical research would be intimately linked. The flow of information would not be linear from clinical research to clinical practice; it would be circular, with information from clinical practice feeding back to clinical researchers in order to generate new knowledge and

---

[4] John Frenzel, Chief Medical Information Officer, The University of Texas MD Anderson Cancer Center; Daniel R. Masys, Affiliate Professor, Biomedical and Health Informatics, University of Washington; Stephen Palmer, Director, Office of e-Health Coordination, Texas Health and Human Services Commission; Adam Schickedanz, IOM Fellow and Pediatrics Resident, University of California, San Francisco; and Peter Yu, Director of Cancer Research, Palo Alto Medical Foundation.

hypotheses for testing. The process of developing new knowledge would be built directly into the health care delivery system. A learning health care system would be designed to expect and accommodate a continuous process for updating what constitutes best evidence and clinical practices.

To support this ongoing process, a learning health care system would facilitate the collection and analysis of big datasets, including genomics data and other complex biomarkers. It would promote the rapid translation of evidence into clinical practice via clinical decision support for clinicians. In addition, a learning health care system would provide tools that engage and empower patients in making decisions about their own care. The achievement of these aims would require payers to create reimbursement incentives that support a system of learning and a health care system that adopts a culture of learning (IOM, 2007, 2010, 2012a). Table 6-1 summarizes fundamental characteristics of the ideal learning health care system.

TABLE 6-1 Characteristics of a Learning Health Care System

Science and Informatics
> *Real-time access to knowledge* – A learning health care system continuously and reliably captures, curates, and delivers the best available evidence to guide, support, tailor, and improve clinical decision making and care safety and quality.
> *Digital capture of the care experience* – A learning health care system captures the care experience on digital platforms for real-time generation and application of knowledge for care improvement.

Patient-Clinician Partnership
> *Engaged, empowered patients* – A learning health care system is anchored in patient needs and perspectives, and promotes the inclusion of patients, families, and other caregivers as vital members of the continuously learning care team.

Incentives
> *Incentives aligned for value* – In a learning health care system, incentives are actively aligned to encourage continuous improvement, identify and reduce waste, and reward high-value care.
> *Full transparency* – A learning health care system systematically monitors the safety, quality, processes, prices, costs, and outcomes of care, and makes information available for care improvement, informed choices, and decision making by clinicians, patients, and their families.

Culture
> *Leadership-instilled culture of learning* – A learning health care system is stewarded by leadership committed to a culture of teamwork, collaboration, and adaptability in support of continuous learning as a core aim.
> *Supportive system competencies* – In a learning health care system, complex care operations and processes are constantly refined through ongoing team training and skill building, systems analysis and information development, and creation of the feedback loops for continuous learning and system improvement.

SOURCE: IOM, 2012a, p. 138.

Many elements which are essential to a learning health care system are already in place for cancer care (Abernethy et al., 2010; IOM, 2010). As mentioned above, the HITECH Act created new incentives for physicians and hospitals to adopt EHRs, which are "real-time patient-centered records . . . [that] contain information about a patient's medical history, diagnoses, medications, immunization dates, allergies, radiology images, and lab and test results" (ONC, 2013d). The Centers for Medicare & Medicaid Services (CMS) is developing meaningful use standards to ensure that EHRs are not just digital versions of paper medical charts that statically record information, but rather, information systems that support clinical decision making, advance clinical processes and workflow, and facilitate data capture and sharing between clinicians and health organizations (ONC, 2013e; Yu, 2011).

Each meaningful use stage requires more demanding standards for EHR use: collecting and using data (Stage 1); using health IT to improve and coordinate care (Stage 2); and capitalizing on clinical decision support and data collection to improve health outcomes (Stage 3) (ONC, 2013e). Stage 1 of meaningful use has been fully implemented by the clinicians and hospitals participating in the CMS program. Clinicians and hospitals will have to comply with Stage 2 starting in 2014, and the comment period for Stage 3 has ended, with Stage 3 standards scheduled to be implemented in 2016. In response to these standards, many academic and community cancer centers are implementing EHR systems that will ultimately enable them to collect data in real-time on every patient.

There are numerous other potential sources of data for a learning health care system in cancer. These include cancer registries, which capture important information on new cancer diagnoses, including the incidence and types of cancer, the anatomic location, stage at diagnosis, planned first course of treatment, and outcome of treatment and clinical management. This information is somewhat limited (i.e., registries only capture a narrow range of health outcomes, initial treatments, and a small segment of the cancer patient population), but could be broadened through a learning health care system. Some of the major cancer registries in the United States include (1) the National Cancer Institute's (NCI's) Surveillance, Epidemiology, and End Results program, which captures cancer incidence and survival data from 28 percent of the U.S. population using data provided by high-quality state and local cancer registries; (2) the Centers for Disease Control and Prevention's (CDC's) National Program of Cancer Registries, which supports statewide, population-based cancer registries from 45 states and the District of Columbia, Puerto Rico, and the U.S. Pacific Island jurisdictions, and covers 96 percent of the population; and (3) the Commission on Cancer's (CoC's) National Cancer Database, which aggregates cancer registry data from approximately 1,500 CoC-accredited institutions (ACoS, 2013; CDC, 2012; NCI, 2013c).

A learning health care system for cancer care would also be supported by a robust infrastructure for clinical trials on cancer; namely, the NCI National Clinical Trials Network (NCI, 2013d). Data from these trials could feed into a learning health care system to provide insights into new and existing cancer treatments. In addition, many biorepositories for cancer are linked with clinical data, genetic data, and environmental data, which could generate new knowledge in a learning health care system (Etheredge, 2013).

A learning health care system for cancer care, as envisioned by the committee, does not yet exist. There are, however, many ongoing efforts to develop prototypes and small-scale learning health care systems that will help demonstrate that the committee's vision is feasible. Table 6-2 provides a description of several ongoing efforts to develop this type of system: CancerLinQ and the Sentinel Initiative are national efforts to create a learning health care system, and Kaiser Permanente's HealthConnect is an example of a learning health care system within an integrated health care organization.

A number of other integrated health care organizations are also creating learning health care systems, including the Department of Veterans Affairs, Intermountain Healthcare, and Group Health (Greene et al., 2012; Starr, 2013; VA, 2013). The Patient-Centered Outcomes Research Institute (PCORI) is investing $68 million to support the development of a National Patient-Centered Clinical Research Network (PCORI, 2013a; Selby et al., 2013). In addition, the Center for Learning Health Care at Duke University is an academic initiative facilitating continuous learning (DCRI, 2013). Efforts to implement key components of a learning health care system are discussed in the next sections of this chapter.

Patient Needs

A learning health care system facilitates patient engagement. As discussed in Chapter 3, the committee's conceptual framework envisions a high-quality cancer care system that actively engages patients in their care and supports them in making informed medical decisions that are consistent with their needs, values, and preferences.

Several characteristics of a learning health care system are important to patient engagement, including patients' online access to their EHRs, clinicians' notes, care plans, and relevant clinical information about their conditions (Walker et al., 2011). The system would allow patients to self-report their health status, side effects of treatment, and other experiences as they happen (Cheng et al., 2011). Many mobile devices, such as smart-

TABLE 6-2 Examples of Efforts to Develop Learning Health Care Systems

Organization	Description
CancerLinQ	CancerLinQ is the American Society of Clinical Oncology's (ASCO's) initiative to create a learning health care system for oncology practices. It will curate and analyze data from electronic health records (EHRs), clinical trials, and clinical practice guidelines. It is in the early stages of development. A demo of the program was presented at the ASCO Quality Symposium in 2012 using data from breast cancer patients.
Kaiser Permanente's HealthConnect	In 2002, Kaiser Permanente contracted with Epic Systems Corporation to create and implement HealthConnect. This is an integrated EHR system that stores information from multiple systems within Kaiser Permanente and presents a longitudinal patient record. The information captured includes demographics, progress notes, active/historical problems, medication records, vital signs, medical history, immunization, preventive health milestones, lab data, and radiology reports. It is designed to allow clinicians to easily document patient encounters, diagnoses and procedures, and clinical notes. It also allows patients and clinicians to electronically message each other. MyHealthManager gives patients the opportunity to see and access their health record. It supports the clinical workforce by providing decision support, capturing quality metrics data, informing clinicians of their concordance with clinical practice guidelines, and including a robust search method of previous treatments and outcomes. HealthConnect encompasses an advanced clinical decision support system for oncology, including 230 standardized protocols for the major adult cancers as well as alerts when patients are eligible for clinical trials. The EHR system captures the goals of therapy and also monitors for potential medication errors and drug interactions.
Sentinel Initiative	The Food and Drug Administration announced the Sentinel Initiative in 2008. The goal of this system is to monitor patient safety in the United States. Initially, this program will rely on EHR and administrative data that medical practices, hospitals, delivery systems, health plans, and insurance agencies routinely collect to monitor safety. Eventually, it may also use data from disease registries, vital statistics registries, and repositories of genomics data. The Mini-Sentinel pilot is up and running. It includes 17 data partners and encompasses data from nearly 100 million people. Participating organizations use a distributed data network that allows them to retain their data and provide the centralized network with a standardized data summary.

SOURCES: ASCO, 2013a; FDA, 2011, 2013; KP, 2011a; Platt et al., 2009; Wallace, 2007.

phones and tablets, could assist with this monitoring process and send patients reminders to take their medications at the correct time or report information to their clinicians (Cheng et al., 2011; West, 2012). The result of these self-reports would be captured in the patients' EHRs, which the cancer care team would monitor. If any of the patient-reported information warrants special attention by the cancer care team, the team would get an electronic notice to follow up with the patient, thus reducing the likelihood of patients needlessly suffering from adverse events or severe symptoms.

The benefits of these elements are supported by the evidence. Reminder systems triggered from data in patients' EHRs can lead to patients' improved adherence to treatment protocols and screening recommendations (Din et al., 2005; Nease et al., 2008; Sequist et al., 2009; Shea et al., 1996). In a study where patients were invited to read their clinicians' notes, patients accessed their EHRs regularly and reported that this was a positive experience; the clinicians reported this had a minimal impact on their workflow (Delbanco et al. 2012).

Moreover, studies show that clinicians value patient-reported information, patients are willing to self-report their symptoms, and collecting patient-reported outcomes leads to patients who are more satisfied with their care as well as improvements in symptom management and patients' overall quality of life (Abernethy et al., 2009; Basch and Abernethy, 2011; Basch et al., 2005, 2007; Detmar et al., 2002a,b; Greenhalgh and Meadows, 1999; Snyder et al., 2010; Taenzer et al., 2000; Velikova et al., 2004). In addition, patients are more likely to accurately report sensitive information, such as answering sexuality-related questions, in an electronic reporting system than during live encounters with their cancer care team (Dupont et al., 2009).

A learning health care system would also facilitate patient-clinician communication through electronic messaging and appointment scheduling. Patients would be able to email or message their clinicians in real time, have their questions answered, their EHR updated with any pertinent information, and schedule follow-up office visits. Patients value this feature because it can save them time and visits to their clinicians' offices, and has the potential to improve care (Chen et al., 2009; Din et al., 2005).

At Group Health Cooperative of Puget Sound, for example, about two-thirds of the patients communicate with their care team electronically (Cohn, 2013). Unfortunately, clinicians in many health care systems have been slow to adopt electronic communication due to the challenges of incorporating patient-reported outcomes into the delivery system, the time it takes busy clinicians to review and respond to electronic communications, and the current reimbursement system's failure to reward these services (Feeny, 2013; Wallwiener et al., 2009). Incentivizing clinicians to quickly respond to patients through an electronic system will require new models of team-based cancer care (see Chapter 4) and reimbursement (see Chapter 8).

A learning health care system would also provide patients with educational material and decision aids at key times during their course of treatment. Currently, clinicians may provide patients with overwhelming amounts of information about their treatment without sensitivity to when a patient will actually need critical information. Smart use of patient portals within a learning health care system would push information and decision aids to patients at specific times (e.g., when patients schedule certain types of appointments) and provide patients with information about their prognosis, treatment options, treatment effects and side effects, advance care planning, and anticipated cost of care in a time-sensitive manner.

In addition, as discussed below in more detail, patients would benefit from a learning health care system's ability to improve the coordination of care, enhance researchers' and clinicians' ability to generate new knowledge to inform clinical practice, and facilitate the process of making quality metrics transparent and publicly available.

Clinical Workforce Needs

The committee's conceptual framework envisions an adequately staffed, trained, and coordinated workforce for cancer care (see Chapter 4). This includes competent, trusted, interprofessional cancer care teams that are aligned with patients' needs, values, and preferences, and that provide care coordinated with patients' primary/geriatrics and specialist care teams. A learning health care system can make this vision a reality by improving the workforce's knowledge of clinical research and best care practices, and by promoting care coordination.

An integral element of a learning health care system is clinical decision support, which can be defined as a system that provides clinicians with "person-specific information, intelligently filtered or presented at appropriate times, to enhance health and health care" (ONC, 2013b). Decision support is important in clinical practice because the amount of new evidence clinical researchers are generating each year "exceed(s) the bounds of unaided human cognition" (Masys, 2002, p. 36).

Research suggests that clinical decision support can influence treatment selection and the ordering of tests, prevent medication errors, and ensure the safe dosage of drugs (Kralj et al., 2003; Neilson et al., 2004; Potts et al., 2004; Schedlbauer et al., 2009). It can also be used to guide clinicians' decisions about molecularly targeted medicine (Pulley et al., 2012). The Agency for Healthcare Research and Quality conducted a systematic review of clinical decision support systems and identified the following list of characteristics as important in making these systems successful at improving care:

- Automatic provision of decision support as part of the clinician's workflow
- Provision of decision support at the time and location of decision making
- Provision of a recommendation, not just an assessment
- Integration with the charting or order entry system to support workflow
- Promotion of action rather than inaction
- Elimination of the need for additional clinical data entry
- Justification of decision support via research evidence
- Local clinician involvement in development
- Provision of decision support results to patients, as well as clinicians (Lobach et al., 2012)

Clinical decision support is particularly important in cancer care due to the complexity of the disease, the diverse treatment options available, and the enormous body of research relevant to clinical care. Clinicians working in cancer would benefit from clinical decision support that provides guidance on the specific options for therapeutic interventions and diagnostic tests, flags potential patient safety concerns (e.g., drug-drug interactions at time of prescribing), and identifies patients who need preventive services or who are at risk for certain adverse side effects.

Because much of the research on clinical decision support has been conducted in areas of health care outside of cancer, additional research needs to be conducted to identify the most effective design features and timing of clinical decision support for the workforce providing cancer care (Clauser et al., 2011; Pearce and Trumble, 2006). In addition, the content of the clinical decision support should be kept current and continually updated with the results of new clinical trials and observational studies. Masys has argued that a learning health care system should meet this requirement by including a "national cancer course guidance infrastructure," analogous to the Federal Aviation Administration's course guidance database (see Box 6-1).

Many EHR vendors are seeking to include clinical decision support for cancer care in their products. For example, Epic Systems Corporation, one of the major EHR vendors, has a medical oncology module that provides information on diagnostic staging, treatment options, chemotherapy dosing schedules, and personalized treatment planning (KP, 2011a). A number of cancer centers are also working with IBM to train the

BOX 6-1
A National Cancer Course Guidance Infrastructure

Efforts to improve the consistency and safety of health care have drawn on the experience and process of other high-risk industries, and parallels between commercial aviation and health care have been cited since the first of the Institute of Medicine Quality Chasm reports, *To Err Is Human*, was published in 1999 (IOM, 1999). One of the most dramatic transformations in aviation has been the supplementation of paper charts and narrative text for critical aspects of flight with an electronic course guidance infrastructure. The U.S. Federal Aviation Administration maintains a series of continuously updated databases of system routes, safe approach paths, destinations, and topographic coordinate data, which is available for downloading by users and commercial developers of navigation systems and autopilots (FAA, 2013). When downloaded onto plug-in media, these data give each aircraft a set of "evidence-based" guidance that, when linked to real-time global positioning system data and other forms of radio navigation, enable autopilot-equipped aircraft to fly complex route patterns, departures, and arrivals with precise, second-by-second automated course monitoring and guidance.

These data have transformed the task of piloting an aircraft from one of eye-hand coordination and physical manipulation of controls into a task of selecting a destination, choosing an appropriate route, entering that plan into the systems that control the aircraft's vertical and lateral movement, and then monitoring whether the flight is proceeding according to the plan. Pilots retain the legal responsibility for the safe conduct of all of the events from takeoff to touchdown, and frequently encounter circumstances that require the plan to be revised as the journey progresses. But the actual flight path taken does not require their minute-by-minute, hands-on movement of the flight controls, and the hundreds of individual control inputs needed in the correct sequence are part of the electronic interaction between the database's representation of the ideal course and the actual course being flown. From the pilot's perspective, this electronic infrastructure dramatically reduces the burden of reading, remembering, and translating a flight plan into physical actions in a safety-critical environment.

Cancer care has a long history of being guided by clinical practice guidelines, wherein diagnostic and therapeutic protocols include dozens of carefully sequenced clinical observations and interventions that require an orchestrated team effort; that effort commonly requires the members of the team to process human-readable documents and manually translate them into a time-sensitive, patient-specific plan. Thus, cancer care is well positioned to take advantage of guidance technologies analogous to those used in aviation. The infrastructure for implementing patient-specific clinical decision support exists and is operational at a small number of leading health centers in the United States. To achieve broad implementation and the benefits of a learning health care system at a national scale, additional research, development, deployment, and evaluation are needed in the following areas:

1. Standards for clinical decision support "modules" that encode the recognition logic (as represented in data recorded in electronic health record [EHR] systems) of the clinical condition for which evidence-based guidance is available. This specification for recognizing when the guidance applies would be packaged together electronically with the educational information to be displayed to clinicians, patients, and families when a decision needs to be made. That information would include the actionable options available, and the specification for the sequence of events that constitute the plan actually chosen (e.g., the computer-interpretable schema of a multi-agent chemotherapy regimen and its monitoring parameters), along with the downstream parameters that would constitute evidence of a successful or unsuccessful health outcome.

2. A public library of clinical decision support hosted by a neutral and respected source, from which health care organizations could download decision support modules, and to which they could upload their observed experience using them. Although federal entities such as the U.S. National Library of Medicine would be potential clearinghouses for the health care course guidance data, a community-based Wikipedia-like resource hosted by a not-for-profit entity is a feasible alternative. The Agency for Healthcare Research and Quality's Clinical Decision Support Consortium (Middleton, 2009), for example, might serve in a dissemination and data exchange role.

3. Standards and software tools for importing electronic guidance data into the decision support components of EHR systems, along with easy-to-use visualization and editing tools that would enable local practice committees to understand, modify, and implement organization-wide guidance for care.

4. Standards and software tools for collecting data on the organizational experience of using the decision support modules, the subsequent health outcomes of individual cases where the guidance was accepted, along with outcomes where the guidance was given, but not implemented by providers, and methods for uploading that aggregate within-organization experience back to the Public Library of decision support. Within the Public Library, those experiences of organizations using the same decision support infrastructure would be pooled together.

SOURCE: Personal communication, D. Masys, University of Washington, August 9, 2012.

Watson Computer to help clinicians with complex diagnostic and treat-ment decisions in oncology (Cohn, 2013; Kohn, 2012). This is the same computer that went on *Jeopardy!* and beat several human champions. IBM sold the technology supporting the Watson Computer to WellPoint Inc. and Citigroup Inc., and these groups expect it to generate revenue by 2015 (Jinks, 2013).

A learning health care system would also support clinicians' decision making in circumstances where there is little to no evidence about the benefits and harms of various treatment options. For example, Hoffman and Podgurski (2011, p. 425) proposed using health IT to enable "per-sonalized comparisons of treatment effectiveness." In their framework, a clinician would be able to search the deidentified EHRs of a cohort of pa-tients who are clinically similar to a patient in question for potential treat-ments and health outcomes. This feature would enable clinicians to use previous patients' experiences in the health care system to guide future care. Frankovich and colleagues operationalized this concept using EHRs from Stanford University to identify the best way to treat a 13-year-old girl with systemic lupus erythematous (Frankovich et al., 2011). For that case, clinicians conducted a search of other EHRs in less than 4 hours and developed a treatment plan. In a learning health care system, this type of search would become regular practice.

In addition to guiding clinical decisions, a learning health care sys-tem would facilitate a coordinated cancer care workforce (Bitton et al., 2012; Forti et al., 2005; Galligioni et al., 2009). The use of health IT to co-ordinate care is particularly important for cancer because of the diverse professional teams providing care and the multiple transitions in care between primary care/geriatrics care teams, the cancer care team, and other specialist care teams. A learning health care system would provide individual members of the cancer care team with a mechanism for easily sharing information with each other, as well as with the primary care/geriatrics care team.

As cancer care becomes increasingly based on clinical practice guide-lines, nonphysician professionals will likely play a larger role in routine cancer care. For example, ASCO envisions nurse practitioners and physi-cian assistants using clinical decision support embedded in a learning health care system to deliver the majority of cancer care in the future. The oncologist's role would evolve to focus on managing the care teams, overseeing the development of care plans, collaborating with primary care/geriatrics care teams, and overseeing complex cases (ASCO, 2013b). Such a change in the provision of cancer care would address the projected workforce shortages (see Chapter 4) and would require a heightened level of coordination between the team of professionals providing the care. A learning health care system would support this shift by enabling improved communication, assigning tasks, and monitoring and updating patients' care plans.

A learning health care system would also enhance clinicians' abilities to recruit patients to clinical trials. As noted in Chapter 5, very few adults with cancer participate in clinical trials and the individuals who do participate are often unrepresentative of the broader population with the disease. A computerized notification system that identifies trials for potentially eligible patients would improve this situation. For example, Kaiser Permanente has embedded alerts into its EHR system that notify clinicians and patients of potentially relevant trials (KP, 2011a). The challenges to creating an effective clinical trial notification system include keeping the list of potential trials current, using consistent terminology for categorizing trials (e.g., "stage IV" vs. "metastatic"), and including the location of the trials (Monaco et al., 2005).

A learning health care system would support the clinical workforce by enhancing communication between clinicians and insurance companies. One estimate found that the average U.S. physician spends 3 hours each week interacting with insurers (Casalino et al., 2009). IBM's Watson, for example, includes a button that allows clinicians to send a treatment proposal to an insurance company for rapid reimbursement approval (Cohn, 2013). The Patient Protection and Affordable Care Act[5] supports electronic communication between payers and clinicians by requiring uniform standards and operating rules for electronic transactions (CMS, 2013).

Finally, learning health care system would also monitor and capture data from clinical encounters, provide clinicians with a report on the concordance of their care with clinical practice guidelines, and inform clinicians about how their performance compares to that of their peers. As discussed in more detail below in the section on Challenges, extracting and analyzing data in a learning health care system is an incredibly complex process and will likely require advances in IT, natural language processing, and analytics in order to become reality.

Cancer Research Needs

In Chapter 5, the committee acknowledges the role that health IT could play in improving the evidence base for high-quality cancer care. A learning health care system would allow researchers to conduct powerful new types of observational studies by utilizing all of the data captured during real-world clinical encounters and integrating it with data cap-

---

[5] Patient Protection and Affordable Care Act, Public Law 111-148, 111th Congress, 2nd Sess. (March 23, 2010).

tured from other sources (e.g., cancer registries, clinical trials, administrative claims databases).

Most datasets currently available for observational studies are small and at risk of bias. The larger databases are narrow in scope (e.g., administrative databases and adverse event reporting systems) and cannot be used to answer broad clinical questions. A learning health care system would address these shortcomings by pooling data from multiple sources to create a very large database (or a number of integrated databases) that would include a diverse population in terms of gender, geography, ethnicity, age, educational level, socioeconomics, and disease/health characteristics. Such a database would provide an enormous quantity of data about older adults and individuals with comorbidities from real-life clinical encounters that researchers would be able to analyze. For example, researchers have used the Department of Veterans Affairs' National Surgical Quality Improvement Program database to pool an enormous numbers of patients (+300,000) to examine the effects of perioperative anemia and polychemia on postoperative outcomes in older veterans (Wu et al., 2007). It would also capture data on the off-label use of cancer drugs and facilitate the Food and Drug Administration's surveillance of drugs on the market that were granted accelerated approval (Abernethy et al., 2010).

To reach its full potential for research, a learning health care system would need to enable researchers to link patient-level data across databases and time, collect data relevant to the quality of cancer care (e.g., functional status, comorbidities), and allow patients to enter information into their EHR about their symptoms. This type of observational research has many advantages over clinical trials because it can be conducted quickly, is less expensive, and analyzes real-world clinical practice.

In addition, a learning health care system would facilitate genomic research by providing researchers with the large numbers of patients necessary to understand the biological complexity of cancer. As noted in Chapter 2, there has been a trend in cancer treatment toward molecular targeted interventions, particularly because collecting molecular data on individual patients has become less expensive and clinicians' understanding of molecular medicine has rapidly increased. A learning health care system would allow researchers to identify patients for clinical trials who have the relevant molecular markers. Researchers would also be able to augment clinical trial data by using EHRs to gather additional patient characteristics and fill in missing clinical details.

For example, in the United Kingdom, the Patient Pathway Manager integrates patient data from EHRs with research data. Researchers are then able to correlate demographic and clinical information (e.g., age, diagnosis, staging, treatment, time of treatment) with study data. The system protects patient privacy by providing different levels of access to patient data for authorized clinical staff and researchers (Newsham et al., 2011). Similarly, there are a number of large biorepositories that link individual genetic data to EHRs, such as Kaiser Permanente's biobank, the Department of Veterans Affairs' Million Veteran Bank, The National Human Genome Research Institute's Electronic Medical Records and Genomics (eMERGE) Network, and the United Kingdom's National Biobank (KP, 2011b; Kupersmith and O'Leary, 2012; McCarty et al., 2011; Wellcome Trust, 2013).

Quality Metrics Development Needs

The committee's conceptual framework for high-quality cancer care requires a system that will measure and assess progress in improving the delivery of cancer care, publicly report that information, and develop innovative strategies for performance improvement (see Chapter 7). A learning health care system, that collects, analyzes, and reports on quality data in real-time, is essential for achieving this goal. It would facilitate the capture of clinical and patient-reported data in EHRs, allowing researchers to measure both the proficiency of care and patients' experiences with care. It would also allow the translation of meaningful quality metrics data back to the point of care to inform clinicians about their performance and to foster improvement. Through such a process, the cancer care team would learn about the concordance of their care with clinical practice guidelines and how their care compares to the care provided by their colleagues. Providing this information to the cancer care team could, in and of itself, drive improved care through clinicians' desire for self-improvement and assurance that they are providing comparable or better care than their colleagues (Lamb et al., 2013). In addition, a learning health care system would offer the necessary infrastructure for transparently reporting quality metrics in a way that meets the needs of clinicians, patients, and payers. These changes require that a learning health care system go beyond simply documenting care processes and that clinicians apply any knowledge gained to improve the quality of care.

Few EHR systems, however, currently capture quality metrics data reliably. Much of the information that would feed into those metrics is unstructured within clinicians' notes (Jha, 2011). Advances in natural language processing could address this problem by enabling computers to analyze the context of words and phrases within clinicians' notes, making the information for quality metrics available electronically (Murff et al., 2011). EHR systems could also lead to clinical data having more standardized content and structure for use in assessing quality metrics.

In addition, Section 601(b) of the Taxpayer Relief Act of 2012 could increase the volume of data collected for quality metrics. This provision creates an incentive for clinicians to submit more data on the quality of care to existing disease registries (including cancer registries).

As discussed in Chapter 7, a major challenge to the collection of quality metrics is that stakeholders in cancer care do not agree about which metrics should be collected. Very little information exists about what outcome measures are important to patients in their decision-making processes. Plus, outcomes that are important to patients may not always be the same as those that are important to clinicians. The complexity of the disease, the diverse treatment options available, and their variability in the potential complications and outcomes of care further complicates the identification of appropriate data to capture. Nevertheless, it is important that the learning health care IT system capture information about the committee's components for a high-quality cancer care delivery system (i.e., the delivery of patient-centered communication and shared decision making, team-based care, evidence-based care, and accessible and affordable care).

Several quality metrics reporting systems currently use health IT. The CoC's Rapid Quality Reporting System Project is a Web-based quality metrics tool that provides hospital-level data on adherence to National Quality Forum–endorsed quality of cancer care measures for breast and colorectal cancers (CoC, 2013). Similarly, ASCO is redesigning its Quality Oncology Practice Initiative (QOPI) to utilize advances in health IT. Through a pilot program with U.S. Oncology, ASCO concluded that EHRs could be used to automatically collect and report data to QOPI rather than relying on manual chart abstraction and retrospective analyses of data reported by clinicians. However, this would require adapting many of QOPI's quality metrics to utilize data that clinicians are capturing in their EHRs (ASCO, 2012). The University of Kentucky also recently developed a model system that enables EHRs to report cancer cases directly to the state's cancer registry in real time (Perry, 2012). Similarly, the CDC is working to automate EHR reporting to cancer registries across the United States (CDC, 2013).

Payer Needs

The committee's conceptual framework states that payers should align reimbursement to reward delivery models that are patient centered and provide high-value care based on measured health outcomes. A learning health care system would make the true cost of cancer care delivery more transparent by systematically collecting data on utilization, patient out-of-pocket costs, reimbursement, and costs to the health care system. It would also integrate this data with quality and outcomes of care data, information which is important for patients, their families, and clinicians in making informed medical decisions (see discussion in Chapter 3). A learning health care system would inform payers' pricing for bundled payments and other reimbursement reforms currently being piloted for cancer (see Chapter 8). In addition, the system's ability to capture quality metrics data would allow payers to identify and reward high-performing clinicians and health care organizations.

CHALLENGES

There are implementation challenges, technical challenges, and ethical oversight challenges to achieving the committee's vision for a learning health care system for cancer care. Each of these challenges is explored below.

Implementation Challenges

The *Best Care* consensus report recognized that clinicians' concerns about the impact of a learning health care system on their workflow could be a major challenge to implementation (IOM, 2012a). It noted that time pressures, stresses, and inefficiencies in the practice of medicine limit clinicians' ability to focus on new initiatives, including the creation of a learning health care system. The sheer number of quality improvement initiatives being implemented by various stakeholders in the health care system can be overwhelming. Thus, initiatives that focus on only incremental improvements to the health care system and add to a clinician's daily workload are unlikely to succeed. The success of a learning health care system will depend on major changes in the environment, context, and systems in which clinicians practice so that they are motivated to participate in this new system of learning and quality improvement. Currently, health IT is often hard to use, does not integrate well with existing workflows, and adds to the time it takes to see patients and to record clinical data (Campbell et al., 2009; Hesse et al., 2010; McDonnell et al., 2010).

For a learning health care system to work, all of the stakeholders involved will need to change their culture to one that values continuous learning. Some clinicians are likely to be resistant to switching from a paper-based system to an electronic system of recording and accessing their patients' data. Additionally, organizations from multiple sectors of the cancer community might be resistant to sharing their data. Likewise, clinicians and the institutions for which they work may not want to share their data because they could lose their competitive advantage, which is gained from the knowledge they generate during their own provision of care. Researchers, too, are often focused on individual achievement and publication rather than on collaborating and sharing data. Similarly, developers of new drugs and devices are likely to be protective of their intellectual property, and EHR vendors have a disincentive to develop interoperable systems that would allow the learning health care system to integrate their data because they do not want to lose market share of their products. Patients may be concerned about the privacy and security of their data in an electronic system and may not want or have the capacity to use IT to communicate with their clinicians and other sectors of the health care system (Kean et al., 2012).

The cost of implementing a learning health care system is also prohibitive. It is very expensive for a health care organization to implement sophisticated EHR systems that have the capacity to feed into a learning health care system. The costs of implementation include software and IT infrastructure costs, as well as considerable personnel and training costs. Health IT experts need to customize the health IT systems for the local environments. In addition, health care organizations need to spend time and money to train the users of the health IT system in best practices. Clinicians and health care organizations often pay the costs of implementing health IT systems, yet it is the payers and patients who benefit from the expected gains in quality and efficiency of care. Thus, there is a disconnect between the parties who pay to implement health IT and the parties who benefit the most from its implementation (Hillestad et al., 2005).

The recent increase in clinicians' and hospitals' adoption of EHRs suggests that meaningful use has been effective at offsetting some of these costs. In 2012, the proportion of office-based physicians who used EHR systems was 72 percent, up from 48 percent in 2009. Sixty-six percent of office-based physicians reported that they planned to apply, or already had applied, for meaningful use incentives, and 27 percent of these physicians had computerized systems that met the requirements for Stage 1 of meaningful use (Hsiao and Hing, 2012). However, organizations in many care settings, such as long-term acute care hospitals and rehabilitation hospitals, are excluded from the HITECH Act and are not adopting health IT at major rates (Wolf et al., 2012). In addition, the meaningful use incentives are temporary. Clinicians and hospitals will eventually be penalized through lower reimbursement rates for failing to adopt EHRs that meet the requirements for meaningful use.

Technical Challenges

The technology currently exists for many of the applications within a learning health care system; however, many technological challenges will need to be addressed to achieve its full potential. Interoperability is one area that will need to be addressed. In a learning health care system, organizations need to be able to transfer information from one entity to another in a way that is timely, accurate, secure, and transparent (Abernethy et al., 2010). This includes EHR systems communicating with each other, as well as EHRs communicating with other critical databases (e.g., Medicare databases and cancer registries). Conversely, health care organizations have routinely adopted health IT systems customized to local institutional needs, which are unable to communicate with other organizations.

The Bipartisan Policy Center found that the "level of health information exchange in the U.S. is extremely low" (BPC, 2012, p. 5). The Direct Project has attempted to address this problem by developing standards and documentation to support the transfer of data from one health care institution to another (Direct Project, 2013). Health information exchanges may also help address this obstacle by providing services that enable organizations to share their data (ONC, 2013c). Additional investments will be required to improve interoperability.

In addition, a number of issues with health care data are likely to create technological challenges for a learning health care system, including the ability to efficiently handle the large quantity of data collected, especially in the age of molecularly targeted medicine. In order for data within a learning health care system to improve the quality of cancer care, clinicians, researchers, quality metrics developers, and payers must be able to effectively extract, use, and analyze the data. This will require input and forethought from data scientists who are skilled at organizing and handling large datasets and in developing IT infrastructure that supports these functions. Unfortunately, there are not enough adequately trained data scientists in health care and it can be difficult to identify individuals with the required skills (Davenport and Patil, 2012). Thus, the quantity of data within a learning health care system could become unmanageable, and it may be difficult for the stakeholders in a learning health care system to effectively extract data necessary for improving the quality of cancer care.

The success of a learning health care system will also depend upon the collection of the right data. Much of the current data that clinicians collect do not relate to important aspects of the quality of care. For example, EHR systems often do not capture data on the patients' experiences with care, patients' ultimate clinical outcomes, or patients' transition from primary cancer treatment to survivorship care (IOM and NRC, 2005; Kean et al., 2012). As mentioned above, many stakeholders disagree about which metrics are important in a high-quality cancer care system and little is known about which metrics patients' value.

The lack of uniformity among data is an additional challenge. Data are often collected in a free-text format rather than a structured format, making the information difficult to aggregate and analyze (Kean et al., 2012). Also, it can be difficult for organizations to share their data across settings because current health care systems use different vocabularies, definitions, and infrastructures. Despite the many ongoing efforts to standardize data definitions, such as the Systematized Nomenclature of Medicine Clinical Terms (Snowmed CT), researchers, clinicians, and industry often define medical terms differently (e.g., disease classifications, symptoms). In addition, many of the standardized codes are not detailed enough for research purposes, especially for cancer, where the disease can be defined by its molecular characteristics (West, 2011). Data definitions will need to be standardized in a way that recognizes the health care system's evolving knowledge of diseases and advances in treatment.

Another technological challenge to a learning health care system is the use of appropriate analytic methods. Data captured in a learning health care system may be less accurate and more subject to bias than data collected in clinical trials. Thus, researchers need new analytic methods to adjust and account for these limitations (IOM, 2012a). PCORI is funding methodological research in this area (PCORI, 2013b). For example, it sponsored an IOM workshop on conducting observational studies in a learning health care system to identify analytic methods for improving the validity and reliability of results from such studies (IOM, 2013).

Ethical Oversight Challenges

The major regulations that govern the ethical oversight of a learning health care system in the United States include (1) the Health Insurance Portability and Accountability Act (HIPAA) Privacy Rule, which protects the privacy of personally identifiable health information by restricting the types of allowable uses and disclosures of data; (2) the HIPAA Security Rule, which requires health care organizations to securely store any personally identifiable health information that is in electronic format; and (3) the Common Rule, which governs human subject research by requiring institutional review board (IRB) oversight and research participants' informed consent.

The IOM has concluded that these regulations often create unnecessary barriers to clinical research and do not protect research participants as well as they should (IOM, 2009, 2012a). It recommended streamlining and revising the existing research regulations to improve care, promote the capture of clinical data, and generate knowledge. A number of ethicists have reached similar conclusions and recommended changes to the existing oversight paradigm (Faden et al., 2013; Platt et al., 2013; Selker et al., 2011).

Members of the IOM's Roundtable on Value & Science-Driven Health Care have proposed exempting many of the activities of a learning health care system from these regulations by classifying the actions as quality improvement and clinical effectiveness assessments rather than research (Platt et al., 2013; Selker et al., 2011). They argue that the creation of generalizable knowledge is a necessary and routine aspect of health care delivery. The amount of oversight required should be commensurate with the level of risk imposed on the patient by the activity. In quality improvement and effectiveness assessments, the biggest risk to patients is that their data might be misused or inappropriately released. However, patients are unlikely to be exposed to risks that exceed those of usual care. Thus, the authors argue that institutions should designate these activities as a type of continuous improvement reviewed through normal institutional systems and exempt them from research oversight (i.e., they should not be overseen by an IRB and patient consent should not be required).

Similarly, in a recent Hastings Center Report, Faden and colleagues argued that the current regulatory distinction between research and clinical practice is antiquated. They stated that a new ethical foundation should be developed that facilitates both care and research, is likely to benefit patients, and provides oversight that is commensurate with risk and burden (Faden et al., 2013; Kass et al., 2013). They believe that a growing number of health care activities cannot be classified as either research or clinical practice. By definition, learning health care systems are designed to "simultaneously deliver the care patients need while capturing the experience of clinical practice in a systematic way that produces generalizable knowledge to improve care for both present and future patients" (Kass et al., 2013, p. S6).

This proposal has been met with a variety of reactions, ranging from strong support to others finding the approach too radical and arguing for maintaining a distinction between research and clinical care (Grady and Wendler, 2013; Kupersmith, 2013; Largent et al., 2013; Menikoff, 2013; Puglisi, 2013; Selby and Krumholz, 2013). Regardless of which approach is taken, developers of a learning health care system will need to ensure that the system is ethically sound and complies with all relevant regulations.

PATH TO IMPLEMENTATION

Although the challenges to creating a learning health care IT system for cancer are formidable, there are many steps that stakeholders can take to move toward the development of such a system. The *Best Care* consensus report outlines recommendations for establishing the digital infrastructure and data utility necessary for continuous learning (see Box 6-2). It recognizes that the creation of a learning health care system will require an effort on the part of many stakeholders, including health care delivery organizations, clinicians, the U.S. Department of Health and Human Services (HHS), payers, patients, researchers, health IT vendors,

---

BOX 6-2
IOM Recommendations on the Foundational
Elements of a Learning Health Care System

Recommendation 1: The Digital Infrastructure

Improve the capacity to capture clinical, care delivery process, and financial data for better care, system improvement, and the generation of new knowledge. Data generated in the course of care delivery should be digitally collected, compiled, and protected as a reliable and accessible resource for care management, process improvement, public health, and the generation of new knowledge.

Strategies for progress toward this goal:

- *Health care delivery organizations* and *clinicians* should fully and effectively employ digital systems that capture patient care experiences reliably and consistently, and implement standards and practices that advance the interoperability of data systems.
- *The National Coordinator for Health Information Technology, digital technology developers,* and *standards organizations* should ensure that the digital infrastructure captures and delivers the core data elements and interoperability needed to support better care, system improvement, and the generation of new knowledge.
- *Payers, health care delivery organizations,* and *medical product companies* should contribute data to research and analytic consortia to support expanded use of care data to generate new insights.
- *Patients* should participate in the development of a robust data utility; use new clinical communication tools, such as personal portals, for self-management and care activities; and be involved in building new knowledge, such as through patient-reported outcomes and other knowledge processes.
- The *Secretary of Health and Human Services* should encourage the development of distributed data research networks and expand the availability of

---

and other stakeholders. These recommendations continue to be relevant and, if followed, would facilitate the development of a learning health care IT system for cancer.

In addition, there are steps that stakeholders in cancer care should take to facilitate the development of a learning health care IT system for cancer. The committee believes that clinicians, through their professional organizations, should take a lead role in creating a learning health care system for cancer. Having clinicians guide the development process will help ensure that the resulting system is seamlessly integrated into clinical practice so that clinicians can easily participate and contribute patient departmental health data resources for translation into accessible knowledge that can be used for improving care, lowering costs, and enhancing public health.

- *Research funding agencies and organizations*, such as the *National Institutes of Health*, the *Agency for Healthcare Research and Quality*, the *Veterans Health Administration*, the *Department of Defense*, and the *Patient-Centered Outcomes Research Institute*, should promote research designs and methods that draw naturally on existing care processes and that also support ongoing quality improvement efforts.

Recommendation 2: The Data Utility

Streamline and revise research regulations to improve care, promote the capture of clinical data, and generate knowledge. Regulatory agencies should clarify and improve regulations governing the collection and use of clinical data to ensure patient privacy but also the seamless use of clinical data for better care coordination and management, improved care, and knowledge enhancement.

Strategies for progress toward this goal:

- The *Secretary of Health and Human Services* should accelerate and expand the review of the Health Insurance Portability and Accountability Act and institutional review board policies with respect to actual or perceived regulatory impediments to the protected use of clinical data, and clarify regulations and their interpretation to support the use of clinical data as a resource for advancing science and care improvement.
- *Patient and consumer groups, clinicians, professional specialty societies, health care delivery organizations, voluntary organizations, researchers,* and *grantmakers* should develop strategies and outreach to improve understanding of the benefits and importance of accelerating the use of clinical data to improve care and health outcomes.

SOURCE: IOM, 2012a.

data. Moreover, professional organizations are already taking the lead in developing a learning health care system for cancer through ASCO's CancerLinQ project. **These groups should continue to design and implement the digital infrastructure and analytics necessary to enable continuous learning in cancer care.** This process should involve consultation with the other stakeholders discussed in this chapter (patients, researchers, quality metrics developers, and payers) to help ensure that the final product also meets their needs.

As in other countries, the federal government has a role to play in developing a learning health care system for cancer (BCG, 2012). HHS, because of its role in promoting health in the United States, should take the lead, with ONC and the NCI involved in the development process. ONC, charged with coordinating nationwide efforts to implement and use advances in health IT to improve quality of care (ONC, 2013a), has the technical expertise necessary to contribute to setting standards and developing the IT infrastructure required for this system.

Similarly, the NCI, with its focus on cancer research and training (NCI, 2013b), has demonstrated an interest in supporting the development of health IT through its caBIG initiative (Cancer Biomedical Informatics Grid), which was designed to enable researchers, clinicians, and patients to share data and knowledge through an informatics grid. This program started a dialogue among cancer researchers on the interoperability of clinical and research software tools, developing standards for data exchange and interoperability, and disseminating research tools to the community.

The program was criticized, however, as being too focused on technology, expanding without clear objectives, lacking flexibility, utilizing an unsustainable business model, and lacking independent scientific oversight (IOM, 2012b). The NCI ended this initiative due to these problems, but has continued to support informatics infrastructure development via a new National Cancer Informatics Program and an Informatics Working Group of National Cancer Advisory Board, which is considering the NCI's future role in developing an IT infrastructure (NCI, 2013a). This Working Group and NCI Director Harold Varmus have expressed the belief that the NCI's investment in health IT should extend to clinical practice, and not be limited to research as it has been in the past.[6] **Thus, HHS, including ONC and the NCI, should support the development and integration of a learning health care IT system for cancer.** This support could be both intellectual and financial.

The committee is concerned that many stakeholders will be reluctant to provide data to the learning health care system. As described above, many clinicians and institutions use their data to achieve a competitive advantage. **Thus, the committee recommends that CMS and other payers create incentives for clinicians to participate in this learning health care system for cancer care, as it develops.**

These incentives could be structured similar to the meaningful use standards for the adoption of EHRs. Payers could provide cancer care teams with bonus payments for being early participants in a learning health care system and allowing the data in their EHR system to automatically feed into the learning health care system. Ultimately, sharing clinical

---

[6] Personal communication, D. Masys, University of Washington, August 9, 2012.

data will require less cost and effort on the part of the cancer care team because the learning health care system will automate this process. Thus, as in meaningful use, payers could change the incentives into penalties for cancer care teams at a later date if they fail to share their data with this system. The new payment models, discussed in Chapter 8, could also include incentives for clinicians to participate in a learning health care system for cancer.

SUMMARY AND RECOMMENDATIONS

The committee's conceptual framework for a high-quality cancer care delivery system calls for implementation of a learning health care IT system: a system that "learns" by collecting data on care outcomes and cost in a systematic manner, analyzing the captured data both retrospectively and through prospective studies, implementing the knowledge gained from these analyses into clinical practice, evaluating the outcomes of the changes in care, and generating new hypotheses to test and implement into clinical care. A learning health care IT system is a key requirement for implementing the components of the committee's conceptual framework for high-quality cancer care.

In the committee's conceptual framework (see Figure S-2), a learning health care IT system supports patient-clinician interactions by providing patients and clinicians with the information and tools necessary to make well-informed medical decisions. It plays an integral role in developing the evidence base from research (e.g., clinical trials and CER) and by capturing data from real-world care settings that researchers can then analyze to generate new knowledge. Further, it is used to collect and report quality metrics data, implement performance improvement initiatives, and allow payers to identify and reward high-quality care.

Many of the elements needed to create a learning health care system are already in place for cancer, including EHRs, cancer registries, a robust infrastructure for cancer clinical trials, and biorepositories that are linked with clinical data. Unfortunately, they are incompletely implemented, have functional deficiencies, and are not integrated in a way that creates a true learning health care system. In addition, relevant regulations that govern clinical care and research could pose a challenge to a learning health care system. The learning system will either need to comply with the relevant regulations or, alternatively, the regulations may need to be updated to accommodate such a system.

Recommendation 7: A Learning Health Care Information Technology System for Cancer

Goal: Develop an ethically sound learning health care information technology system for cancer that enables real-time analysis of data from cancer patients in a variety of care settings.

To accomplish this:

- **Professional organizations should design and implement the digital infrastructure and analytics necessary to enable continuous learning in cancer care.**
- **The U.S. Department of Health and Human Services should support the development and integration of a learning health care IT system for cancer.**
- **The Centers for Medicare & Medicaid Services and other payers should create incentives for clinicians to participate in this learning health care system for cancer, as it develops.**

REFERENCES

Abernethy, A. P., J. E. Herndon, 2nd, J. L. Wheeler, J. M. Day, L. Hood, M. Patwardhan, H. Shaw, and H. K. Lyerly. 2009. Feasibility and acceptability to patients of a longitudinal system for evaluating cancer-related symptoms and quality of life: Pilot study of an e/tablet data-collection system in academic oncology. *Journal of Pain and Symptom Management* 37(6):1027-1038.

Abernethy, A. P., L. M. Etheredge, P. A. Ganz, P. Wallace, R. R. German, C. Neti, P. B. Bach, and S. B. Murphy. 2010. Rapid-learning system for cancer care. *Journal of Clinical Oncology* 28(27):4268-4274.

ACoS (American College of Surgeons). 2013. *National Cancer Data Base.* http://www.facs.org/cancer/ncdb/index.html (accessed March 4, 2013).

AHRQ (Agency for Healthcare Research and Quality). 2012. *Enabling patient-centered care through health information technology.* http://effectivehealthcare.ahrq.gov/index.cfm/search-for-guides-reviews-and-reports/?productid=1158&pageaction=displayproduct (accessed February 20, 2013).

ASCO (American Society of Clinical Oncology). 2012. *Starting down the path toward electronic QOPI: ASCO and U.S. Oncology collaborate in quality measurement.* http://www.ascopost.com/issues/march-1-2012/starting-down-the-path-toward-electronic-qopi-asco-and-us%C2%A0oncology-collaborate-in-quality-measurement.aspx (accessed February 21, 2013).

———. 2013a. *CancerLinQ: Building a transformation in cancer care.* http://www.asco.org/ASCOv2/Practice+%26+Guidelines/Quality+Care/CancerLinQ+-+Building+a+Transformation+in+Cancer+Care (accessed March 7, 2013).

———. 2013b. *Shaping the future of oncology: Envisioning cancer care in 2030.* http://www.asco.org/ASCOv2/Department%20Content/Communications/Downloads/Shaping Future-lowres.pdf (accessed February 19, 2013).

Basch, E., and A. P. Abernethy. 2011. Supporting clinical practice decisions with real-time patient-reported outcomes. *Journal of Clinical Oncology* 29(8):954-956.

Basch, E., D. Artz, D. Dulko, K. Scher, P. Sabbatini, M. Hensley, N. Mitra, J. Speakman, M. McCabe, and D. Schrag. 2005. Patient online self-reporting of toxicity symptoms during chemotherapy. *Journal of Clinical Oncology* 23(15):3552-3561.

Basch, E., A. Iasonos, A. Barz, A. Culkin, M. G. Kris, D. Artz, P. Fearn, J. Speakman, R. Farquhar, H. I. Scher, M. McCabe, and D. Schrag. 2007. Long-term toxicity monitoring via electronic patient-reported outcomes in patients receiving chemotherapy. *Journal of Clinical Oncology* 25(34):5374-5380.

BCG (Boston Consulting Group). 2012. *Progress toward value-based health care.* https://www.bcg perspectives.com/content/articles/health_care_public_sector_progress_toward_value_based_health_care (accessed February 14, 2013).

Bitton, A., L. A. Flier, and A. K. Jha. 2012. Health information technology in the era of care delivery reform: To what end? *Journal of the American Medical Association* 307(24):2593-2594.

BPC (Bipartisan Policy Center). 2012. *Transforming health care: The role of health IT.* http://bipartisanpolicy.org/sites/default/files/Transforming%20Health%20Care.pdf (accessed March 7, 2013).

Bush, G. W. 2004. *State of the Union Address to the 108th Congress, second session, January 20, 2004.* http://georgewbush-whitehouse.archives.gov/infocus/bushrecord/documents/Selected_Speeches_George_W_Bush.pdf (accessed February 25, 2013).

Campbell, E. M., K. P. Guappone, D. F. Sittig, R. H. Dykstra, and J. S. Ash. 2009. Computerized provider order entry adoption: Implications for clinical workflow. *Journal of General Internal Medicine* 24(1):21-26.

Casalino, L. P., S. Nicholson, D. N. Gans, T. Hammons, D. Morra, T. Karrison, and W. Levinson. 2009. What does it cost physician practices to interact with health insurance plans? *Health Affairs (Millwood)* 28(4):w533-w543.

CDC (Centers for Disease Control and Prevention). 2012. *National Program of Cancer Registries: About the program.* http://www.cdc.gov/cancer/npcr/about.htm (accessed February 20, 2013).

———. 2013. *Advancing e-cancer reporting and registry operations.* http://www.cdc.gov/cancer/npcr/informatics/aerro/index.htm (accessed March 7, 2013).

Chen, C., T. Garrido, D. Chock, G. Okawa, and L. Liang. 2009. The Kaiser Permanente electronic health record: Transforming and streamlining modalities of care. *Health Affairs (Millwood)* 28(2):323-333.

Cheng, C., T. H. Stokes, and M. D. Wang. 2011. Caremote: The design of a cancer reporting and monitoring telemedicine system for domestic care. *Conference Proceedings: 333d Annual International Conference of the IEEE EMBS* 2011:3168-3171.

Cimino, J. J. 2013. Improving the electronic health record: Are clinicians getting what they wished for? *Journal of the American Medical Association* 309(10):991-992.

Clauser, S. B., E. H. Wagner, E. J. Aiello Bowles, L. Tuzzio, and S. M. Greene. 2011. Improving modern cancer care through information technology. *American Journal of Preventive Medicine* 40(5 Suppl 2):S198-S207.

CMS (Centers for Medicare & Medicaid Services). 2013. *Operating Rules and Standards for EFT and Remittance Advice.* http://www.cms.gov/Regulations-and-Guidance/HIPAA-Administrative-Simplification/Affordable-Care-Act/OperatingRulesandStandardsforEFTandRemittanceAdviceERA.html (accessed June 18, 2013).

CoC (Commission on Cancer). 2013. *Rapid quality reporting system.* http://www.facs.org/cancer/ncdb/rqrs.html (accessed February 20, 2013).

Cohn, J. 2013. *The robot will see you now.* http://www.theatlantic.com/magazine/archive/2013/03/the-robot-will-see-you-now/309216/1/ (accessed March 4, 2013).

Davenport, T. H., and D. J. Patil. 2012. *Data scientist: The sexiest job of the 21st century.* http://hbr.org/2012/10/data-scientist-the-sexiest-job-of-the-21st-century/ar/1 (accessed February 19, 2013).

DCRI (Duke Clinical Research Institute). 2013. *Center for Learning Health Care.* https://www.dcri.org/outcomes/center-for-learning-health-care (accessed March 7, 2013).

Delbanco, T., J. Walker, S. K. Bell, J. D. Darer, J. G. Elmore, N. Farag, H. J. Feldman, R. Mejilla, L. Ngo, J. D. Ralston, S. E. Ross, N. Trivedi, E. Vodicka, and S. G. Leveille. 2012. Inviting patients to read their doctors' notes: A quasi-experimental study and a look ahead. *Annals of Internal Medicine* 157(7):461-470.

Detmar, S. B., M. J. Muller, J. H. Schornagel, L. D. Wever, and N. K. Aaronson. 2002a. Health-related quality-of-life assessments and patient-physician communication: A randomized controlled trial. *Journal of the American Medical Association* 288(23):3027-3034.

———. 2002b. Role of health-related quality of life in palliative chemotherapy treatment decisions. *Journal of Clinical Oncology* 20(4):1056-1062.

Din, F. M., Y. Tao, S. Malhotra, J. L. Zimmerman, and R. Kukafka. 2005. Improving patient compliance with best practices guidelines: A web based automated and personalized reminders system. *AMIA Annual Symposium Proceedings*:939.

Direct Project. 2013. *Overview.* http://directproject.org/content.php?key=overview (accessed February 21, 2013).

Dupont, A., J. Wheeler, J. E. Herndon, 2nd, A. Coan, S. Y. Zafar, L. Hood, M. Patwardhan, H. S. Shaw, H. K. Lyerly, and A. P. Abernethy. 2009. Use of tablet personal computers for sensitive patient-reported information. *Journal of Supportive Oncology* 7(3):91-97.

Eddy, D. M. 2007. Linking electronic medical records to large-scale simulation models: Can we put rapid learning on turbo? *Health Affairs (Millwood)* 26(2):w125-w136.

Etheredge, L. M. 2007. A rapid-learning health system. *Health Affairs (Millwood)* 26(2):w107-w118.

———. 2013. *Rapid learning for precision medicine: A big data to knowledge (bd2k) initiative.* http://healthaffairs.org/blog/2013/02/21/rapid-learning-for-precision-medicine-a-big-data-to-knowledge-bd2k-initiative/?zbrandid=4337&zidType=CH&zid=15606499&zsubscriberId=1021390268&zbdom=http://npc.informz.net (accessed February 25, 2013).

FAA (Federal Aviation Administration). 2013. *Coded instrument flight procedures.* http://www.faa.gov/air_traffic/flight_info/aeronav/productcatalog/DigitalProducts/nfd (accessed March 26, 2013).

Faden, R. R., N. E. Kass, S. N. Goodman, P. Pronovost, S. Tunis, and T. L. Beauchamp. 2013. An ethics framework for a learning health care system: A departure from traditional research ethics and clinical ethics. *Hastings Center Report* 43(s1):S16-S27.

FDA (Food and Drug Administration). 2011. *Mini-sentinel.* http://mini-sentinel.org/default.aspx (accessed February 12, 2013).

———. 2013. *FDA's Sentinel Initiative.* http://www.fda.gov/safety/FDAsSentinelInitiative/ucm2007250.htm (accessed February 12, 2013).

Feeny, D. 2013. Health-related quality-of-life data should be regarded as a vital sign. *Journal of Clinical Epidemiology* 66(7):706-709.

Forti, S., M. Galvagni, E. Galligioni, and C. Eccher. 2005. A real time teleconsultation system for sharing an oncologic web-based electronic medical record. *AMIA Annual Symposium Proceedings*:959.

Frankovich, J., C. A. Longhurst, and S. M. Sutherland. 2011. Evidence-based medicine in the EMR era. *New England Journal of Medicine* 365(19):1758-1759.

Galligioni, E., F. Berloffa, O. Caffo, G. Tonazzolli, G. Ambrosini, F. Valduga, C. Eccher, A. Ferro, and S. Forti. 2009. Development and daily use of an electronic oncological patient record for the total management of cancer patients: 7 years experience. *Annals of Oncology* 20(2):349-352.

Grady, C., and D. Wendler. 2013. Making the transition to a learning health care system. *Hastings Center Report* 43(1):S32-S33.

Greene, S. M., R. J. Reid, and E. B. Larson. 2012. Implementing the learning health system: From concept to action. *Annals of Internal Medicine* 157(3):207-210.

Greenhalgh, J., and K. Meadows. 1999. The effectiveness of the use of patient-based measures of health in routine practice in improving the process and outcomes of patient care: A literature review. *Journal of Evaluation in Clinical Practice* 5(4):401-416.

Hesse, B. W., C. Hanna, H. A. Massett, and N. K. Hesse. 2010. Outside the box: Will information technology be a viable intervention to improve the quality of cancer care? *Journal of the National Cancer Institute Monograph* 2010(40):81-89.

Hillestad, R., J. Bigelow, A. Bower, F. Girosi, R. Meili, R. Scoville, and R. Taylor. 2005. Can electronic medical record systems transform health care? Potential health benefits, savings, and costs. *Health Affairs (Millwood)* 24(5):1103-1117.

Hoffman, S., and A. Podgurski. 2011. Improving health care outcomes through personalized comparisons of treatment effectiveness based on electronic health records. *Journal of Law, Medicine, & Ethics* 39(3):425-436.

Hsiao, C., and E. Hing. 2012. *Use and characteristics of electronic health record systems among office-based physician practices: United states, 2001-2012.* http://www.cdc.gov/nchs/data/databriefs/db111.htm (accessed February 13, 2013).

IOM (Institute of Medicine). 1999. *To err is human: Building a safer health system.* Washington, DC: National Academy Press.

———. 2001. *Crossing the quality chasm: A new health system for the 21st century.* Washington, DC: National Academy Press.

———. 2007. *The learning healthcare system: Workshop summary.*Washington, DC: The National Academies Press.

———. 2009. *Beyond the HIPAA Privacy Rule: Enhancing privacy, improving health through research.* Washington, DC: The National Academies Press.

———. 2010. *A foundation for evidence-driven practice: A rapid learning system for cancer care: Workshop summary.* Washington, DC: The National Academies Press.

———. 2011a. *Digital infrastructure for the learning health system: The foundation for continuous improvement in health and health care: Workshop series summary.* Washington, DC: The National Academies Press.

———. 2011b. *Health IT and patient safety: Building safer systems for better care.* Washington, DC: The National Academies Press.

———. 2012a. *Best care at lower cost: The path to continuously learning health care in America.* Washington, DC: The National Academies Press.

———. 2012b. *Informatics needs and challenges in cancer research: Workshop summary.* Washington, DC: The National Academies Press.

____. 2013. *Observational studies in a learning health system: Workshop summary.* Washington, DC: The National Academies Press.

IOM and NRC (National Research Council). 1999. *Ensuring quality cancer care.* Washington, DC: National Academy Press.

———. 2005. *From cancer patient to cancer survivor: Lost in transition.* Washington, DC: The National Academies Press.

Jha, A. K. 2011. The promise of electronic records: Around the corner or down the road? *Journal of the American Medical Association* 306(8):880-881.

Jinks, B. 2013. *IBM's watson to help memorial sloan-kettering with cancer.* http://www.bloomberg.com/news/2012-03-22/ibm-s-watson-to-help-memorial-sloan-kettering-with-cancer-care.html (accessed March 12, 2013).

Kass, N., R. Faden, S. Goodman, P. Pronovost, S. Tunis, and T. Beauchamp. 2013. The research-treatment distinction: A problematic approach for determining which activities should have ethical oversight. *Hastings Center Report* 43(s1):S4-S15.

Kean, M. A., A. P. Abernethy, A. M. Clark, W. S. Dalton, B. H. Pollock, L. N. Shulman, and S. B. Murphy. 2012. Achieving data liquidity in the cancer community: Proposal for a coalition of stakeholders. *Discussion Paper.* http://www.iom.edu/Global/Perspectives/2012/DataLiquidityCancerCommunity.aspx (accessed February 19, 2013).

Kellermann, A. L., and S. S. Jones. 2013. What it will take to achieve the as-yet-unfulfilled promises of health information technology. *Health Affairs (Millwood)* 32(1):63-68.

Kohn, M. S. 2012. *Analytics in support of health care transformation.* http://iom.edu/Global/Perspectives/2012/AnalyticsHealthTransformation.aspx?utm_medium=etmail&utm_source=Institute%20of%20Medicine&utm_campaign=12.14.12+Perspective+Alert&utm_content=New%20Perspectives&utm_term=Non-profit (accessed March 4, 2013).

KP (Kaiser Permanente). 2011a. *Kaiser Permanente HealthConnect: HIMSS Davies Award 2011.* Oakland, CA: Kaiser Permanente.

———. 2011b. Kaiser Permanente, UCSF scientists complete NIH-Funded genomics project involving 100,000 people. http://www.dor.kaiser.org/external/news/press_releases/Kaiser_Permanente,_UCSF_Scientists_Complete_NIH-Funded_Genomics_Project_Involving_100,000_People (accessed June 28, 2013).

Kralj, B., D. Iverson, K. Hotz, and F. D. Ashbury. 2003. The impact of computerized clinical reminders on physician prescribing behavior: Evidence from community oncology practice. *American Journal of Medical Quality* 18(5):197-203.

Kupersmith, J. 2013. Advances in the research enterprise. *Hastings Center Report* 43(1):S43-S44.

Kupersmith, J., and T. O'Leary. 2012. *The million veteran program: Building VA's mega-database for genomic medicine.* http://healthaffairs.org/blog/2012/11/19/the-million-veteran-program-building-vas-mega-database-for-genomic-medicine (accessed February 25, 2013).

Kupersmith, J., J. Francis, E. Kerr, S. Krein, L. Pogach, R. M. Kolodner, and J. B. Perlin. 2007. Advancing evidence-based care for diabetes: Lessons from the Veterans Health Administration. *Health Affairs (Millwood)* 26(2):w156-w168.

Lamb, G. C., M. A. Smith, W. B. Weeks, and C. Queram. 2013. Publicly reported quality-of-care measures influenced Wisconsin physician groups to improve performance. *Health Affairs (Millwood)* 32(3):536-543.

Largent, E., S. Joffe, and F. Miller. 2013. A prescription for ethical learning. *Hastings Center Report* 43(1):S28-S29.

Liang, L. 2007. The gap between evidence and practice. *Health Affairs (Millwood)* 26(2): w119-w121.

Lobach, D., G. D. Sanders, T. J. Bright, A. Wong, R. Dhurjati, E. Bristow, L. Bastian, R. Coeytaux, G. Samsa, V. Hasselblad, J. W. Williams, L. Wing, M. Musty, and A. S. Kendrick. 2012. *Enabling health care decisionmaking through clinical decision support and knowledge management. Evidence report no. 203., AHRQ publication no. 12-e001-ef.* Rockville, MD: Agency for Healthcare Research and Quality.

Lumpkin, J. R. 2007. Archimedes: A bold step into the future. *Health Affairs* 26(2):w137-w139.

Mandl, K. D., and I. S. Kohane. 2012. Escaping the EHR trap: The future of health IT. *New England Journal of Medicine* 366(24):2240-2242.

Masys, D. R. 2002. Effects of current and future information technologies on the health care workforce. *Health Affairs (Millwood)* 21(5):33-41.

McCarty, C. A., R. L. Chisholm, C. G. Chute, I. J. Kullo, G. P. Jarvik, E. B. Larson, R. Li, D. R. Masys, M. D. Ritchie, D. M. Roden, J. P. Struewing, and W. A. Wolf. 2011. The eMERGE network: A consortium of biorepositories linked to electronic medical records data for conducting genomic studies. *BMC Medical Genomics* 4:13.

McDonnell, C., K. Werner, and L. Wendel. 2010. *Electronic health record usability: Vendor practices and perspectives, AHRQ publication no. 09(10)-0091-3-ef.* Rockville, MD: Agency for Healthcare Research and Quality.

Menikoff, J. 2013. The unbelievable rightness of being in clinical trials. *Hastings Center Report* 43(1):S30-S31.

Middleton, B. 2009. The clinical decision support consortium. *Studies in Health Technology & Informatics* 150:26-30.

Monaco, V., S. A. Jacobs, A. M. Arnold, and M. B. Simon. 2005. Providing PDA-based clinical trial listings to oncologists. *AMIA Annual Symposium Proceedings*:1056.

Murff, H. J., F. FitzHenry, M. E. Matheny, N. Gentry, K. L. Kotter, K. Crimin, R. S. Dittus, A. K. Rosen, P. L. Elkin, S. H. Brown, and T. Speroff. 2011. Automated identification of postoperative complications within an electronic medical record using natural language processing. *Journal of the American Medical Association* 306(8):848-855.

NCI (National Cancer Institute). 2013a. *Announcement: New national cancer informatics program.* https://cabig.nci.nih.gov/ncip_announcement (accessed March 12, 2013).

———. 2013b. *NCI mission statement.* http://www.cancer.gov/aboutnci/overview/mission (accessed March 5, 2013).

———. 2013c. *Overview of the SEER program.* http://seer.cancer.gov/about/overview.html (accessed June 13, 2012).

———. 2013d. *Transforming the NCI clinical trials enterprise.* http://transformingtrials.cancer.gov (accessed March 12, 2013).

Nease, D. E., Jr., M. T. t. Ruffin, M. S. Klinkman, M. Jimbo, T. M. Braun, and J. M. Underwood. 2008. Impact of a generalizable reminder system on colorectal cancer screening in diverse primary care practices: A report from the prompting and reminding at encounters for prevention project. *Medical Care* 46(9 Suppl 1):S68-S73.

Neilson, E. G., K. B. Johnson, S. T. Rosenbloom, W. D. Dupont, D. Talbert, D. A. Giuse, A. Kaiser, and R. A. Miller. 2004. The impact of peer management on test-ordering behavior. *Annals of Internal Medicine* 141(3):196-204.

Neumann, P. J. 2007. Challenges ahead for federal technology assessment. *Health Affairs (Millwood)* 26(2):w150-w152.

Newsham, A. C., C. Johnston, G. Hall, M. G. Leahy, A. B. Smith, A. Vikram, A. M. Donnelly, G. Velikova, P. J. Selby, and S. E. Fisher. 2011. Development of an advanced database for clinical trials integrated with an electronic patient record system. *Computers in Biology and Medicine* 41(8):575-586.

NRC (National Research Center). 2009. *Computational technology for effective health care: Immediate steps and strategic direction.* Washington, DC: The National Academies Press.

ONC (Office of the National Coordinator for Health Information Technology). 2013a. *About ONC.* http://www.healthit.gov/newsroom/about-onc (accessed February 26, 2013).

———. 2013b. *Clinical decision support.* http://www.healthit.gov/policy-researchers-implementers/clinical-decision-support-cds (accessed February 14, 2013).

———. 2013c. *Health information exchange.* http://www.healthit.gov/providers-professionals/health-information-exchange (accessed July 30, 2013).

———. 2013d. *Learn EHR basics.* http://www.healthit.gov/providers-professionals/learn-ehr-basics (accessed May 16, 2013).

———. 2013e. *What is meaningful use?* http://www.healthit.gov/policy-researchers-implementers/meaningful-use (accessed March 7, 2013).

Pawlson, L. G. 2007. Health information technology: Does it facilitate or hinder rapid learning? *Health Affairs (Millwood)* 26(2):w178-w180.

PCAST (President's Council of Advisors on Science and Technology). 2010. *Realizing the full potential of health information technology to improve healthcare for americans: The path forward.* http://www.whitehouse.gov/sites/default/files/microsites/ostp/pcast-health-it-report.pdf (accessed February 14, 2013).

PCORI (Patient-Centered Outcomes Research Institute). 2013a. *Patient-Centered Outcomes Research Institute to invest up to $68 million to develop a national patient-centered clinical research network.* http://www.pcori.org/2013/national-patient-centered-research-network (accessed April 25, 2013).

———. 2013b. *Research methodology.* http://www.pcori.org/research-we-support/methodology/ (accessed March 7, 2013).

Pearce, C., and S. Trumble. 2006. Computers can't listen: Algorithmic logic meets patient centredness. *Australian Familiy Physician* 35(6):439-442.

Perlin, J. B., and J. Kupersmith. 2007. Information technology and the inferential gap. *Health Affairs (Millwood)* 26(2):w192-w194.

Perry, A. 2012. *UK initiates first cancer reporting model of its kind in U.S.* http://uknow.uky.edu/content/uk-initiates-first-cancer-reporting-model-its-kind-us (accessed February 19, 2013).

Platt, R. 2007. Speed bumps, potholes, and tollbooths on the road to panacea: Making best use of data. *Health Affairs (Millwood)* 26(2):w153-w155.

Platt, R., M. Wilson, K. A. Chan, J. S. Benner, J. Marchibroda, and M. McClellan. 2009. The new Sentinel Network: Improving the evidence of medical-product safety. *New England Journal of Medicine* 361(7):645-647.

Platt, R., C. Grossman, and J. P. Selker. 2013. Evaluation as part of operations: Reconciling the Common Rule and continuous improvement. *Hastings Center Report* 43(1):S37-S39.

Potts, A. L., F. E. Barr, D. F. Gregory, L. Wright, and N. R. Patel. 2004. Computerized physician order entry and medication errors in a pediatric critical care unit. *Pediatrics* 113(1):59-63.

Puglisi, T. 2013. Reform within the Common Rule? *Hastings Center Report* 43(1):S40-S42.

Pulley, J. M., J. C. Denny, J. F. Peterson, G. R. Bernard, C. L. Vnencak-Jones, A. H. Ramirez, J. T. Delaney, E. Bowton, K. Brothers, K. Johnson, D. C. Crawford, J. Schildcrout, D. R. Masys, H. H. Dilks, R. A. Wilke, E. W. Clayton, E. Shultz, M. Laposata, J. McPherson, J. N. Jirjis, and D. M. Roden. 2012. Operational implementation of prospective genotyping for personalized medicine: The design of the Vanderbilt Predict Project. *Clinical Pharmacology & Therapeutics* 92(1):87-95.

RAND Health. 2005. *Health information technology: Can HIT lower costs and improve quality?* http://www.rand.org/content/dam/rand/pubs/research_briefs/2005/RAND_RB9136.pdf (accessed February 25, 2013).

Schedlbauer, A., V. Prasad, C. Mulvaney, S. Phansalkar, W. Stanton, D. W. Bates, and A. J. Avery. 2009. What evidence supports the use of computerized alerts and prompts to improve clinicians' prescribing behavior? *Journal of the American Medical Informatics Association* 16(4):531-538.

Selby, J., and H. Krumholz. 2013. Ethical oversight: Serving the best interests of patients. *Hastings Center Report* 43(1):S34-S36.

Selby, J. V., H. M. Krumholz, R. E. Kuntz, and F. S. Collins. 2013. Network news: Powering clinical research. *Science Translational Medicine* 5(182):182fs113.

Selker, H., C. Grossmann, A. Adams, D. Goldmann, C. Dezil, G. Meyer, V. Roger, L. A. Savitz, and R. Platt. 2011. The Common Rule and continuous improvement in health care: A learning health system perspective. *Commentary.* http://www.iom.edu/Global/Perspectives/2012/CommonRule.aspx?page=3 (accessed February 15, 2013).

Sequist, T. D., A. M. Zaslavsky, R. Marshall, R. H. Fletcher, and J. Z. Ayanian. 2009. Patient and physician reminders to promote colorectal cancer screening: A randomized controlled trial. *Archives of Internal Medicine* 169(4):364-371.

Shea, S., W. DuMouchel, and L. Bahamonde. 1996. A meta-analysis of 16 randomized controlled trials to evaluate computer-based clinical reminder systems for preventive care in the ambulatory setting. *Journal of the American Medical Informatics Association* 3(6):399-409.

Slutsky, J. R. 2007. Moving closer to a rapid-learning health care system. *Health Affairs (Millwood)* 26(2):w122-w124.

Snyder, C. F., A. L. Blackford, J. R. Brahmer, M. A. Carducci, R. Pili, V. Stearns, A. C. Wolff, S. M. Dy, and A. W. Wu. 2010. Needs assessments can identify scores on HRQOL questionnaires that represent problems for patients: An illustration with the supportive care needs survey and the qlq-c30. *Quality of Life Research* 19(6):837-845.

Starr, R. 2013. Deloitte: *Alliance around big data and analytics*. http://www.big4.com/deloitte/deloitte-alliance-around-big-data-and-analytics/?zbrandid=4337&zidType=CH&zid=1 5757612&zsubscriberId=1021390268&zbdom=http://npc.informz.net (accessed March 7, 2013).

Stewart, W. F., N. R. Shah, M. J. Selna, R. A. Paulus, and J. M. Walker. 2007. Bridging the inferential gap: The electronic health record and clinical evidence. *Health Affairs (Millwood)* 26(2):w181-w191.

Taenzer, P., B. D. Bultz, L. E. Carlson, M. Speca, T. DeGagne, K. Olson, R. Doll, and Z. Rosberger. 2000. Impact of computerized quality of life screening on physician behaviour and patient satisfaction in lung cancer outpatients. *Psychooncology* 9(3):203-213.

Tunis, S. R., T. V. Carino, R. D. Williams, 2nd, and P. B. Bach. 2007. Federal initiatives to support rapid learning about new technologies. *Health Affairs (Millwood)* 26(2):w140-w149.

VA (Department of Veterans Affairs). 2013. *VistA*. http://www.ehealth.va.gov/VistA.asp (accessed February 12, 2013).

Velikova, G., L. Booth, A. B. Smith, P. M. Brown, P. Lynch, J. M. Brown, and P. J. Selby. 2004. Measuring quality of life in routine oncology practice improves communication and patient well-being: A randomized controlled trial. *Journal of Clinical Oncology* 22(4):714-724.

Walker, J., S. G. Leveille, L. Ngo, E. Vodicka, J. D. Darer, S. Dhanireddy, J. G. Elmore, H. J. Feldman, M. J. Lichtenfeld, N. Oster, J. D. Ralston, S. E. Ross, and T. Delbanco. 2011. Inviting patients to read their doctors' notes: Patients and doctors look ahead: Patient and physician surveys. *Annals of Internal Medicine* 155(12):811-819.

Wallace, P. J. 2007. Reshaping cancer learning through the use of health information technology. *Health Affairs (Millwood)* 26(2):w169-w177.

Wallwiener, M., C. W. Wallwiener, J. K. Kansy, H. Seeger, and T. K. Rajab. 2009. Impact of electronic messaging on the patient-physician interaction. *Journal of Telemedicine & Telecare* 15(5):243-250.

Wellcome Trust. 2013. *UK biobank*. http://www.wellcome.ac.uk/Funding/Biomedical-science/Funded-projects/Major-initiatives/UK-Biobank/index.htm (accessed February 25, 2013).

West, D. 2011. *Enabling personalized medicine through health information technology: Advancing the integration of information*. http://www.brookings.edu/research/papers/2011/01/28-personalized-medicine-west (accessed February 15, 2013).

———. 2012. *How mobile devices are transforming healthcare*. http://www.brookings.edu/research/papers/2012/05/22-mobile-health-west (accessed February 12, 2013).

Wolf, L., J. Harvell, and A. K. Jha. 2012. Hospitals ineligible for federal meaningful-use incentives have dismally low rates of adoption of electronic health records. *Health Affairs (Millwood)* 31(3):505-513.

Wu, W., T. L. Schifftner, W. G. Henderson, C. B. Eaton, R. M. Poses, G. Uttley, S. C. Sharma, M. Vezeridis, S. F. Khuri, and P. D. Friedmann. 2007. Preoperative hematocrit levels and postoperative outcomes in older patients undergoing noncardiac surgery. *Journal of the American Medical Association* 297(22):2481-2488.

Yamin, C. K., S. Emani, D. H. Williams, S. R. Lipsitz, A. S. Karson, J. S. Wald, and D. W. Bates. 2011. The digital divide in adoption and use of a personal health record. *Archives of Internal Medicine* 171(6):568-574.

Yasnoff, W. A., L. Sweeney, and E. H. Shortliffe. 2013. Putting health IT on the path to success. *JAMA* 309(10):989-990.

Yu, P. P. 2011. The evolution of oncology electronic health records. *Cancer Journal* 17(4):197-202.

7

Translating Evidence into Practice, Measuring Quality, and Improving Performance

Ahigh-quality cancer care delivery system should translate evidence into practice, measure quality, and improve the performance of clinicians. To arrive at a high-quality cancer care delivery system that does just that, clinicians need tools and initiatives that assist them with quickly incorporating new medical knowledge into routine care. Clinicians also need to be able to measure and assess progress in improving the delivery of cancer care, publicly report that information, and develop innovative strategies for further performance improvement.

In the figure illustrating the committee's conceptual framework (see Figure S-2), knowledge translation and performance improvement are part of a cyclical process that measures the outcomes of patient-clinician interactions, implements innovative strategies to improve care, evaluates the impact of those interventions on the quality of care, and generates new hypotheses for investigation. Clinical practice guidelines (CPGs), quality metrics, and performance improvement initiatives are all tools supportive of that cyclical process. CPGs and performance improvement strategies enhance the translation of evidence into practice. Specifically, CPGs translate research results into clinical recommendations for clinicians, and performance improvement initiatives systematically bring about a change in the delivery of care that reflects the best available evidence. Quality metrics evaluate health care clinicians' performance and practices by comparing actual clinical practices against recommended practices, and identifying areas that could be improved.

A high-quality cancer care delivery system's focus on quality metrics and CPGs is consistent with the Institute of Medicine's (IOM's) 1999 report

Ensuring Quality Cancer Care, which recommended improving clinicians' use of systematically developed guidelines and increasing the measurement and monitoring of cancer care using a core set of quality measures (IOM and NRC, 1999). Despite those recommendations, the translation of research findings into practice in the current cancer care system has been slow and incomplete, and many challenges plague the system for measuring and assessing performance. CPGs, for example, are often developed by fragmented processes that lack transparency (IOM, 2011c). Serious limitations in the evidence base supporting CPGs can result in different guidelines being developed on the same topic with conflicting advice to clinicians. Performance improvement initiatives are generally modest, localized efforts, and because they are tailored to unique local circumstances, are difficult to translate to the national level. Similarly, there are many challenges and pervasive gaps in existing measures that impede the development of cancer quality metrics.

The previous chapters discussed the importance of improving the scientific evidence base to guide the clinical decision making of patients and their health care clinicians, as well as the role of a learning health care information technology (IT) system for cancer in accomplishing this goal. This chapter discusses how to ensure that this evidence is translated into practice, that quality is measured, and that the system monitors and assesses its performance. The majority of the chapter focuses on cancer quality metrics. The committee commissioned a background paper on this topic and identified a great need for improvement in the metrics development process. The remainder of the chapter focuses on CPGs and performance improvement initiatives. The committee relied heavily on the IOM's previous work on CPGs to derive the evidence base for the guideline portion of this chapter (IOM, 2008, 2011c). The committee identifies one recommendation for improving cancer quality metrics.

CANCER QUALITY METRICS[1]

Cancer quality measures provide objective descriptors of the consequences of care and transform the nebulous concept of "good medicine" into a measurable discipline. These measures serve a number of roles in assessing quality of care by providing a standardized and objective means of measurement. For example, quality assurance measures assess a clinician's or an organization's performance for purposes of compliance, accreditation, and payment. Performance improvement metrics, however,

---

[1] This section of the chapter was adapted from a background paper by Tracy Spinks, MD Anderson Cancer Center and Consultant, IOM Committee on Improving the Quality of Cancer Care: Addressing the Challenges of an Aging Population (2012).

are designed to identify gaps in care with the objective of closing those gaps. Typically these measures are implemented in a collaborative, rather than a punitive, environment. They can drive improvements in care by informing patients and influencing clinician behavior and reimbursement. Appropriately selected quality measures may be used prospectively to influence decision making and care planning and to align the mutual interests of patients, caregivers, clinicians, and payers. Moreover, they can provide insights into practice variations between clinicians and document changes over time within a given practice setting.

There are many unique considerations in measuring the quality of cancer care. As discussed in earlier chapters, the complexity of cancer care has exceeded that of many other common chronic conditions. Cancer comprises hundreds of different types of diseases and subtypes and includes multiple stages of disease (e.g., precancer, early-stage disease, metastatic disease). Cancer care often occurs in multiple phases—an acute phase, a chronic phase, and an end-of-life phase—requiring different treatments and approaches to care over time. The multiple treatment modalities and combination strategies during the acute treatment phase demand coordinated teams of professionals with multiple skill sets. Treatment during the chronic phase also requires coordination between various care teams. Additionally, patients and clinicians must make difficult treatment decisions due to the toxicity of many of the treatment options. Quality measures in cancer need to reflect and account for these complex characteristics of the disease.

The National Quality Forum (NQF), the Agency for Healthcare Research and Quality (AHRQ), the American Society of Clinical Oncology (ASCO), and the American College of Surgeons' (ACoS's) Commission on Cancer (CoC) have developed[2] or endorsed[3] a number of quality measures specific to or applicable to cancer for use in performance improvement and national mandatory reporting programs in the United States. These measures broadly fall into two categories: disease-specific measures (e.g., measures specific to breast cancer), and cross-cutting measures, which apply to a variety of cancers. Additionally, the Patient Protection and Affordable Care Act[4] outlined six categories of measures for use in federal reporting of cancer care by the nation's eleven cancer centers not

---

[2] An organization develops a quality measure by investing time and resources to create a new variable to measure.

[3] An organization endorses a quality measure by publicly expressing support or approval for the measure.

[4] Patient Protection and Affordable Care Act, Public Law 111-148, 111th Congress, 2nd Sess. (March 23, 2010).

TABLE 7-1 Examples of Quality Metrics Projects Relevant to Cancer Care

Organization	Description
Assessing Care of Vulnerable Elders (ACOVE)	ACOVE quality measures were developed by health services researchers at RAND Corporation in 2000 to assess care provided to vulnerable older adults (defined as those most likely to die or become severely disabled in the next 2 years). The measures reflect the complexity of measuring the quality of care for older adults, who often have multiple comorbidities and substantial variation in treatment preferences. They cover the broad range of health care issues that older adults experience, including primary care, chronic obstructive pulmonary disease, colorectal cancer, breast cancer, sleep disorders, and benign prostatic hypertrophy.
National Cancer Data Base (NCDB)	The Commission on Cancer (CoC) is a multidisciplinary consortium dedicated to increasing survival and improving quality of life in cancer patients through research, education, standard setting, and quality assessments. Currently, more than 1,500 cancer programs meet the criteria for CoC accreditation (ACoS, 2011d), which requires a review of the scope, organization, and activity of the cancer program and compliance with 36 specific standards (ACoS, 2011c). Since 1996, all CoC-accredited cancer programs have been required to submit data to the NCDB, a joint program of CoC and the American Cancer Society. The cases submitted to the NCDB represent approximately 70 percent of all newly diagnosed cancer cases in the United States and are summarized in various clinician-level reports to facilitate performance improvement, create benchmarks for comparative purposes, and identify trends in cancer care, such as survival and cancer incidence.

paid under the Prospective Payment System (PPS)[5]: outcomes, structure, process, costs of care, efficiency, and patients' perspectives on care. Existing measures are largely process oriented, although there are some measures of outcomes, structure, and patients' perceptions of care. The activities of major organizations involved in quality metrics in cancer are summarized in Table 7-1.

---

[5] The Prospective Payment System is used by Medicare to reimburse providers for services based on predetermined prices.

TABLE 7-1 Continued

Organization	Description
National Quality Forum (NQF)	The NQF was formed in 1999 in response to a specific recommendation of the President's Advisory Commission to create a nonprofit, public-private partnership that would develop a national strategy for measuring and reporting on health care quality to advance national aims in health care. In 2009, the NQF was awarded a contract with the U.S. Department of Health and Human Services (HHS) to endorse health care quality measures for use in public reporting in the United States. To date, the NQF has endorsed more than 60 cancer-specific measures that were developed by the American Society of Clinical Oncology (ASCO), the American Academy of Medicine's (AMA's) Physician Consortium for Performance Improvement, the American Society for Radiation Oncology, and the American Urological Association. These include more than 40 disease-specific measures that assess screening, diagnosis and staging, and initial cancer treatment (e.g., measures that assess concordance with treatment guidelines for breast cancer). The NQF has also endorsed broader cross-cutting measures that focus on end-of-life issues, such as symptom management and overutilization of care.
National Quality Measures Clearinghouse (NQMC)	The Agency for Healthcare Research and Quality established the NQMC in 2002 to serve as a Web-based repository of evidence-based health care quality measures and to promote widespread access to these measures among health care clinicians, health plans, purchasers, and other interested stakeholders. As of June 2013, the NQMC included 370 cancer-specific measures that assess screening, initial treatment, and end-of-life care. Of note, the NQMC includes many NQF-endorsed measures as well as cancer-specific measures that were developed outside of the United States, such as in Australia and the United Kingdom. The NQMC also includes a database of 95 cancer-specific measures currently used by the various agencies within HHS, including the Medicare Fee-For-Service Physician Feedback Program, the Meaningful Use Electronic Health Record Incentive Program, and the Hospital Outpatient Quality Reporting Program.

continued

TABLE 7-1 Continued

Organization	Description
National Surgical Quality Improvement Program (NSQIP)	The Department of Veterans Affairs (VA) developed NSQIP in 1994 to monitor and improve the quality of surgical interventions in all VA medical centers. The American College of Surgeons expanded NSQIP in 2004 to serve as a private-sector quality improvement program for surgical care. The program is intended to assist hospitals in capturing and reporting 30-day morbidity and mortality outcomes for all major inpatient and outpatient surgical procedures. Examples of measures include surgical site infection, urinary tract infection, surgical outcomes in older adults, colorectal surgery outcomes, and lower-extremity bypass. The measures are captured using a site's Surgical Clinical Reviewer who reviews patients' medical charts, and if necessary, may contact patients by letters or phone.
Physician Consortium for Performance Improvement (PCPI)	PCPI, a national, physician-led initiative convened by the AMA, has developed evidence-based health care quality measures for use in the clinical setting. The NQF has endorsed more than 20 cancer-specific measures developed by PCPI, including cross-cutting measures for pain and disease-specific measures for breast, prostate, and other cancers.
Quality Oncology Practice Initiative (QOPI)	ASCO began work on its QOPI Program in 2002 to fill the void in oncology quality measurement. ASCO made the QOPI Program available to its member physicians as a voluntary practice-based program in 2006. This program provides tools and resources to oncology practices for quality measurement, benchmarking, and performance improvement and currently has more than 800 registered member practices. ASCO also offers a 3-year certification through its QOPI Certification Program, which is available to outpatient medical or hematology oncology practices in the United States. QOPI certification is awarded to practices that meet data submission requirements, minimum performance on a subset of QOPI measures, and compliance with certification standards developed by ASCO and the Oncology Nursing Society. As of June 2013, there are 190 QOPI-certified oncology practices across the country.

SOURCES: ACoS, 2011a,b,c,d, 2013; AHRQ, 2012b,c,d,e; AMA, 2012; ASCO, 2012b,c,e, 2013; Bilimoria et al., 2008; Jacobson et al., 2008; Kizer, 2000; McNiff, 2006; Menck et al., 1991; NQF, 2012b,d, 2013c; President's Advisory Commission on Consumer Protection and Quality in the Health Care Industry, 1998; RAND, 2010.

Challenges in Cancer Quality Measurement

There is minimal empirical support that publicly reporting health care quality measures has triggered meaningful improvements in the effectiveness, safety, and patient-centeredness of care (Shekelle et al., 2008; Werner et al., 2009). At best, experts have noted "pockets of excellence on specific measures or in particular services at individual health care facilities" (Chassin and Loeb, 2011, p. 562). Because cancer care has largely been excluded from public reporting, it is unclear whether these findings will hold true for cancer care in the future; however, some studies examining the impact of quality reporting in cancer care have noted improvements in care.

Blayney and colleagues studied the impact of implementing the ASCO Quality Oncology Practice Initiative (QOPI) at the University of Michigan's Comprehensive Cancer Center between 2006 and 2008. They found that physicians changed their behavior when provided with oncology-specific quality data, especially in the areas of treatment planning and management (Blayney et al., 2009). Between 2009 and 2011, Blayney and colleagues expanded their focus and evaluated the impact of implementing QOPI at multiple oncology practices. They concluded that physician participation in the voluntary reporting program increased when the costs of data collection were defrayed by Blue Cross Blue Shield of Michigan. At the same time, they found that providing physicians with access to the quality reports was insufficient to trigger measurable improvements in care across participating practices (Blayney et al., 2012). In a separate study, Wick and colleagues studied the impact of participation in the ACoS's National Surgical Quality Improvement Program (NSQIP) on surgical site infection rates following colorectal surgery at the Johns Hopkins Hospital. They observed a 33.3 percent reduction in the surgical site infection rate during the 2-year period studied (July 2009 to July 2011) (Wick et al., 2012).

There is no federal program that requires clinicians to report data on core cancer measures. Existing programs are primarily voluntary and favor "measures of convenience," which are easy to report but lack meaning for patients (Spinks et al., 2011, p. 669). These measures are generally clinician-oriented, reflect existing fragmentation in care, and lack a clear method for triggering improvements. Most measures focus on short-term outcomes in care. Thus, there are serious deficiencies in cancer quality measurement in the United States, including (1) pervasive gaps in existing cancer measures, (2) challenges intrinsic to the measure development process, (3) a lack of consumer engagement in measure development and reporting, and (4) the need for data to support meaningful, timely, and actionable performance measurement. This chapter discusses each of these issues below.

Gaps in Existing Cancer Measures

No current quality reporting program or set of measures adequately assesses cancer care in a comprehensive, patient-oriented way. A recent report by the NQF-convened Measure Applications Partnership (MAP), which provides input to the Secretary of Health and Human Services (HHS) on the selection of measures for use in federal reporting, noted that cancer care measures are largely disease specific, process focused, and measured at the clinician level. These measures support operational improvement, but they are limited in their ability to induce wide-scale improvements in care, and provide limited insight into overall health care quality (MAP and NQF, 2012). For example, process measures are useful for establishing minimum standards for delivery systems to achieve and are simple to validate. Unfortunately, they do not reliably predict outcomes and they rarely are able to account for patient preferences of what constitutes a desirable care. Thus, it is important that process measures be supplemented by additional measures of outcome, structure, efficiency, cost, and patient perception of their care. Table 7-2 provides a summary of the benefits and drawbacks of the various types of measures used in cancer care.

All phases of the cancer care continuum—from prevention and early detection, to treatment, survivorship, and end-of-life care—need new measures. While NQF-endorsed measures and those included in the National Quality Measures Clearinghouse (NQMC) focus on screening and initial cancer treatment, few measures address post-treatment follow-up and the long-term consequences of care, such as survivorship care, disease recurrence, and secondary cancers. Assessments of end-of-life care, including overuse of therapeutic treatment at the end of life, are included in both measure sets, but could be expanded (AHRQ, 2012c; NQF, 2012d). The QOPI measure set primarily addresses treatment and includes a few measures related to prevention and diagnosis, as well as more than 25 measures evaluating end-of-life care (ASCO, 2012d). All of these measure sets, however, could better assess palliative care and hospice care referral patterns and the associated quality of life for cancer patients requiring these services. The MAP report emphasized survivorship care (by stage and cancer type), palliative care, and end-of-life care as priorities for enhancing quality measurement across the continuum of care (MAP and NQF, 2012).

Existing cancer measures also often fail to address all of the relevant dimensions of cancer care, such as access to care and care coordination, evaluation and management of psychosocial needs, patient and family engagement (especially shared decision making and honoring patient preferences), management of complex comorbidities, and advance care

TABLE 7-2 Types of Quality Metrics Used in Cancer Care

Type	Description	Benefits	Challenges
Structure	Measures the settings in which clinicians deliver health care, including material resources, human resources, and organizational structure (e.g., types of services available, qualifications of clinicians, and staffing hierarchies)	Identifies core infrastructure needed for high-quality care	Difficult to compare across settings of variable sizes and resources; implications for patients' outcomes not always clear
Process	Measures the delivery of care in defined circumstances (e.g., screening the general populations, psychosocial evaluations of all newly diagnosed patients, care planning before starting chemotherapy)	Encourages evidence-based care and is generally straightforward to measure	Need to consider patient choices that differ from standard of care and contraindications; implications for patients' outcomes not always clear
Clinical Outcome	Measures personal health and functional status as a consequence of contact with the health care system (e.g., survival, success of treatment)	Allows assessment of ultimate endpoints of care	Need to risk adjust for comorbidities; difficult to compare across settings with variable populations
Patient-Reported Outcome	Measures patients' perceived physical, mental, and social well-being based on information that comes directly from the patient (e.g., quality of life, time to return to normal activity, symptom burden)	Integrates the patient's "voice" into the medical record	Some outcomes are outside the scope of clinical care (e.g., social well-being)
Patients' Perspective on Care	Measures patients' satisfaction with the health care they received	Gathers data on patients' experience throughout the health care delivery cycle	Need to account for patients' limitations in assessing technical aspects of care

continued

TABLE 7-2 Continued

Type	Description	Benefits	Challenges
Cost	Measures the resources required for the health care system to deliver care and the economic impact on patients, their families, and governmental and private payers	Allows parties to weigh the relative values of potential treatment options, when combined with outcome measures	Difficult to measure the true cost of care given the range of prices and expenses in medical care; costs vary according to perspective (patients, payer, society, etc.); need to distinguish between costs and charges
Efficiency	Measures the time, effort, or cost to produce a specific output in the health care system (e.g., time to initiate therapy after diagnosis, coordination of care)	Reflects important determinants of patients' outcomes and satisfaction with care and is a major driver of cost	Need to correlate with outcome measures; need to account for patient characteristics and preferences
Cross-Cutting	Measures issues that cross cancer or disease types (e.g., patient safety, care coordination, equity, and patients' perspective on care)	Aligns with measurement of other cancers or conditions and reflects true multidisciplinary nature of cancer care	Difficult to capture the unique characteristics of cancer
Disease-Specific	Measures issues within a specific cancer type (e.g., clinicians' concordance with clinical practice guidelines for breast, prostate, and colon cancer)	Reflects diversity of cancer and tumor biology	Need to account for stage of disease at presentation and comorbidities

NOTE: The basis of quality measurement centers on the three major elements of quality measurement: outcome, processes and structure (Donabedian, 1980). These elements have been expanded in recent years to include concepts of efficiency, cost, and patient-reported outcomes. The types of measures are interrelated and overlapping. For example, a measure can be disease-specific and a process or outcome measure, or a patient-reported outcome and a clinical outcome.

planning for cancer patients. There are a number of NQF-endorsed measures, as well as measures in the NQMC and QOPI, that focus on the short-term physical consequences of cancer and its treatment (AHRQ, 2012c; ASCO, 2012d; NQF, 2012d). In addition, Cancer Care Ontario conducted a recent performance improvement project that included developing measures to assess the integration and coordination of palliative care services in cancer care (Dudgeon et al., 2009). However, management of complex comorbidities and the functional, emotional, and social consequences of the disease, and other high-quality measures, are largely unaddressed by current measures (Bishop, 2013; Spinks et al., 2011).

There are also gaps in measures that assess care planning and care coordination, which is particularly problematic because cancer care is rarely confined to one hospital or physician. Cancer patients tend to move between multiple care settings—primary care teams, cancer care teams, community and specialty hospitals, and potentially emergency centers, long-term care facilities, and hospice care (MAP and NQF, 2012). Existing cancer measures are limited by where a patient receives cancer care because many oncology practices and hospitals lack the infrastructure and sophistication to measure the quality of care they deliver. Moreover, NQF requires its endorsed measures to be validated in a specific disease or care setting, thus limiting the applicability of the measures in persons with multiple comorbidities or who traverse multiple care settings. In addition, the measurement of care is fragmented and rarely focused on the overall patient experience. Few measurement systems integrate a patient's experience across care settings.

Quality metric development has also thus far failed to prioritize less common cancers. Although NQF has endorsed and AHRQ has included in the NQMC a number of disease-specific measures, including measures for more common cancers, such as breast and prostate cancers, as well as measures for less common cancers, such as pancreatic cancer and multiple myeloma, these measures are not evenly distributed across the diseases. There are few or no measures for other rare cancers, such as brain and ovarian cancers (AHRQ, 2012c; NQF, 2012d). QOPI, for example, includes disease-specific measures for breast, colorectal, lung, and gynecologic cancers, and non-Hodgkin lymphoma, but does not address prostate cancer or many other rare cancers (ASCO, 2012d).

The IOM's 1999 report on the quality of cancer care recommended that patients undergoing technical procedures be treated in high-volume facilities (IOM and NRC, 1999). A large body of evidence shows that patients undergoing high-risk surgeries at high-volume facilities have better health outcomes and short-term survival than patients treated in low-volume facilities (Birkmeyer et al., 2003; Finks et al., 2011; Finlayson et al., 2003; Ho et al., 2006). Even with their strong track record, however, high-volume facilities currently lack the capacity to treat all cancer patients who require highly skilled procedures (Finks et al., 2011; Spinks et al., 2012). Thus, it will be necessary to establish additional quality measures that identify high-quality, lower volume facilities and clinicians.

ACoS's NSQIP, the American Board of Medical Specialties Maintenance of Certification Evaluation of Performance in Practice, the Joint Commission Ongoing Professional Practice Evaluation, and some payer-driven pay-for-performance initiatives are implementing programs for clinicians at low-volume facilities to transparently attain, verify, and maintain competence in highly technical procedures. These programs should be continually employed to help patients identify competent clinicians, regardless of the size of the program in which they practice (Spinks et al., 2012).

The challenges to developing meaningful and comprehensive quality measurements are amplified in older adults with cancer. Older adults have been underrepresented in quality measurement for cancer care for several reasons: their underrepresentation in clinical trials (see Chapter 5), conflicting recommendations and clinician beliefs regarding cancer screening and therapeutic treatment for this population, increased sensitivity to treatment-related toxicities, and multiple comorbidities (see discussion on older adults in Chapter 2). As a result, existing quality measures may not apply directly to older adults with cancer, and in some cases, existing quality measures may be clinically inappropriate for older adults with cancer. Process-based measures are traditionally developed based on guidelines for patients with a single disease (i.e., cancer), which do not address the complexities of caring for many older patients who have multiple, complex conditions and receive care across multiple settings over time.

Challenges Associated with the Measure Development Process

Many of the cancer measurement gaps stem from challenges associated with the measure development process. The NQF, AHRQ, and other organizations have adopted stringent guidelines for the evaluation of health care quality measures, such as scientific acceptability, usability, importance, and feasibility. These guidelines help ensure meaningful quality metrics that measure what they are intended to and help inform the decisions of patients, payers, and federal and state agencies. While this approach is generally well suited for process-based measures that evaluate the technical aspects of care (e.g., guideline adherence), it is not particularly suitable for evaluating other measures that assess the interpersonal aspects of care, outcomes, patients' perspectives on care, and other non-process-oriented measures. In addition, quality measures often do not account for the appropriateness of some processes of care measures in special circumstances (e.g., advanced dementia, short life expectancy).

A lack of national coordination and oversight seriously compromises the measurement development process. Many independent groups, capable of funding the testing and validation of their own measures, have developed discipline-specific quality metrics, which reflects the fragmentation in health care delivery. In its 2011 report *For the Public's Health: The Role of Measurement in Action and Accountability*, the IOM noted that this process had produced an abundance of overlapping health care measure sets that vary in quality and application, confuse health care decision makers, and lead to further fragmentation in an already splintered field (IOM, 2011a). For example, the NQF has endorsed two measures related to hormonal therapy for hormone receptor positive breast cancer: *NQF measure #0220—Adjuvant hormonal therapy*; and *NQF measure #0387— Oncology: Hormonal therapy for stage IC through IIIC, ER/PR positive breast cancer* (NQF, 2012a,e). Both measures, based on National Comprehensive Cancer Network's (NCCN's) CPGs for breast cancer patients, have slight, but meaningful differences (e.g., patient population, care setting, and/or data source). This lack of coordination has contributed to pervasive gaps in measures, as discussed above.

Efforts by organizations, such as the NQF, to create parsimonious families of quality measures have reduced measure fragmentation to a limited degree. These organizations have prioritized the development of measures that fill crucial gaps in cancer measurement and apply to certain diseases and dimensions of care. Because these organizations lack the authority to ensure that measure developers implement their recommendations, however, minimal progress has been made in filling persisting gaps.

These groups are also working to harmonize existing measures. In its 2010 publication *Guidance for Measure Harmonization—A Consensus Report*, the NQF provided specific guidance to measure developers and NQF project steering committees. Outlined in the report were seven principles for measuring harmonization as well as considerations for harmonizing overlapping and related measures (NQF, 2010). Additionally, when submitting measures to the NQF for potential endorsement, measure developers must attest that the measure has been harmonized with existing measures (NQF, 2012c).

Compared with the scientific evidence supporting measurement of the technical aspects of cancer care (Schneider et al., 2004), there is a major void in the body of evidence supporting measure development for other dimensions of care—most notably, access to care and care coordination; patient and family engagement (including shared decision making and honoring patient preferences); management of complex comorbidities; quality-of-life issues during and after treatment; reintegration into society (e.g., return to work); and the costs of care. In Chapter 5, the committee makes several recommendations for improving the breadth and depth of information collected in clinical research. If these recommendations are implemented, the scientific evidence available to inform measurement development should improve.

Many process-of-care measures assess adherence to disease- and stage-specific CPGs. Despite the ubiquity of these guidelines, wide variations in adherence have been observed for certain diseases, for selected clinicians, and within cancer programs (Foster et al., 2009; Romanus et al., 2009). The voluntary nature of guideline adherence drives some variation, while a patient's prior cancer treatment, comorbidities, and preferences may also influence guideline adherence (Spinks et al., 2012). Respecting individual patient needs, values, and preferences is at the heart of patient centeredness and is the foundation for the shift toward patient-driven, personalized cancer care (see discussion in Chapter 3). Thus, measures of clinicians' adherence to guidelines must account for patient preferences in assessing performance without penalizing clinicians for honoring patients' preferences. These measures should address patients who opt for care that differs from recommendations for screening and treatment (Kahn et al., 2002).

Several process-of-care measures "credit" physicians for recommending guideline-based treatment to their cancer patients, even when the patient does not receive the treatment due to medical contraindications or patient preference (e.g., *NQF measure #0220—Adjuvant hormonal therapy*) (NQF, 2012a), which is appropriate in many instances. It is important that measures be transparent and distinguish between concordant and recommended care. These delineations can identify areas where disparities in access to care exist and can be used to understand the relationship between the long-term outcomes and the use of evidence-based guidelines (NQF, 2012c)

Clinician attribution can also challenge the development of quality measures. Health care quality measures should assess aspects of care that may be influenced by individual clinicians (IOM, 2001), specifically for the purposes of accountability and reimbursement. In the current health care delivery system, where patients often move between multiple care settings and multiple clinicians are influencing patient outcomes, attribution of health care outcomes has become daunting. The shift to an "episode of care" framework, where quality is assessed and costs are accumulated across clinicians for a specific condition or disease or a designated period of time, could make the assessment of clinician attribution even more complicated because it will be unclear which clinician is responsible for each health outcome (Krumholz et al., 2008).

Understandably, clinicians may be reticent to be held accountable for the outcomes of care where multiple health care clinicians are engaged in its delivery. When resource use for any one patient is evaluated across multiple clinicians, these concerns may be amplified (Hussey and McGlynn, 2009). Thus, measure developers should adopt adequate precautions to ensure that measures are attributed to the individuals, groups, or organizations responsible for the decisions, outcomes, and costs of care (Krumholz et al., 2008). Cancer care plans, as recommended in Chapter 3, should indicate who is responsible for each element of care provision, thereby making attribution easier. In assessing whether appropriate care was received, quality measures should account for the complications of treating asymptomatic disease, inappropriate or inadequate prior care, and patient preferences that differ from clinician recommendations (Kahn et al., 2002).

A number of risk-adjustment strategies, which account for factors that influence clinical outcomes (e.g., patient demographics, severity of illness, comorbid conditions), have been developed to support equitable comparisons across clinicians and to assess variations in patient outcomes. Because these models are not specific to cancer, however, they ignore some primary drivers of cancer outcomes: cancer type and stage, tumor markers, functional status and well-being, previous treatment, and patient adherence with treatment regimens (Kahn et al., 2002). Although a number of efforts (most recently by the University Health System Consortium) have been initiated to enhance existing risk-adjustment methodologies for more meaningful comparisons of cancer care (UHC, 2012), the utility of these models is limited by the availability, quality, and completeness of data to support risk adjustment.

Traditional risk-adjustment models utilize administrative claims data, which are widely available, but fail to capture many important variables, such as functional status, patient adherence with treatment regimens, socioeconomic status, and education level. Thus, standardized definitions, data collection, and reporting methods should be adopted for these outcomes drivers. Additionally, as risk-adjustment models are refined, risk adjustments should not mask disparities in care (Deutsch et al., 2012; NQF, 2012c; Weissman et al., 2011). Weismann and colleagues recommended stratifying outcomes by socioeconomic status and other demographic factors, where possible, rather than adjusting for these factors (Weissman et al., 2011).

A similar problem exists in comparing measures across care settings, especially measures of patients' survival. Recently, a number of academic cancer centers began publishing their 3- and 5-year survival outcomes on the Internet, usually comparing their outcomes to national statistics or community-based data (Goldberg, 2011). Although survival outcomes data are critically important to patients, interpreting comparative survival outcomes data are complicated because of the great variability in cancer care delivery organizations' patient populations and approaches to staging and labeling cancers (Berry, 2011). NQF's MAP has had formal discussions about how to publicly report survival outcomes in a way that allows meaningful comparisons (NQF, 2012f). However, considerable work needs to be done to achieve this goal.

Finally, small sample sizes can create problems for the measure development process. As part of that process, developers perform statistical testing to ensure that the measure results are statistically valid. Small sample sizes—which arise from measuring rare diseases, the increasing specificity of many measures, and measuring at the clinician level where an individual clinician may only see a small number of patients with a specific condition of interest (Higgins et al., 2011; MAP and NQF, 2012)— make it difficult to validate results. Cross-cutting measures that focus more broadly on patient safety, care coordination, and patients' perspectives on care can help to overcome the limitations of small sample sizes (MAP and NQF, 2012). Use of these measures would create opportunities for assessing the quality of care across a much larger population, particularly for patients with rarer diseases that have not been addressed by existing disease-specific measures.

Lack of Consumer Engagement in Quality Measurement

Publicly reporting health care quality measures has been championed as a means of guiding patients to high-quality and efficient health care. The HHS National Strategy for Performance Improvement in Health Care (or National Quality Strategy) has identified public reporting as a policy lever for improving patients' access to high-quality and affordable care in the United States (National Priorities Partnership, 2011). Furthermore, Hibbard and Sofaer proposed that consumer use of comparative performance reports might influence health care quality by enabling patients to seek out and obtain high-quality health care and encouraging performance improvement among health care clinicians to protect their reputations and maintain their market share (Hibbard and Sofaer, 2010).

This consumer-driven health care model assumes that patients, when provided with health care quality data, will seek care from high-quality and low-cost clinicians (Harris and Beeuwkes Buntin, 2008). Research suggests that patients have a strong interest in information on clinician quality (Harris and Beeuwkes Buntin, 2008), but rarely use health care quality data in choosing a clinician (Faber et al., 2009; Totten et al., 2012). For example, the Henry J. Kaiser Family Foundation, together with AHRQ, conducted a series of patient surveys in 2000, 2004, and 2006 to assess the national perception of health care quality, patients' exposure to and use of health care quality information, and patients' experience with poor care coordination and medical errors. In the 2006 study, only 36 percent of respondents reported viewing information on the quality of health plans, hospitals, and doctors within the prior year, and only 20 percent of respondents reported using this information to make health care decisions. Exposure to and usage of information on health plans was highest (29 percent and 12 percent, respectively) while exposure to and usage of information on physicians was lowest (12 percent and 7 percent, respectively) (KFF and AHRQ, 2006).

In 2010, AHRQ began publishing its "Best Practices in Public Reporting" series to guide public and private organizations in making public reports of health care quality data clearer, more meaningful, and actionable for patients. The first report in this series—*Best Practices in Public Reporting No. 1: How to Effectively Present Health Care Performance Data to Consumers*—outlined several challenges to consumers' use of health care quality data, including differing definitions of quality among patients and clinical experts, and consumer difficulty with understanding and interpreting quality measures. The report also noted that clinical quality measures are often not meaningful to patients and are frequently misinterpreted. For example, patients may not associate high rates of hospital readmissions with poor care or harm by clinicians. Additionally, patients erroneously may equate more efficient, lower cost care with poor care (Hibbard and Sofaer, 2010). This type of misinterpretation may be common across all segments of society, but is likely more concentrated among individuals with poor health literacy, a characteristic that is disproportionately high among older adults and individuals with limited education, poor English proficiency, lower socioeconomic status, or mental or physical disabilities (IOM, 2011b).

Although most publishers of health care quality data have adopted a philosophy that "if you build it, they will come," there is a dearth of consumer engagement in developing these reports; fundamental differences in perceptions of quality and value of health care by patients, clinicians, health plans, and state and federal agencies are likely contributors. Research suggests that patients place a high value on clinicians who are responsive to their individual needs, access to and choice of clinicians and services, and treatments that maximize their quality of life and productivity. Clinicians evaluate care in terms of their ability to draw on their medical expertise to achieve optimal patient outcomes, while health plans and state and federal agencies tend to equate quality of care with efficiency, appropriate utilization of diagnostic and therapeutic technologies, and high patient satisfaction. While there are some commonalities among these divergent perspectives (e.g., none of these stakeholder groups is indifferent to patient harm), balancing their diverse perspectives continues to challenge quality measurement, especially in public reporting (IOM and NRC, 1999; McGlynn, 1997).

Additionally, consumer reactions to variations in health care costs and quality of care may vary considerably from consumer reactions to corresponding changes in other sectors of the economy, which often reflect trade-offs between costs and quality of goods and services. Limited supply (e.g., one hospital in the geographic region), the absence of information, passive behavior on the part of patients, and insurance coverage, which often shields patients from fluctuations in health care costs, have been suggested as contributing factors. Without access to accurate and timely cost and quality information, patients may err in their assessments of quality of care, and health care costs will lack sensitivity to quality of care (Pauly, 2011; Usman, 2011).

To reach patients effectively, quality and cost data should be collected and reported with patient needs in mind. Measure developers and reporting agencies will need to work closely with patients and their caregivers to understand their evolving informational needs and at what point in the cancer care continuum giving patients that information will be appropriate. Additionally, measure developers and reporting agencies should accommodate patient preferences regarding the format and delivery mechanism of this information so that it is understandable and useful for patients facing health care decisions. By bridging the gulf between patients and measure developers and reporting agencies, patient advocacy groups could play a key role in consumer-driven, patient-centered quality reporting.

Meaningful, Timely, and Actionable Performance Data

The widespread need for and general absence of meaningful, timely, and actionable performance data to support quality measurement and performance improvement is well documented (Anderson et al., 2012; IOM and NRC, 1999, 2000; MAP and NQF, 2012; Russell, 1998). Despite that recognition, during the past two decades, there has been little advancement in data collection and reporting to support better performance data. More than ever, the health care system in the United States has proved itself to be capable of documenting its persistent deficiencies, but it has failed to produce actionable performance data to mobilize real and lasting change (Davies, 2001). This absence of progress provides a sharp contrast to the technical and technological changes observed in health care delivery and health care technology for cancer care.

Electronic health records (EHRs) could improve the speed and ease of data collection and reporting. As described in Chapter 6, the Health Information Technology for Economic and Clinical Health (HITECH) Act of 2009 has triggered substantial increases in EHR adoption among health care clinicians through a series of incentive payments and penalties. However, EHRs were not designed as quality measurement and reporting systems and they often lack interoperability—the ability for data systems to exchange data to support health care delivery, decision making, and care coordination across multiple clinicians (Anderson et al., 2012). Moreover, patient-reported outcomes and other critical data elements are not routinely captured in EHRs or are not captured in a discrete and reportable format. Preliminary assessments of EHR-generated quality measures suggest that major work will be required to ensure the accuracy and validity of quality data obtained from EHRs (Parsons et al., 2012).

Manual chart abstraction and data entry remain a primary mechanism of data collection for quality measurement. In a 2012 hospital staffing survey published by The Advisory Board Company, respondents reported that a large proportion of quality data was obtained through manual abstraction: approximately 55 percent of respondents indicated that 80 percent to 100 percent of their quality data was obtained manually. In contrast, approximately 3 percent of respondents reported obtaining up to 25 percent of their quality data through manual abstraction. Survey respondents also noted a mean of 3.7 full-time employee equivalents responsible for data abstraction to support quality reporting, with a mean of 2.5 full-time employee equivalents dedicated to the Centers for Medicare & Medicaid Services' (CMS') inpatient and outpatient quality reporting programs (The Advisory Board Company, 2012). Staffing for these activities is costly, especially for smaller community hospitals, and it seems likely that these costs are passed onto patients and payers through increased charges.

Also problematic is the substantial delay that frequently occurs when manual data collection is required. For many cancer registries, including the NCI's Surveillance, Epidemiology, and End Results program and the ACoS CoC's National Cancer Data Base, several months may lapse between diagnosis and data submission, and the data are usually not available for review until many months to years later (ACoS, 2011d; NCI, 2012; Schneider et al., 2004). While these registries are rich national data sources on cancer incidence, treatment, and outcomes, delays limit their utility for real-time and actionable quality reporting. Likewise, retrospective outcomes studies, traditionally conducted on an ad hoc basis following treatment completion for a cohort of patients, require lengthy manual chart abstraction and data analysis. These studies, too, are limited in their ability to influence health care delivery because of their lengthy turnaround time.

A learning cancer IT system for cancer, as recommended by the committee (see Chapter 6), would provide a structured data system that collects and reports data to support more real-time quality assessments and informed decision making by patients, their caregivers, clinicians, payers, and federal and state agencies. Such a system would capture patient-reported data, integrate this information with data in EHRs and other sources, and support robust data analytics and real-time decision-making support.

Clinicians will also play a crucial role in advancing the quantity and quality of data collected for reporting purposes. Clinicians need to agree on many complex decisions, such as

- Which data collection activities should be automated?
- Is prospective or retrospective data collection more appropriate for a given data collection activity?
- Which data elements must be collected by physicians, and which data elements may be collected in a more economical fashion by other members of the clinical staff without sacrificing the quality of the data?

Clinicians may need to sacrifice some degree of autonomy and personal preference to utilize and benefit from emerging technologies, such as structured dictation and clinical documentation. They may need to adopt standardized documentation styles and terminology to facilitate structured data collection and reporting, and to support data sharing with each other. Advances in natural language processing, however, could potentially reduce this need by allowing computers to analyze and capture the context of words and phrases within clinicians' notes (Murff et al., 2011).

The transition from manual to automated data collection will require increased accuracy and specificity at the data collection point. EHRs and other IT systems cannot report accurately on patient characteristics or health care delivery that is not documented or is documented improperly. Recent research supports the intuitive notion that clinician workflow and documentation practice have a strong influence on EHR-based quality measures (Parsons et al., 2012). Thus, the quality and completeness of the data entered may constrain the utility, quality, and accuracy of automated reporting. Improved clinician workflow and documentation, together with IT advancements, could promote the availability of meaningful, timely, and actionable performance data for cancer quality measurement and reporting.

The Path Forward

The current independent efforts to develop cancer metrics have left patients, payers, clinicians, and state and federal agencies without an effective method to assess and improve the quality of cancer care delivery in America. Thus, to advance quality measurement in cancer care and improve the quality of cancer care, **the committee identified the goal of** creating a national quality reporting program for cancer care as part of a learning health care system (see Chapter 6) (Recommendation 8).

The committee considered a number of stakeholders as potential leaders in accomplishing this goal. For example, several organizations have attempted to influence quality measurement for cancer care, including the IOM, RAND Corporation, NQF, AHRQ, and, most recently, two NQF-convened public-private partnerships (the MAP and the NPP) (NQF, 2013a,b). These organizations have expended substantial effort to expand this discipline, but they lack the authority to enforce their recommendations and the resources to fund the tremendous body of research that is needed. They also are not focused exclusively on cancer care. Additionally, professional organizations including the ACoS and ASCO, have instituted voluntary reporting programs through which program participants have demonstrated improvements in cancer care. The work of these organizations reflects some collaboration but their activities have been siloed to a large degree.

CMS, together with its parent agency HHS, have also attempted to influence quality measurement for cancer care through various mandatory reporting programs, including the Physician Quality Reporting System (CMS, 2012) and, most recently, a mandatory reporting program for the nation's eleven cancer centers that are not paid under the PPS (Spinks et al., 2011). However, CMS has not provided strategic direction for cancer quality metrics. It has generally proposed an ever-growing list of process-oriented measures (or measures of short-term outcomes), which frequently are reported from administrative claims databases or patient sampling and are, therefore, relatively inexpensive to produce (Pronovost and Lilford, 2011). This approach fits the federal timetable under which CMS operates and its quest for provider accountability, but these timelines are too brief and CMS' focus on the Medicare population is too narrow to implement an effective and influential national reporting program for cancer care.

In order to advance the development of a national quality reporting program for cancer, **the committee recommends that HHS work with professional organizations to create and implement a formal long-term strategy for publicly reporting quality measures for cancer care that leverages existing efforts.** The long-term strategy should focus on the needs of all individuals diagnosed with or at risk for developing cancer. The committee believes that clinicians, through their professional organizations, should be the primary actors because a clinician-led process will help ensure that the resulting reporting program is acceptable to practicing clinicians and reflects of key quality issues in cancer care. Moreover, these organizations are already in the process of developing quality metrics for their members. The committee believes that HHS should play a convening role in order to improve the coordination of the work of professional organizations. In the past, these organizations have collaborated on an ad hoc basis but more systematic collaboration would speed progress toward this goal.

A key component of developing a formal long-term strategy for quality measures for cancer will be **prioritizing, funding, and directing the development of meaningful quality measures, with a focus on outcome measures, and with performance targets for use in publicly reporting the performance of institutions, practices, and individual clinicians.** These measures should target gaps in cross-cutting, nontechnical measures as well as measures for specific types of cancers that have largely been excluded from previous measure development efforts. The measures should also incorporate the components of the committee's conceptual framework at the level of institutions or oncology practices, including measuring the effectiveness of

- patient-clinician communication and shared decision making in supporting patients and caregivers in making informed medical decisions consistent with their needs, values, and preferences, as well as advance care planning, the provision of palliative care and psychosocial support across the continuum of care, and timely referral to hospice care at the end of life (see Chapter 3);
- team-based cancer care that prioritizes patient-centered care and coordination with a patient's primary care/geriatrics care team and other care teams (Chapter 4);
- evidence-based cancer care that is concordant with clinical practice guidelines and consistent with patients' needs, values, and preferences (Chapter 5);
- clinician participation in the learning health care system and the national quality reporting program (Chapters 6 and 7); and
- efforts to improve the accessibility and affordability of cancer care (Chapter 8).

To be successful, stakeholders will need to make uncomfortable adjustments, such as adopting shared accountability across clinicians, increasing the transparency of traditionally proprietary cost data, and requiring patients to accept greater responsibility for their outcomes of care. While data availability will be an important consideration, it should not be the sole factor in measure selection. The committee's goals of improving the breadth and depth of information collected in clinical research (see Chapter 5) will help fill in some of the knowledge gaps surrounding cancer care, such as management of complex comorbidities, quality-of-life issues during and after treatment, and the cost of care. A formal tool could be developed to assist with prioritizing and selecting measures for development.

HHS should also work with professional organizations to implement a coordinated, transparent reporting infrastructure that meets the informational needs of all stakeholders, with an emphasis on transparency and reporting data that are meaningful and understandable to patients and can be used to guide their health care decisions. Achieving this recommendation will likely require the development of a learning health care IT system for cancer care, as discussed in Chapter 6. A learning health care IT system could facilitate the collection of reliable data in EHRs as part of clinicians' day-to-day workflow. These data could then be aggregated to assess individual and organizational performance, and made publicly available to inform patients and other decision makers. The committee recognizes that implementation of this recommendation will present considerable challenges (e.g., technological, financial, and cultural). However, the need for a robust reporting infrastructure is great, given that independent efforts to develop cancer metrics have left patients, clinicians, payers, and the government without an effective mechanism to assess and improve the quality of cancer care delivery in the United States.

CLINICAL PRACTICE GUIDELINES

Clinical research leads to improvements in the quality of care only if these research results are translated into practice. Clinicians use CPGs to synthesize research findings into actionable steps for providing care. The IOM has defined CPGs as "statements that include recommendations intended to optimize patient care that are informed by a systematic review of the evidence and an assessment of the benefits and harms of alternative care options" (IOM, 2011c, p. 4). CPGs are often used to inform the development of quality metrics and decision support tools in EHRs (see Chapter 6). Clinicians' adherence to CPGs may be measured as part of an outcomes-based reimbursement system (see Chapter 8). The major organizations that develop CPGs in cancer are ASCO, the American Society for Radiation Oncology, and NCCN, as well as the U.S. Preventive Services Task Force, which establishes recommendations on cancer screening and prevention. The activities of these organizations are summarized in Table 7-3.

The translation of evidence into CPGs is not straightforward or consistent. As mentioned in Chapter 5, the evidence base supporting clinical decisions is often incomplete, with few or no studies addressing many questions that are important to patients and clinicians. There is also great variability in the quality of individual scientific studies and in the sys-

TABLE 7-3 Examples of Organizations That Establish Clinical Practice Guidelines in Cancer

Organization	Description
American Society for Radiation Oncology (ASTRO)	ASTRO is a professional organization that represents radiation oncologists, medical physicists, dosimetrists, radiation therapists, radiation oncology nurses and nurse practitioners, biologists, physician assistants, and practice administrators. It develops clinical practice guidelines (CPGs) for these radiation oncology clinicians.
American Society of Clinical Oncology (ASCO)	ASCO was founded in 1964 as a nonprofit professional organization that represents clinicians from all of the oncology disciplines and subspecialties. It convenes expert panels to develop CPGs for methods of cancer treatment and care. Many of ASCO's guidelines are developed in partnership with other specialty societies, such as the American Society of Hematology and the College of American Pathologists. The manual for generating these guidelines is updated regularly to reflect changes in methodology standards.
National Comprehensive Cancer Network (NCCN)	NCCN is a coalition of 23 cancer centers. It develops CPGs that address preventive, diagnostic, treatment, and supportive services. The guidelines are developed and updated through informal consensus by expert panels, composed of clinicians and oncology researchers from the 23 NCCN member institutions.
U.S. Preventive Services Task Force (USPSTF)	The U.S. Public Health Services convened the USPSTF in 1984, and since 1998, it has been sponsored by the Agency for Healthcare Research and Quality. The USPSTF consists of a panel of private-sector experts, and its recommendations are regarded as the gold standard for clinical preventive services. It has produced recommendations on screening for bladder, breast, cervical, colorectal, lung, oral, ovarian, pancreatic, prostate, skin, testicular, and thyroid cancer, as well as some recommendations on cancer prevention.

SOURCES: ASCO, 2012a; ASTRO, 2013; IOM, 2008; NCCN, 2012; USPSTF, 2012.

tematic reviews upon which CPGs should be based. In addition, the CPG development process is often fragmented, lacking in transparency, and plagued by potential conflicts of interest in the membership of the CPG panels that may bias the resulting product. In response to these criticisms, the IOM convened a committee to develop standards for trustworthy guidelines (IOM, 2011c). The recommendations of this committee are summarized in Box 7-1. In general, the guidelines committee concluded that to be trustworthy, CPGs should be based on a systematic review of the evidence; be developed by a knowledgeable and multidisciplinary panel; consider patient subgroups and patient preferences; be developed

BOX 7-1
IOM Standards for Developing Trustworthy
Clinical Practice Guidelines (CPGs)

1. Establishing Transparency
   1.1 The processes by which a CPG is developed and funded should be detailed explicitly and publicly accessible.

2. Management of Conflict of Interest (COI)
   2.1 Prior to selection of the guideline development group (GDG), individuals being considered for membership should declare all interests and activities that would potentially result in COI with development group activity by written disclosure to those convening the GDG:
      • Disclosure should reflect all current and planned commercial (including services from which a clinician derives a substantial proportion of income), noncommercial, intellectual, institutional, and patient-public activities pertinent to the potential scope of the CPG.
   2.2 Disclosure of COIs within GDG:
      • All COI of each GDG member should be reported and discussed by the prospective development group prior to the onset of his or her work.
      • Each panel member should explain how his or her COI could influence the CPG development process or specific recommendations.
   2.3 Divestment
      • Members of the GDG should divest themselves of financial investments they or their family members have in, and not participate in marketing activities or advisory boards of, entities whose interests could be affected by CPG recommendations.
   2.4 Exclusions
      • Whenever possible, GDG members should not have COI.
      • In some circumstances, a GDG may not be able to perform its work without members who have COI, such as relevant clinical specialists who receive a substantial portion of their incomes from services pertinent to the CPG.
      • Members with COI should represent not more than a minority of the GDG.
      • The chair or co-chairs should not be a person(s) with COI.
      • Funders should have no role in CPG development.

3. GDG Composition
   3.1 The GDG should be multidisciplinary and balanced, comprising a variety of methodological experts and clinicians, and populations expected to be affected by the CPG.
   3.2 Patient and public involvement should be facilitated by including (at least at the time of clinical question formulation and draft CPG review) a current or former patient, and a patient advocate or patient/consumer organization representative in the GDG.

continued

BOX 7-1 Continued

3.3 Strategies to increase effective participation of patient and consumer representatives, including training in appraisal of evidence, should be adopted by GDGs.

4. CPG–Systematic Review Intersection
   4.1 CPG developers should use systematic reviews that meet standards set by the IOM's Committee on Standards for Systematic Reviews of Comparative Effectiveness Research.
   4.2 When systematic reviews are conducted specifically to inform particular guidelines, the GDG and systematic review team should interact regarding the scope, approach, and output of both processes.

5. Establishing Evidence Foundations and Rating Strength of Recommendations
   5.1 For each recommendation, the following should be provided:
   • An explanation of the reasoning underlying the recommendation, including
     o A clear description of potential benefits and harms.
     o A summary of relevant available evidence (and evidentiary gaps), description of the quality (including applicability), quantity (including completeness), and consistency of the aggregate available evidence.
     o An explanation of the part played by values, opinion, theory, and clinical experience in deriving the recommendation.
   • A rating of the level of confidence in (certainty regarding) the evidence underpinning the recommendation.
   • A rating of the strength of the recommendation in light of the preceding bullets.
   • A description and explanation of any differences of opinion regarding the recommendation.

6. Articulation of Recommendations
   6.1 Recommendations should be articulated in a standardized form detailing, precisely, the recommended action, and under what circumstances it should be performed.

using a transparent process; provide ratings of both the quality of evidence and strength of recommendations; and be updated regularly.

Few CPGs in oncology meet the IOM's standards for trustworthiness. Kung and colleagues (2012) reviewed the adherence of CPGs archived in the National Guidelines Clearinghouse to IOM standards. They found that the average CPG only satisfied 8 out of the 18 standards reviewed (44.4 percent) and fewer than half of the CPGs met more than 50 percent

6.2 Strong recommendations should be worded so that compliance with the recommendation(s) can be evaluated.

7. External Review
7.1 External reviewers should comprise a full spectrum of relevant stakeholders, including scientific and clinical experts, organizations (e.g., health care, specialty societies), agencies (e.g., federal government), patients, and representatives of the public.
7.2 The authorship of external reviews submitted by individuals and/or organizations should be kept confidential unless that protection has been waived by the reviewer(s).
7.3 The GDG should consider all external reviewers' comments and keep a written record of the rationale for modifying or not modifying a CPG in response to reviewers' comments.
7.4 A draft of the CPG at the external review stage or immediately following it (i.e., prior to the final draft) should be made available to the general public for comment. Reasonable notice of impending publication should be provided to interested public stakeholders.

8. Updating
8.1 The CPG publication date, date of pertinent systematic evidence review, and proposed date for future CPG review should be documented in the CPG.
8.2 Literature should be monitored regularly following CPG publication to identify the emergence of new, potentially relevant evidence and to evaluate the continued validity of the CPG.
8.3 CPGs should be updated when new evidence suggests the need for modification of clinically important recommendations. For example, a CPG should be updated if new evidence shows that a recommended intervention causes previously unknown substantial harm; that a new intervention is significantly superior to a previously recommended intervention from an efficacy or harms perspective; or that a recommendation can be applied to new populations.

SOURCE: IOM, 2011c.

of the IOM standards. Oncology CPGs were slightly above average, satisfying a median of 9.5 out of the 18 (52.8 percent) standards reviewed, with just over half meeting more than 50 percent of the standards.

In a separate study, Reames and colleagues (2013) scored CPGs and consensus statements addressing the screening, evaluation, or management of the four leading causes of cancer mortality in the United States (non-small-cell lung, breast, prostate, and colorectal cancers) on their consistency with the IOM's standards for CPGs published between 2005 and 2010. None of the 168 CPGs included in the study met all of the IOM's standards; the average was 2.8 out of the 8 standards assessed. The CPGs were most compliant with the standards addressing transparency in the development process, articulation of the recommendations, and use of external review. The CPGs were least likely to comply with the standards requiring that CPGs be based on a systematic review of the evidence, involve patients and the public in the development process, or specify a process for making updates. In addition, Norris and colleagues found that most CPG developers have failed to develop conflict of interest policies consistent with the IOM's recommendations (Norris et al., 2012).

The committee acknowledges the considerable challenges to implementing the IOM's standards for trustworthy CPGs. The standards are stringent, resource intensive, and require major investments in time and human resources. Because of the importance of CPGs to improving the quality of cancer care and translating evidence into clinical practice, however, **the committee endorses the IOM's recommendations on producing trustworthy CPGs and encourages developers of CPGs in oncology to strive to meet these standards.**

PERFORMANCE IMPROVEMENT INITIATIVES

Quality measurement and CPGs are essential components of improving performance in health care. As discussed above, quality metrics provide insights into which aspects of health care require improvement and may be used to assess the success of performance improvement initiatives. They can also be used by individual clinicians to assess their performance and improve the care they provide (Blayney et al., 2009). CPGs are a type of performance improvement initiative that help clinicians stay abreast of an ever increasing evidence base and apply that information to their clinical practice. Although necessary, these activities, in the absence of other levers, are insufficient to drive meaningful improvements in health care (Berwick et al., 2003; Davies, 2001; IOM, 2011a).

To be successful, health care organizations must foster a culture of change through a variety of activities, such as those discussed in this report. Those activities include improving patient engagement, decision making, and communication (see Chapter 3); ensuring that personnel have sufficient training, appropriate licensure and certifications, and are empowered to contribute to performance improvement initiatives (see Chapter 4); investing in learning health care IT systems to collect data on quality of care, making this data transparent to the entire organization, and providing clinical decision support (see Chapter 6); and creating incentives that encourage clinicians and provider organizations to ad-

TABLE 7-4 Examples of Performance Improvement Strategies

Type	Description
Audit and Feedback	Clinician performance tracking and reviews, comparison with national/state quality report cards, publicly released performance data, and benchmark outcome data
Clinical Decision Support	Information technology provides clinicians with access to evidence-based clinical practice guidelines
Clinician and Patient Education	Classes, parent and family education, pamphlets, and other media
Clinician Reminder Systems	Prompts in electronic health records
Facilitated Relay of Clinical Data to Clinicians	Patient data transmitted by telephone call or fax from outpatient specialty clinics to primary care clinicians
Financial Incentives	Performance-based bonuses and alternative reimbursement systems for clinicians, positive or negative financial incentives for patients, changes in professional licensure requirements
Organizational Changes	Continuous performance improvement programs, lean and Six Sigma approaches, shifting from paper-based to computer-based record keeping, long-distance case discussion between professional peers, etc.
Patient Reminder Systems	Telephone calls or postcards from clinicians to their patients
Patient Safety Initiatives	Checklists, safety incident reporting, close call reporting, and root-cause analysis
Promotion of Disease Self-Management	Workshops, materials such as blood pressure or glucose monitoring devices

SOURCE: Adapted from AHRQ, 2012a.

minister high-quality care rather than a high volume of care (e.g., patient-centered medical homes, care pathways, accountable care organizations) (see Chapter 8).

Performance improvement initiatives, which are conducted at the local level, have been described as "systematic, data-guided activities designed to bring about immediate, positive change in the delivery of health care in a particular setting," as well as across settings (Baily, 2006, p. S5). These activities are interrelated and overlapping with quality improvement and patient safety initiatives. Table 7-4 provides examples of performance improvement initiatives. Because these efforts are implemented in a single organization or health system, they can be undertaken immediately without action on a national or system level and can be tailored to the unique circumstances of the local environment. Experts have noted, however, that traditional approaches to performance improvement—clinician practice peer review, public reporting of quality measures, continuous performance improvement and total quality management, and regulatory and legislatively imposed reforms and penalties—lack the pace, breadth, magnitude, coordination, and sustainability to transform health care delivery (Chassin and Loeb, 2011; Davies, 2001).

Leadership is needed to create an institutional culture that values high-quality care, a key component of successful performance improvement initiatives. The aviation industry has long recognized the importance of embedding performance improvement initiatives in cultures that value inquiry and quality, and that have strong leaders dedicated to facilitating the necessary changes (Helmreich, 2000). Health care organizations have successfully applied this approach to performance improvement through efforts aimed at improving patient safety, such as by using checklists to reduce human error, and could apply them more broadly to improve quality in other areas of care (Gawande, 2009; Hudson, 2003; Longo et al., 2005; Pronovost et al., 2003).

In addition, health care organizations have rushed to adopt Six Sigma and "lean" systems approaches to reduce variation and waste in health care. These robust industrial performance improvement tools are most effective within organizations that have an embedded safety culture, senior leadership dedicated to organizational change, and clear mechanisms for identifying quality and safety issues and triggering performance improvement initiatives (Chassin and Loeb, 2011). Also important is leadership's commitment to funding these activities, which often consume substantial organizational resources (Pryor et al., 2011). Without these organizational characteristics, it is unlikely that performance improvement initiatives will lead to improved patient outcomes and sustained improvements in care delivery.

SUMMARY AND RECOMMENDATIONS

A high-quality cancer care delivery system should translate evidence into clinical practice, measure quality, and improve clinician performance. This involves developing CPGs to assist clinicians in quickly incorporating new medical knowledge into routine care. Also critical are measuring and assessing a system's progress in improving the delivery of cancer care, publicly reporting the information gathered, and developing innovative strategies to further facilitate performance improvement. In the figure illustrating the committee's conceptual framework (see Figure S-2), knowledge translation and performance improvement are part of a cyclical process that measures the outcomes of patient-clinician interactions and implements innovative strategies to improve the accessibility, affordability, and quality of care

CPGs translate evidence into practice by synthesizing research findings into actionable steps clinicians can take when providing care. The development of CPGs is not straightforward or consistent because the evidence base supporting clinical decisions is often incomplete and includes studies and systematic reviews of variable quality. In addition, organizations that develop CPGs often use fragmented processes that lack transparency and they are plagued by conflicts of interest. The committee endorses the standards in the 2011 IOM report *Clinical Practice Guidelines We Can Trust* to address these problems and produce trustworthy CPGs.

Performance improvement initiatives can also be used to translate evidence into practice. These tools have been described as "systematic, data-guided activities designed to bring about immediate, positive change in the delivery of health care in a particular setting," (Baily, 2006, p. 55) as well as across settings. They can improve the efficiency, patient satisfaction, health outcomes, and costs of cancer care. These efforts are typically implemented in a single organization or health system; as a result, they often lack the pace, breadth, magnitude, coordination, and sustainability to transform health care delivery nationwide.

Cancer care quality measures provide a standardized and objective means for assessing the quality of cancer care delivered. Measuring performance has the potential to drive improvements in care, inform patients, and influence clinician behavior and reimbursement. There are currently serious deficiencies in cancer care quality measurement in the United States, including pervasive gaps in existing measures, challenges in the measure development process, lack of consumer engagement in measure development and reporting, and the need for data to support meaningful, timely, and actionable performance measurement. A number of groups representing clinicians who provide cancer care, including ASCO and ACoS, have instituted voluntary reporting programs, through which program participants have demonstrated improvements. HHS has also attempted to influence quality measurement for cancer care through various mandatory reporting programs.

Recommendation 8: Quality Measurement

Goal: Develop a national quality reporting program for cancer care as part of a learning health care system.

To accomplish this, the U.S. Department of Health and Human Services should work with professional societies to:

- Create and implement a formal long-term strategy for publicly reporting quality measures for cancer care that leverages existing efforts.
- Prioritize, fund, and direct the development of meaningful quality measures for cancer care with a focus on outcome measures and with performance targets for use in publicly reporting the performance of institutions, practices, and individual clinicians.
- Implement a coordinated, transparent reporting infrastructure that meets the needs of all stakeholders, including patients, and is integrated into a learning health care system.

REFERENCES

ACoS (American College of Surgeons). 2011a. *About ACS NSQIP.* http://site.acsnsqip.org/about (accessed April 25, 2013).
———. 2011b. *About the CoCc.* http://www.facs.org/cancer/coc/cocar.html (accessed August 15, 2012).
———. 2011c. *How are cancer programs accredited?* http://www.facs.org/cancer/coc/howacc.html (accessed August 15, 2012).
———. 2011d. *National Cancer Data Base.* http://www.facs.org/cancer/ncdb/index.html (accessed August 15, 2012).
———. 2013. *Measures.* http://site.acsnsqip.org/program-specifics/program-options/measures-option (accessed June 28, 2013).
The Advisory Board Company. 2012. *Clinical Advisory Board Member Survey results: Staffing models for supporting quality reporting.* http://www.advisory.com/~/media/Advisory-com/Research/CAB/Resources/2012/2012%20Staffing%20Models%20Survey%20Results.pdf (accessed August 15, 2012).
AHRQ (Agency for Healthcare Research and Quality). 2012a. *Closing the quality gap series: Quality improvement interventions to address health disparities.* http://www.effective healthcare.ahrq.gov/search-for-guides-reviews-and-reports/?pageaction=display product&productID=1242&ECem=120827 (accessed December 21, 2012).
———. 2012b. *Measures sought for National Quality Measures Clearinghouse.* http://www.ahrq.gov/qual/nqmcmeas.htm (accessed August 15, 2012).
———. 2012c. *National Quality Measures Clearinghouse measures by topic.* http://www.quality measures.ahrq.gov/browse/by-topic.aspx (accessed August 15, 2012).
———. 2012d. *National Quality Measures Clearinghouse: About.* http://www.qualitymeasures.ahrq.gov/about/index.aspx (accessed August 15, 2012).
———. 2012e. *National Quality Measures Clearinghouse, U.S. Department of Health and Human Services: Measure inventory.* http://www.qualitymeasures.ahrq.gov/hhs-measure-inventory/browse.aspx (accessed August 15, 2012).
AMA (American Medical Association). 2012. *Resources.* http://www.ama-assn.org/ama/pub/physician-resources/physician-consortium-performance-improvement.page (accessed August 15, 2012).

Anderson, K. M., C. A. Marsh, A. C. Flemming, H. Isenstein, and J. Reynolds. 2012. An environmental snapshot—Quality measurement enabled by health IT: Overview, possibilities, and challenges. http://healthit.ahrq.gov/sites/default/files/docs/page/NRCD1PTQ%20Final%20Draft%20Background%20Report%2007102012_508compliant.pdf (accessed August 15, 2012).

ASCO (American Society of Clinical Oncology). 2012a. *Clinical practice guidelines.* http://www.asco.org/ASCOv2/Practice+%26+Guidelines/Guidelines/Clinical+Practice+Guidelines (accessed December 20, 2012).

———. 2012b. *Geographic distribution.* http://qopi.asco.org/GeographicDistribution (accessed August 15, 2012).

———. 2012c. *QOPI certified practices.* http://qopi.asco.org/certifiedpractices (accessed October 1, 2012).

———. 2012d. *QOPI summary of measures, fall 2012.* http://qopi.asco.org/Documents/QOPIFall12MeasuresSummary_002.pdf (accessed August 15, 2012).

———. 2012e. *Who can apply?* http://qopi.asco.org/whocanapply (accessed August 15, 2012).

———. 2013. *Certification.* http://qopi.asco.org/certification.html (accessed June 26, 2012).

ASTRO (American Society for Radiation Oncology). 2013. *Guidelines.* https://www.astro.org/Clinical-Practice/Guidelines/Index.aspx (accessed March 27, 2013).

Baily, M. A., M. Bottrell, J. Lynn, and B. Jennings. 2006. *Hastings Center Report* 36(4):S1-S40.

Berry, D. A. 2011. Comparing survival outcomes across centers: Biases galore. *Cancer Letter* 37(11):7-10.

Berwick, D. M., B. James, and M. J. Coye. 2003. Connections between quality measurement and improvement. *Medical Care* 41(1):I30-I38.

Bilimoria, K. Y., A. K. Stewart, D. P. Winchester, and C. Y. Ko. 2008. The National Cancer Database: A powerful initiative to improve cancer care in the Uunited States. *Annals of Surgical Oncology* 15(3):683-690.

Birkmeyer, J. D., T. A. Stukel, A. E. Siewers, P. P. Goodney, D. E. Wennberg, and F. L. Lucas. 2003. Surgeon volume and operative mortality in the United States. *New England Journal of Medicine* 349(22):2117-2127.

Bishop, T. F. 2013. Pushing the outpatient quality envelope. *Journal of the American Medical Association* 1-2.

Blayney, D. W., K. McNiff, D. Hanauer, G. Miela, D. Markstrom, and M. Neuss. 2009. Implementation of the Quality Oncology Practice Initiative at a university comprehensive cancer center. *Journal of Clinical Oncology* 27(23):3802-3807.

Blayney, D. W., J. Severson, C. J. Martin, P. Kadlubek, T. Ruane, and K. Harrison. 2012. Michigan oncology practices showed varying adherence rates to practice guidelines, but quality interventions improved care. *Health Affairs (Millwood)* 31(4):718-728.

Chassin, M. R., and J. M. Loeb. 2011. The ongoing quality improvement journey: Next stop, high reliability. *Health Affairs (Millwood)* 30(4):559-568.

CMS (Centers for Medicare & Medicaid Services). 2012. *Physician Quality Reporting System formerly known as the Physician Quality Reporting Initiative.* http://www.cms.gov/PQRS (accessed August 15, 2012).

Davies, H. T. 2001. Exploring the pathology of quality failings: Measuring quality is not the problem—changing it is. *Journal of Evaluation in Clinical Practice* 7(2):243-251.

Deutsch, A., B. Gage, L. Smith, and C. Kelleher. 2012. *Patient-reported outcomes in performance measurement commissioned paper on PRO-based performance measures for healthcare accountable entities draft #1, September 4, 2012.* http://www.qualityforum.org/WorkArea/linkit.aspx?LinkIdentifier=id&ItemID=71824 (accessed September 15, 2012).

Donabedian, A. 1980. Explorations in Quality Assessment and Monitoring. In *The definition of quality and approaches to its assessment*. Vol. 1. Ann Arbor, MI: Health Administration Press.

Dudgeon, D. J., C. Knott, C. Chapman, K. Coulson, E. Jeffery, S. Preston, M. Eichholz, J. P. Van Dijk, and A. Smith. 2009. Development, implementation, and process evaluation of a regional palliative care quality improvement project. *Journal of Pain and Symptom Management* 38(4):483-495.

Faber, M., M. Bosch, H. Wollersheim, S. Leatherman, and R. Grol. 2009. Public reporting in health care: How do consumers use quality-of-care information? A systematic review. *Medical Care* 47(1):1-8.

Finks, J. F., N. H. Osborne, and J. D. Birkmeyer. 2011. Trends in hospital volume and operative mortality for high-risk surgery. *New England Journal of Medicine* 364(22):2128-2137.

Finlayson, E. V., P. P. Goodney, and J. D. Birkmeyer. 2003. Hospital volume and operative mortality in cancer surgery: A national study. *Archives of Surgery* 138(7):721-725.

Foster, J. A., M. Abdolrasulnia, H. Doroodchi, J. McClure, and L. Casebeer. 2009. Practice patterns and guideline adherence of medical oncologists in managing patients with early breast cancer. *Journal of the National Comprehensive Cancer Network* 7(7):697-706.

Gawande, A. 2009. *The checklist manifesto: How to get things right*. New York: Metropolitan books.

Goldberg, P. 2011. Fox Chase publishes its cancer survival data: The move is partly science, partly marketing. *Cancer Letter* 37(5):1-5.

Harris, K. M., and M. Beeuwkes Buntin. 2008. Choosing a health care provider. *The Synthesis project. Research Synthesis Report* (14).

Helmreich, R. L. 2000. On error management: Lessons from aviation. *British Medical Journal* 320(7237):781-785.

Hibbard, J., and S. Sofaer. 2010. *Best practices in public reporting no. 1: How to effectively present health care performance data to consumers*. http://www.ahrq.gov/qual/pubrptguide1.pdf (accessed August 15, 2012).

Higgins, A., T. Zeddies, and S. D. Pearson. 2011. Measuring the performance of individual physicians by collecting data from multiple health plans: The results of a two-state test. *Health Affairs (Millwood)* 30(4):673-681.

Ho, V., M. J. Heslin, H. Yun, and L. Howard. 2006. Trends in hospital and surgeon volume and operative mortality for cancer surgery. *Annals of Surgical Oncology* 13(6):851-858.

Hudson, P. 2003. Applying the lessons of high risk industries to health care. *Quality & Safety in Health Care* 12(Suppl 1):i7-i12.

Hussey, P., and E. A. McGlynn. 2009. *Why are there no efficiency measures in the National Quality Measures Clearinghouse?* http://www.qualitymeasures.ahrq.gov/expert/expert-commentary.aspx?id=16459 (accessed August 15, 2012).

IOM (Institute of Medicine). 2001. *Envisioning The National Health Care Quality Report*. Edited by M. P. Hurtado, E. K. Swift, and J. M. Corrigan. Washington, DC: National Academy Press.

———. 2008. *Knowing what works in health care: A roadmap for the nation*. Washington, DC: The National Academies Press.

———. 2011a. *For the public's health: The role of measurement in action and accountability*. Washington, DC: The National Academies Press.

———. 2011b. *Health literacy implications for health care reform: Workshop summary*. Washington, DC: The National Academies Press.

———. 2011c. *Clinical practice guidelines we can trust*. Washington, DC: The National Academies Press.

IOM and NRC (National Research Council). 1999. *Ensuring quality cancer care*. Washington, DC: National Academy Press.

————. 2000. *Enhancing data systems to improve the quality of cancer care.* Edited by M. Hewitt and J. V. Simone. Washington, DC: National Academy Press.

Jacobson, J. O., M. N. Neuss, K. K. McNiff, P. Kadlubek, L. R. Thacker, 2nd, F. Song, P. D. Eisenberg, and J. V. Simone. 2008. Improvement in oncology practice performance through voluntary participation in the Quality Oncology Practice Initiative. *Journal of Clinical Oncology* 26(11):1893-1898.

Kahn, K. L., J. L. Malin, J. Adams, and P. A. Ganz. 2002. Developing a reliable, valid, and feasible plan for quality-of-care measurement for cancer: How should we measure? *Medical Care* 40(6 Suppl):III73-III85.

KFF (Kaiser Family Foundation) and AHRQ. 2006. *Update on consumers' views on patient safety and quality information.* www.kff.org/kaiserpolls/pomr092706pkg.cfm (accessed August 15, 2012).

Kizer, K. W. 2000. The National Quality Forum seeks to improve health care. *Academic Medicine* 75(4):320-321.

Krumholz, H. M., P. S. Keenan, J. E. Brush, Jr., V. J. Bufalino, M. E. Chernew, A. J. Epstein, P. A. Heidenreich, V. Ho, F. A. Masoudi, D. B. Matchar, S. L. Normand, J. S. Rumsfeld, J. D. Schuur, S. C. Smith, Jr., J. A. Spertus, and M. N. Walsh. 2008. Standards for measures used for public reporting of efficiency in health care: A scientific statement from the American Heart Association Interdisciplinary Council on Quality of Care and Outcomes Rresearch and the American College of Cardiology Foundation. *Journal of the American College of Cardiology* 52(18):1518-1526.

Kung, J., R. R. Miller, and P. A. Mackowiak. 2012. Failure of clinical practice guidelines to meet Institute of Medicine standards: Two more decades of little, if any, progress. *Archives of Internal Medicine* 172(21):1628-1633.

Longo, D. R., J. E. Hewett, B. Ge, and S. Schubert. 2005. The long road to patient safety. A status report on patient safety systems. *Journal of the American Medical Association* 294(22):2825-2865.

MAP (Measure Applications Partnership) and NQF (National Quality Forum). 2012. *Performance measurement coordination strategy for PPSs-exempt cancer hospitals.* http://www.qualityforum.org/WorkArea/linkit.aspx?LinkIdentifier=id&ItemID=71217 (accessed August 15, 2012).

McGlynn, E. A. 1997. Six challenges in measuring the quality of health care. *Health Affairs (Millwood)* 16(3):7-21.

McNiff, K. 2006. The Quality Oncology Practice Initiative: Assessing and improving care within the medical oncology practice. *Journal of Oncology Practice/American Society of Clinical Oncology* 2(1):26-30.

Menck, H. R., L. Garfinkel, and G. D. Dodd. 1991. Preliminary report of the National Cancer Database. *CA: A Cancer Journal for Clinicians* 41(1):7-18.

Murff, H. J., F. FitzHenry, M. E. Matheny, N. Gentry, K. L. Kotter, K. Crimin, R. S. Dittus, A. K. Rosen, P. L. Elkin, S. H. Brown, and T. Speroff. 2011. Automated identification of post-operative complications within an electronic medical record using natural language processing. *Journal of the American Medical Association* 306(8):848-855.

National Priorities Partnership. 2011. *Input to the Secretary of Health and Human Services on priorities for The National Quality Strategy.* http://www.qualityforum.org/WorkArea/linkit.aspx?LinkIdentifier=id&ItemID=68238 (accessed August 15, 2012).

NCCN (National Comprehensive Cancer Network). 2012. *NCCN guidelines & clinical resources.* http://www.nccn.org/clinical.asp (accessed December 20, 2012).

NCI (National Cancer Institute). 2012. *Surveillance, Epidemiology, and End Results: Overview of the SEER program.* http://seer.cancer.gov/about/overview.html (accessed August 15, 2012).

Norris, S. L., H. K. Holmer, B. U. Burda, L. A. Ogden, and R. Fu. 2012. Conflict of interest policies for organizations producing a large number of clinical practice guidelines. *PloS ONE* 7(5):e37413.

NQF (National Quality Forum). 2010. *Guidance for measure harmonization: A consensus report.* http://www.qualityforum.org/WorkArea/linkit.aspx?LinkIdentifier=id&ItemID=62381 (accessed August 15, 2012).

———. 2012a. *Adjuvant hormonal therapy.* http://www.qualityforum.org/MeasureDetails.aspx?actid=0&SubmissionId=450 (accessed August 15, 2012).

———. 2012b. *Funding.* http://www.qualityforum.org/About_NQF/Funding.aspx (accessed August 15, 2012).

———. 2012c. *National Quality Forum: Measure evaluation criteria, january 2011.* http://www.qualityforum.org/Measuring_Performance/Submitting_Standards/Measure_Evaluation_Criteria.aspx (accessed August 15, 2012).

———. 2012d. *NQF-endorsed standards.* http://www.qualityforum.org/Measures_List.aspx (accessed August 15, 2012).

———. 2012e. *Oncology: Hormonal therapy for stage I through III, ER/PRR positive breast cancer.* http://www.qualityforum.org/MeasureDetails.aspx?actid=0&SubmissionId=631 (accessed August 15, 2012).

———. 2012f. Performance measurement coordination strategy for PPS-exempt cancer hospitals. https://www.qualityforum.org/Publications/2012/06/Performance_Measurement_Coordination_Strategy_for_PPS-Exempt_Cancer_Hospitals.aspx (accessed August 8, 2013).

———. 2013a. *Measure Applications Partnership.* http://www.qualityforum.org/map (accessed August 7, 2013).

———. 2013b. *National Priorities Partnership.* http://www.qualityforum.org/Setting_Priorities/NPP/National_Priorities_Partnership.aspx (accessed August 7, 2013).

———. 2013c. NQF-Endorsed Standards. http://www.qualityforum.org/Measures_List.aspx (accessed June 28, 2013).

Parsons, A., C. McCullough, J. Wang, and S. Shih. 2012. Validity of electronic health record-derived quality measurement for performance monitoring. *Journal of the American Medical Informatics Association* 19(4):604-609.

Pauly, M. V. 2011. Analysis & commentary: The trade-off among quality, quantity, and cost: How to make it—if we must. *Health Affairs (Millwood)* 30(4):574-580.

President's Advisory Commission on Consumer Protection and Quality in the Health Care Industry. 1998. *Quality first: Better health care for all Americans, final report to the President of the United States.* Washington, DC: United States G.P.O.

Pronovost, P. J, and R. Lilford. 2011. Analysis & commentary: A road map for improving the performance of performance measures. *Health Affairs (Millwood)* 30(4):569-573.

Pronovost, P. J., B. Weast, C. G. Holzmueller, B. J. Rosenstein, R. P. Kidwell, K. B. Haller, E. R. Reroli, J. B. Sexton, and H. R. Rubin, 2003. Evalution of the culture of safety: Survey of clinicians and managers in an academic medical center. *Quality & Safety in Health Care* 12:405-410.

Pryor, D., A. Hendrich, R. J. Henkel, J. K. Beckmann, and A. R. Tersigni. 2011. The quality "journey" at ascension health: How we've prevented at least 1,500 avoidable deaths a year—and aim to do even better. *Health Affairs (Millwood)* 30(4):604-611.

RAND. 2010. *About acove.* http://www.rand.org/health/projects/acove/about.html (accessed April 25, 2013).

Reames, B. N., R. W. Krell, S. N. Ponto, and S. L. Wong. 2013. A critical evaluation of oncology clinical practice guidelines. *Journal of Clinical Oncology* 31(20):2563-2568.

Romanus, D., M. R. Weiser, J. M. Skibber, A. Ter Veer, J. C. Niland, J. L. Wilson, A. Rajput, Y. N. Wong, A. B. Benson, S. Shibata, and D. Schrag. 2009. Concordance with NCCN colorectal cancer guidelines and ASCO/NCCN quality measures: An NCCN institutional analysis. *Journal of the National Comprehensive Cancer Network* 7(8):895-904.

Russell, E. 1998. The ethics of attribution: The case of health care outcome indicators. *Social Science & Medicine* 47(9):1161-1169.

Schneider, E. C., J. L. Malin, K. L. Kahn, E. J. Emanuel, and A. M. Epstein. 2004. Developing a system to assess the quality of cancer care: ASCO's national initiative on cancer care quality. *Journal of Clinical Oncology* 22(15):2985-2991.

Shekelle, P. G., Y. W. Lim, S. Mattke, and C. Damberg. 2008. *Does public release of performance results improve quality of care? A systematic review.* London, UK: The Health Foundation.

Spinks, T. E., R. Walters, T. W. Feeley, H. W. Albright, V. S. Jordan, J. Bingham, and T. W. Burke. 2011. Improving cancer care through public reporting of meaningful quality measures. *Health Affairs (Millwood)* 30(4):664-672.

Spinks, T., H. W. Albright, T. W. Feeley, R. Walters, T. W. Burke, T. Aloia, E. Bruera, A. Buzdar, L. Foxhall, D. Hui, B. Summers, A. Rodriguez, R. Dubois, and K. I. Shine. 2012. Ensuring quality cancer care: A follow-up review of the Institute of Medicine's 10 recommendations for improving the quality of cancer care in america. *Cancer* 118(10):2571-2582.

Totten, A. M., J. Wagner, A. Tiwari, C. O'Haire, J. Griffin, and M. Walker. 2012. *Public reporting as a quality improvement strategy. Closing the quality gap: Revisiting the state of the science.* http://www.effectivehealthcare.ahrq.gov/ehc/products/343/1198/Evidencereport208_CQG-PublicReporting_ExecutiveSummary_20120724.pdf (accessed August 15, 2012).

UHC (UnitedHealthcare). 2012. UHC expands and refines risk-adjusted models for pediatrics and oncology—updated models take children's care into account, help simplify cancer patient diagnosis and treatment methods. https://www.uhc.edu/docs/45014734_Press_Release_RiskModel.pdf (accessed August 15, 2012).

Usman, O. 2011. We need more supply-side regulation. *Health Affairs (Millwood)* 30(8):1615; author reply 1615.

USPSTF (U.S. Preventive Services Task Force). 2012. *USPSTF topic guide.* http://www.uspreventiveservicestaskforce.org/uspstopics.htm#Ctopics (accessed December 20, 2012).

Weissman, J. S., J. R. Betancourt, A. R. Green, G. S. Meyer, A. Tan-McGrory, J. D. Nudel, J. A. Zeidman, and J. E. Carrillo. 2011. *Commissioned paper: Healthcare disparities measurement.* Boston, MA: Massachusetts General Hospital and Harvard Medical School. Sponsored by the National Quality Forum, grant funding from Robert Wood Johnson Foundation.

Werner, R. M., R. T. Konetzka, E. A. Stuart, E. C. Norton, D. Polsky, and J. Park. 2009. Impact of public reporting on quality of postacute care. *Health Services Research* 44(4):1169-1187.

Wick, E. C., D. B. Hobson, J. L. Bennett, R. Demski, L. Maragakis, S. L. Gearhart, J. Efron, S. M. Berenholtz, and M. A. Makary. 2012. Implementation of a surgical comprehensive unit-based safety program to reduce surgical site infections. *Journal of the American College of Surgeons* 215(2):193-200.

8

Accessible and Affordable Cancer Care

The committee's vision for a cancer care delivery system is one in which all people with cancer have access to high-quality, affordable cancer care. Underpinning this system are new payment models that reward cancer care teams for providing patient-centered, high-quality care and eliminating wasteful interventions. The committee's conceptual framework (see Figure S-2) illustrates the concept of rewarding clinicians for high-quality care through quality measurement and new payment models that promote accessible, affordable, high-quality cancer care. The focus on improving access to cancer care is consistent with the Institute of Medicine's (IOM's) report *Ensuring Quality Cancer Care*, which recommended enhancing services for the un- and underinsured and conducting studies to assess the reasons why certain segments of the population do not receive appropriate cancer care (IOM and NRC, 1999). The focus on affordability is a major update in this report.

In the current cancer care system, many patients lack access to affordable, high-quality cancer care. There are major disparities in cancer outcomes among individuals who are of lower socioeconomic status, are racial or ethnic minorities, and who are underinsured or lack health insurance coverage (see discussion in Chapter 2). Many of the disparities are exacerbated by these individuals' lack of access to cancer care. Social determinants of health[1] that extend beyond the health care system, such as individuals' education, economic opportunity, and neighborhood and

---

[1] Social determinants of health are defined by the World Health Organization as "the conditions in which people are born, grow, live, work, and age" (WHO, 2013).

community factors, can also drive these disparities (see discussion in Chapter 2).

At the same time, the increased costs of cancer care are negatively impacting patients and their families (Bernard et al., 2011; Shankaran et al., 2012). People with cancer are at higher risk for bankruptcy than people without a cancer diagnosis (Ramsey et al., 2013). In addition, a survey found that more than a third of individuals reported that medical problems were the reason for bankruptcy, even though three out of four families studied had insurance at the onset of illness (Himmelstein et al., 2009). From a system perspective, health care costs, including the costs of cancer care, are on an unsustainable trajectory that could pose serious fiscal consequences for the United States. Drivers of increased cancer spending include the aging population and the associated increase in cancer diagnoses, as well as the diffusion of new innovations into practice that may or may not be supported by evidence of better patient outcomes. In addition, the current fee-for-service reimbursement system encourages a high volume of care, but fails to reward the provision of high-quality care.

This chapter presents the committee's vision for an accessible and affordable high-quality cancer care delivery system. The first half of the chapter discusses access to care, including the importance of health insurance coverage and barriers to care for vulnerable and underserved populations. The second half of the chapter addresses the affordability of cancer care, reviewing the current challenges to delivering affordable cancer care and strategies for improvement, including eliminating waste, encouraging high-quality cancer care through new payment models, and considering changes to benefit design. The committee derived much of the evidence base on access from the IOM's previous work in this area (IOM, 1993, 2001, 2003, 2004, 2009a). Presentations and discussions from the National Cancer Policy Forum workshop *Delivering Affordable Cancer Care in the 21st Century* informed the committee's deliberations on affordability (IOM, 2013a). The committee identifies two recommendations to address the pressing problems of access and affordability.

ACCESSIBLE CANCER CARE

Access to care, or "the timely use of personal health services to achieve the best possible health outcomes" (IOM, 1993, p. 4), is an important aspect of high-quality cancer care (IOM and NRC, 1999). Patients' health insurance status is a factor influencing an individual's ability to access high-quality cancer care. Certain health system, patient, and clinician characteristics can also affect patients' access to care and cancer care outcomes. This section discusses the impact of health insurance coverage on patients' access to care and, more generally, vulnerable and underserved populations' access to care.

Improve Access Through Health Insurance Coverage

Health insurance coverage is a critical way to increase patients' access to cancer care (C-Change, 2008; Goss et al., 2009; IOM, 1993, 2004, 2009a). Health insurance coverage can improve care for individuals by increasing their likelihood of receiving preventive care, obtaining early diagnoses of disease, undergoing timely and appropriate treatment, and taking needed medications. Studies of previously uninsured adults found that when individuals became eligible for Medicare they could better access physician services and hospital care, and their use of effective clinical preventive services increased (reviewed in IOM, 2009a).

The IOM has repeatedly recommended that the United States ensure that all people have health insurance coverage. Most recently, in *America's Uninsured Crisis: Consequences for Health and Health Care*, the IOM recommended that "the President work with Congress and other public and private sector leaders on an urgent basis to achieve health insurance coverage for everyone" (IOM, 2009a, p. 114). That recommendation echoes the earlier report *Insuring America's Health: Principles and Recommendations* (2004), which also recommended that the President and Congress develop a strategy to achieve health insurance coverage for all people. Similarly, the IOM's 1999 report *Ensuring Quality Cancer Care* recommended improving health insurance coverage for the un- and underinsured to ensure entry and equitable treatment within the cancer care system (IOM and NRC, 1999).

A primary goal of the Patient Protection and Affordable Care Act (ACA) is to expand health insurance coverage.[2] Passage of the ACA is expected to result in 25 million people gaining insurance coverage by 2023 through the individual mandate, the expansion of Medicaid, the creation of Health Insurance Marketplaces, and coverage of young adults on their parents' insurance plans (see Chapter 2) (CBO, 2013). In addition, a number of ACA provisions will expand access to cancer care by ensuring that certain health insurance plans cover important benefits, such as preventive care, cancer screenings, and routine costs for clinical trials, and by preventing certain health plans from imposing a lifetime dollar limit on most benefits (see Annex 2-1 for a more detailed description of the ACA). For example, insurance plans being offered through the Health Insurance Marketplaces will be required to cover essential health benefits, although

---

[2] Patient Protection and Affordable Care Act, Public Law 111-148, 111th Congress, 2nd Sess. (March 23, 2010).

the federal government has given states flexibility in determining which health benefits to designate as "essential" (HealthCare.gov, 2013a). Medicare must also cover annual wellness visits without cost sharing and fully cover many services recommended by the U.S. Preventive Services Task Force (Koh and Sebelius, 2010). Moreover, the ACA filled in the Medicare Part D prescription drug coverage gap, often called the "donut hole" (Koh and Sebelius, 2010).

Much of the ACA has not yet been implemented and its full impact on access to cancer care is unknown. The Congressional Budget Office estimates that approximately 90 percent of the nonelderly population will be insured by 2022 (CBO, 2012a) and the ACA could reduce the underinsured population by 70 percent (Schoen et al., 2011).

A number of individuals, however, will likely remain uninsured or underinsured. Due to the Supreme Court ruling on the ACA, states may opt out of the Medicaid expansion provision of the law that increases the eligibility for Medicaid to people with incomes of up to 138 percent of the federal poverty level (FPL).[3] As of June 2013, 23 states and the District of Columbia plan to expand their Medicaid programs, 6 states are undecided, and 21 are not expanding their Medicaid program at this time (KFF, 2013). Although individuals between 100-138 percent of the FPL will be eligible for federal subsidies for coverage through the state health insurance Marketplaces, individuals below 100 percent of the FPL are not eligible for these subsidies (Kenney et al., 2012; Price and Eibner, 2013). Taking into account the states that are not expanding Medicaid, estimates suggest that around 30 million individuals will remain uninsured (CBO, 2013; Nardin et al., 2013). The uneven expansion of Medicaid may perpetuate disparities in access based on state of residence. Many of the remaining uninsured will be working age individuals (around 60 percent will be age 18-44) (Nardin et al., 2013). In addition, underinsurance may persist, placing people at risk for unaffordable health care costs, financial stress, and the inability to access high-quality cancer care (Schoen et al., 2008, 2011).

The ACA includes a number of provisions to monitor the effect of the law's implementation on access to care. This will enable future efforts to improve patients' access to cancer care to be narrowly tailored to address the remaining gaps in health insurance coverage. It will also be important for researchers to study the impact of the ACA on patients' cancer outcomes because patients' outcomes may be influenced by their access to care.

---

[3] *National Federation of Independent Businesses v. Sebelius*, 132 S. Ct. 2566 (June 28, 2012).

Improve Access for Vulnerable and Underserved Populations

Health insurance coverage does not ensure individuals high-quality care (IOM, 2009a; IOM and NRC, 1999). Even after the ACA is fully implemented, it is likely that many cancer patients will continue to experience problems accessing the care they need. This report uses the phrase "vulnerable and underserved" to describe people who may have difficulty accessing high-quality cancer care. Vulnerable and underserved populations include, but are not limited to

- Racial and ethnic minorities
- Older adults
- Individuals living in rural and urban underserved areas
- Uninsured and underinsured individuals
- Populations of lower socioeconomic status

In addition to health insurance coverage, other factors that impact patients' access to cancer care include (1) affordability of care (e.g., financial resources, cost of health care, childcare, transportation, and productivity reduction [absenteeism and presenteeism[4]], as well as loss of employment due to cancer); (2) health care delivery system attributes (e.g., geographic distribution of cancer care facilities, hours of availability for patient care, or strength of service coordination); (3) patient attributes (e.g., perceptions of cancer prevention and treatment, lack of information, health literacy, language, or cultural factors); and (4) clinician attributes (e.g., communication style, cultural and language competencies, and treatment knowledge/expertise) (IOM and NRC, 1999).

The IOM has made numerous recommendations to improve access and care for individuals who are vulnerable and underserved (IOM, 1993, 1999, 2001, 2003, 2004, 2009a; IOM and NRC, 1999). The IOM report *Crossing the Quality Chasm: A New Health System for the 21st Century* (2001) included equity—defined as "providing care that does not vary in quality because of personal characteristics such as gender, ethnicity, geographic location, and socioeconomic status"—as a major domain of high-quality care (IOM, 2001, p. 6). In *Unequal Treatment: Confronting Racial and Ethnic Disparities in Health Care,* the IOM recommended a series of interventions designed to eliminate health care disparities that targeted legal, regulatory, and policy issues; health system issues; patient education and empowerment; cross-cultural education in health professions; data collection and monitoring; and research needs (IOM, 2003). *Ensuring Quality Cancer Care* recommended that the research community focus on under-

---

[4] Presenteeism is attending work while sick.

standing why specific segments of the population (e.g., racial and ethnic minorities and older patients) often do not receive appropriate cancer care (IOM and NRC, 1999). The IOM report *The Unequal Burden of Cancer: An Assessment of NIH Research and Programs for Ethnic Minorities and the Medically Underserved* (1999) recommended improvements to National Institutes of Health (NIH) programs and priority setting to achieve greater involvement of ethnic minorities and medically underserved populations in cancer research.

The federal government has undertaken significant efforts to collect data on the nature and impact of disparities for vulnerable and underserved populations. For example, the U.S. Department of Health and Human Services' (HHS) *Healthy People 2020* (2013a) tracks health outcomes across a number of demographic factors, including race and ethnicity, gender, sexual identity and orientation, disability status or special health care needs, and geographic location. *Healthy People 2020* aims to achieve health equity (defined as the attainment of the highest level of health for all people), eliminate disparities, and improve the health of all groups (HHS, 2010). The Agency for Healthcare Research and Quality (AHRQ) publishes a yearly, congressionally mandated national health care disparities report (AHRQ, 2012b). The most recent report includes more than 250 measures of disparities, including some cancer-specific measures, and found that access did not improve for most vulnerable and underserved populations from 2002 to 2008; of the 250 measures, 50 percent showed no improvement and 40 percent of measures were getting worse (AHRQ, 2012c). Similarly, the NCI's Surveillance, Epidemiology, and End Results (SEER) cancer registry expanded to collect information on diverse populations and it routinely reports cancer statistics by race, ethnicity, age, gender, and geography (NCI, 2013j).

Although the pervasiveness of disparities among vulnerable and underserved populations in the United States has been well documented, less progress has been made in eradicating these disparities (Spinks et al., 2012; Wallerstein et al., 2011).

The ACA includes multiple provisions designed to improve patients' access to care and reduce disparities for vulnerable and underserved populations. These include establishing the Community Health Center Fund and the Prevention and Public Health Fund; reauthorizing the Patient Navigator and Chronic Disease Prevention grants; and expanding funding for the National Health Service Corps (see Annex 2-1 for a description of these programs). The ACA has mandated that all federally funded health care or public health programs collect and report data on race, ethnicity, sex, primary language, and disability status. It also elevated the National Center on Minority Health and Health Disparities to the level of an institute within NIH, granting the center the authority to develop and evaluate all health disparities research conducted and supported by NIH, and to coordinate NIH's health disparities strategic plan and budget (IOM, 2012b; NIH Record, 2010).

Many public and private efforts are also under way to improve patients' access to care and address disparities for vulnerable and underserved populations (see Annex 8-1). For example, HHS created an action plan to reduce health disparities by transforming health care; strengthening infrastructure and workforce; advancing health, safety, well-being, and innovation; and increasing efficiency, transparency, and accountability (HHS, 2011). This plan was designed to complement the efforts of the National Partnership for Action to End Health Disparities, which was established to "mobilize a nationwide, comprehensive, community-driven, and sustained approach to combating health disparities and to move the nation toward achieving health equity" (NPA, 2011, p. 1). Annex 8-1 also describes a number of additional efforts that aim to reduce barriers in access to health care for vulnerable and underserved populations, such as the NCI and C-Change's involvement in patient navigation.

The barriers impeding patients' access to care are often specific to the communities in which the patients live, and thus, the solutions to address those barriers are most likely to emerge from the communities. Some of the most promising efforts to improve access to care for vulnerable and underserved populations involve federal initiatives that focus on supporting community interventions.

The Coordinated Federal Action Plan to Reduce Racial and Ethnic Asthma Disparities exemplifies a federal government effort to facilitate community interventions designed to improve access for vulnerable and underserved populations (President's Task Force on Environmental Health Risks and Safety Risks to Children, 2012). Major components of the plan focus on evaluating partnership models that engage communities, identifying and targeting disparate populations, and providing comprehensive, integrated care at the community level. Similarly, HHS' Million Hearts® Initiative works to prevent heart disease and stroke by improving access and quality of care through cardiovascular disease prevention activities coordinated across the public and private sectors (HHS, 2013b). The Centers for Medicare & Medicaid Services (CMS) and the Centers for Disease Control and Prevention (CDC) are co-leading the Million Hearts® Initiative, along with the American Heart Association, the YMCA, and many other community organizations, with the goal of preventing one million heart attacks and strokes by 2017. In July 2013, President Obama signed an executive order announcing the HIV Care Continuum Initiative to mobilize and coordinate federal efforts to prevent and treat HIV infection (White House, 2013a). Many of the activities of the initiative will involve federal-level support of community-level programs, including capacity building among community health centers, health departments, community-based organizations, and health care organizations (White House, 2013b).

Several organizations discussed in Annex 8-1 are also focusing on community-specific interventions to improve access and reduce disparities. C-Change's Geographic Intervention Project, for example, is developing a community-based process for addressing health care disparities that can be leveraged by other communities. Similarly, the CDC's Racial and Ethnic Approaches to Community Health (REACH) program provides funding for communities to implement and evaluate community-based approaches to improve health (CDC, 2012). REACH is a part of the CDC's Healthy Communities program, which provides tools that support community action and convenes action institutes to help community leaders make policy, system, and environmental changes that aim to prevent chronic disease (CDC, 2011a).

Given the promise of federal initiatives that support community interventions, the committee recommends that HHS develop a national strategy to reduce disparities in access to cancer care for vulnerable and underserved populations by leveraging existing efforts by public and private organizations. As part of this strategy, the committee recommends that HHS (1) support the development of innovative programs, (2) identify and disseminate effective community interventions, and (3) provide ongoing support to existing successful community interventions (Recommendation 9).

An important focus of the national plan should be the dissemination of successful community interventions that improve access to high-quality cancer care for vulnerable and underserved populations. HHS' role in disseminating successful community interventions could help other communities identify potential strategies that could be evaluated for their unique local environment and population. HHS should also help ensure the sustainability of successful community interventions. The committee recognizes that ongoing support will require substantial resources. Savings derived from other changes to the cancer care delivery system recommended by the committee may offset some of these costs.

AFFORDABLE CANCER CARE

The affordability of care is equally important to a high-quality cancer care system. As mentioned in Chapter 2, the United States is currently facing unsustainable growth in the cost of cancer care and the rising costs of cancer care are negatively impacting patients and their families (Bernard et al., 2011; Cohen et al., 2013; Ramsey et al., 2013; Shankaran et al., 2012; Zafar et al., 2013). This section explores the perverse incentives in the current reimbursement system for cancer care and presents three strategies for achieving affordable cancer care, while maintaining or improving the quality of care:

- eliminating waste in the cancer care system by engaging clinicians and payers;
- incentivizing affordable, high-quality cancer care by realigning the reimbursement system to reward high-quality, affordable cancer care; and
- designing insurance benefits that enable patients to take an active role in choosing affordable, high-quality cancer care that aligns with their needs, values, and preferences.

These strategies have the potential to make cancer care more affordable for patients by reducing the incentive for clinicians to provide more (or more expensive) care that does not improve patient outcomes and by lowering patients' cost sharing for high-quality cancer care.

Given the challenges to defining value in cancer care (see Box 8-1), the committee purposefully chose to frame its discussion in terms of high-quality and affordable cancer care.

Challenges in Cancer Care Reimbursement

The most common form of financial reimbursement for health care in the United States is fee-for-service reimbursement.[5] Fee-for-service reimbursement incentivizes the volume of services provided by clinicians or hospitals, but typically overlooks quality or efficiency of care (CEA, 2009; Etheredge, 2009; IOM, 2012a,c, 2013a). For example, the IOM report *Best Care at Lower Cost: The Path to Continuously Learning Health Care in America* concluded that fee-for-service reimbursement does not reward clinicians for the quality of care they provide, and encourages wasteful and ineffective care (IOM, 2012a).

In the cancer care setting, fee-for-service reimbursement incentivizes clinicians to provide patients with interventions, even if there is a lack of evidence to show that those interventions improve patient outcomes. It also incentivizes clinicians to prescribe more expensive chemotherapy and recommend more costly methods of delivering radiation therapy, surgery, or imaging, irrespective of the benefits to patients (IOM, 2013a). One survey found that oncologists derive three-quarters of their practice revenues from chemotherapy drug charges (Akscin et al., 2007).

---

[5] Fee-for-service reimbursement is a financing methodology in which clinicians are reimbursed for each individual procedure or patient encounter (IOM, 2006).

BOX 8-1
Defining Value in Cancer Care

Defining value in health care is challenging. Many definitions and concepts of value have been suggested. The basic premise of value is that it represents the quality of care relative to the cost of care. Value is created in care when outcomes improve and costs are maintained or when costs are reduced and outcomes are not adversely impacted.

Many attempts have been made recently to describe value in cancer care (Feeley et al., 2010; IOM, 2009b; Ramsey and Schickedanz, 2010). A 2009 Institute of Medicine (IOM) workshop on value in cancer care outlined attributes and metrics of value. Based on this workshop, Ramsey and Schickedanz (2010) suggested that "an intervention in cancer care can be described as having value if patients, their families, physicians, and health insurers all agree that the benefits afforded by the intervention are sufficient to support the total sum of resources expended for its use" (p. 2).

Other groups within the IOM have also grappled with how to define value in health care. The Committee on Geographic Variation in Health Care Spending and Promotion of High-Value Health Care defined health care value as equivalent to net benefit: "the amount by which overall health benefit and/or well-being produced by care exceeds (or falls short of) the costs of producing it" (IOM, 2013b, p. 11). The IOM Roundtable on Value & Science-Driven Health Care held a workshop on value in health care, but concluded that "no single consistent definition of value was identified by the participants" (IOM, 2009d, p. xv).

The U.S. Department of Veterans Affairs (VA) has used a value equation in its quality improvement efforts, which is expressed as a ratio of outputs to inputs. Inputs include the financial resources of the VA, while outputs include technical quality of care, access to services, patient functional status, patient satisfaction, and community health (Perlin et al., 2004).

The Affordable Care Act used the term "value" more than 200 times, yet never defined the term. The Agency for Healthcare Research and Quality (2010) refers to improving value by reducing unnecessary costs (waste) and increasing efficiency while maintaining or improving health care quality. The United Kingdom's

---

Previous changes in the way oncologists were reimbursed for chemotherapy administration, such as the enactment of the Medicare Prescription Drug, Improvement, and Modernization Act, have influenced which drugs oncologists prescribe (Jacobson et al., 2006, 2010) (see also Box 8-2). A substantial number of oncologists in fee-for-service practice have reported that their income increases from administering chemotherapy or hematopoietic growth factors (Malin et al., 2013). At the same time, other important aspects of cancer care are not well compensated, such as

National Institute for Clinical Excellence applies the concept that the value of treatment is based on scientific value judgments, including a clinical evaluation and an economic evaluation, and social value judgments, including considerations of efficiency and effectiveness (Rawlins, 2004; Rawlins and Culyer, 2004).

Porter and Teisberg have defined value in health care as the health outcomes per dollar expended (Porter and Teisberg, 2006). This definition is premised on achieving the best possible outcomes as efficiently as possible (Lee, 2010). It places the responsibility for health reform on clinicians and assumes that the purpose of the health care system is not to minimize costs, but to deliver value to patients—in other words, better health per dollar spent (Porter and Teisberg, 2007).

Porter and Teisberg suggested seven essentials of value-based competition in health care delivery, frequently called the value proposition in health care delivery (Feeley et al., 2010):

1. Set the goal as value for patients; not access, equity, volume, convenience, or cost containment.
2. Quality improvement is the key driver of cost containment and value improvement, where quality equals health outcomes.
3. Care delivery should be organized around medical conditions over the full cycle of care.
4. Provider experience, scale, and learning at the medical condition level drive value improvement.
5. Care must be integrated across facilities and geography, rather than duplicating services within stand-alone units.
6. One must measure and report outcomes and costs for every provider for every medical condition.
7. Reimbursement must be aligned with value, and, furthermore, innovation needs to be rewarded.

A crosscutting principle of a value-based delivery system is that there needs to be an information technology platform that enables all aspects of the system to function as efficiently as possible.

cognitive care[6] provided by physicians and support services offered by nurses, psychologists, chaplains, or social workers in cancer care (IOM, 2009b; Smith and Hillner, 2011) (see also Chapter 3). The extent to which oncologists in fee-for-service practice have been using the profit margins on chemotherapy to finance other uncompensated care is unknown, al-

---

[6] Cognitive care refers to evaluation and management services, which entails time spent discussing, for example, prognosis and treatment options (Smith and Hillner, 2011).

BOX 8-2
Medicare Prescription Drug, Improvement,
and Modernization Act

Enacted in 2003, the Medicare Prescription Drug, Improvement, and Modernization Act, also known as the Medicare Modernization Act (MMA), made substantial changes to the way Medicare Part B drugs are reimbursed, and established the Medicare Part D prescription drug benefit (Part D), expanding patient access to oncology drugs.

Most physician-administered oncology drugs, and some of their oral equivalents, are reimbursed under the Medicare Part B benefit. Prior to implementation of the MMA, Medicare paid providers 95 percent of the average wholesale price (AWP) for Part B drugs. A number of studies from the U.S. Government Accountability Office and the Health and Human Services' Office of the Inspector General showed that reimbursing for AWP greatly exceeded clinician costs for these drugs (reviewed in MedPAC, 2003). In order to reduce overpaying for Part B drugs, the MMA changed the reimbursement from AWP to average sales price (ASP) plus a 6 percent administration fee. The year the payment change went into effect, there was an 8 percent decrease in spending (MedPAC, 2011). However, some suggest spending has not decreased as much as anticipated, in part, because drug manufacturers responded by raising their unit prices (IOM, 2013a). From 2006 to 2009, Medicare spending for Part B drugs increased at an average rate of 2.3 percent per year.

The Medicare prescription drug benefit (Part D) improved patients' access to cancer treatment by extending drug coverage to Medicare beneficiaries. In the

---

though Bach asserted that the incentives in cancer care have promoted a culture of buying and selling cancer drugs at the expense of other aspects of cancer care (Bach, 2007).

Similar pressures influence the types of radiation therapy that clinicians provide (IOM, 2013a). Clinicians who own radiation therapy equipment have an incentive to prescribe this treatment over other types of interventions because they are financially rewarded under fee-for-service reimbursement (Bekelman et al., 2013). In addition, clinicians have rapidly diffused many radiation therapy innovations into clinical practice because of high fee-for-service reimbursement. There have been rapid shifts from 3-D conformal radiotherapy to intensity-modulated radiotherapy (IMRT) to proton beam therapy for prostate cancer, for example, even though the new technologies have not been evaluated in prospective comparative trials to determine whether they improve patient outcomes (Sheets et al., 2012; Yeboa et al., 2010). From 2000 to 2008, clinicians' use of IMRT compared to 3-D conformal radiotherapy in prostate cancer increased from 0.15 percent to 95.9 percent (Sheets et al., 2012). From 2006 to 2009, the

cancer setting, Part D provides coverage for non-physician-administered drugs, including self-injectables and oral formulations of drugs. Part D drug benefit plans are required to cover "all or substantially all" drugs in certain therapeutic classes, including cancer (Bach, 2009; Bach and McClellan, 2005; Bowman et al., 2006). Yet, because private insurers administer Part D, each plan determines formulary design, cost-sharing structure, and utilization management tools. For example, a plan may require prior authorization for brand-name cancer drugs but not generic ones, or choose not to cover some brand-name cancer medications at all (Bowman et al., 2006). The Centers for Medicare & Medicaid Services (CMS) monitors formularies to ensure that no one disease or condition is discriminated against (Bach and McClellan, 2005). Bowman and colleagues (2006) found that 75 percent of cancer drugs were included in Part D plans' formularies, and that most of the excluded cancer drugs were brand-name versions in which generic versions were available. However, Part D does not cover drugs that are prescribed for off-label uses unless they are medically necessary.[a] The MMA also created a coverage gap in which beneficiaries had to pay out of pocket when their annual drug costs ranged from approximately $900 to $4,400. The Affordable Care Act narrowed, and will eliminate by 2020, the coverage gap known as the "donut hole".

NOTE: Off-label use is the prescribing of drugs already on the market for an indication, age group, dose, or form of administration that has not been approved by the Food and Drug Administration. A large proportion of oncology drugs are prescribed for off-label purposes (Conti et al., 2013; Soares, 2005).

[a] 42 USCS § 1395w-104(b)(3)(G)(i).

number of Medicare beneficiaries receiving proton beam therapy almost doubled (Jarosek et al., 2012). In an analysis of Medicare patients receiving radiation therapy for prostate cancer, median reimbursement for proton therapy was $32,428 compared to $18,575 for IMRT, despite no difference in side effects at 12 months post-treatment (Yu et al., 2013). The use of brachytherapy in breast cancer offers another example of rapid diffusion of new technology without established evidence of benefit from trials (Smith et al., 2011).

Clinicians have also rapidly deployed surgical innovations into practice. For example, the use of robot-assisted prostatectomies grew substantially from 2005 to 2008 (Barbash and Glied, 2010). In 2011, clinicians used the robotic da Vinci Surgical System to conduct as many as four out of five radical prostatectomies (NCI, 2011). One study found clinicians' use of robotic surgery increased the costs of surgery by about 13 percent and estimated that replacing open surgery with robotic surgery in all procedures would add $2.5 billion annually to health care expenditures (Barbash and Glied, 2010). While the rate of reimbursement is the same for robotic-assisted procedures and their non-robotic-assisted counterparts (e.g., robotic-assisted laparoscopic radical prostatectomy [LRP] and LRP without robotic assistance), the total hospitalization charges for robotic surgeries is higher than the same surgeries without the assistance of a robotic system (Bolenz et al., 2012). Hospitals that have purchased the robotic surgical system profit from increased utilization of this equipment.

Waste is another unintended consequence of fee-for-service reimbursement. The *Best Care at Lower Cost* report estimated that more than $750 billion of health care costs are wasteful (IOM, 2012a). This study categorized waste in U.S. health care spending as unnecessary services, inefficiently delivered services, excess administrative costs, prices that are too high, missed opportunities for prevention, and fraud.

In cancer care, overuse is a persistent problem (Katz and Morrow, 2013a,b; Schnipper et al., 2012). One study found that almost one-quarter of Medicare patients who had negative colonoscopy findings underwent another screening less than 7 years later, a screening interval not supported by current guidelines (Goodwin et al., 2011). In addition, many patients with metastatic non-small-cell lung cancer receive a greater number of treatments or higher doses of palliative radiotherapy than is supported by current evidence (Chen et al., 2013). Futile chemotherapy near the end of life is another example of overuse. The American Society of Clinical Oncology's (ASCO's) Quality Oncology Practice Initiative has included a measure of chemotherapy administration in the last 2 weeks of life as an indication of poor quality cancer care (see Chapter 7 for more information on quality measures).

In addition, fee-for-service reimbursement does not facilitate cancer care coordination because clinicians act as separate entities and are typically reimbursed accordingly (MedPAC, 2012). Failures of care coordination and the fragmentation of health care have been highlighted as critical problems of the cancer care system (see Chapter 4) (IOM, 2011; IOM and NRC, 1999; Spinks et al., 2012). Poor coordination can lead to costly duplication of care and result in patient complications. Fee-for-service reimbursement is especially problematic for patients who have comorbidities that must be managed by both the cancer care team and other specialist care teams.

A number of laws and regulations limit CMS' and private insurers' ability to pay for cancer care in ways that reward clinicians for providing high-quality and affordable care (Bach, 2009; Neumann and Chambers, 2012). State laws, affecting around 74 percent of the U.S. population, require coverage of cancer treatments if their use is recognized in the drug compendia, peer-reviewed literature, or both (Bach, 2009). The information in the compendia, however, is of variable quality and is often not supported by adequate evidence (Abernethy et al., 2010). Similarly, Medicare is required to cover any Part B drug used in a chemotherapy regimen as long as its use is for a medically accepted indication (Bach, 2009). For Part D drug plans, formularies are required to include essentially all drugs "where restricted access would have major or life threatening clinical consequences … such as drugs used in the treatment of cancer" (Bach, 2009, p. 630).

This complex legal and regulatory framework makes it difficult for payers to use comparative effectiveness research evaluating the effectiveness of cancer drugs in reimbursement decisions (Pearson, 2012). Thus, "pharmaceutical firms know that these very expensive new cancer drugs will not be denied coverage by Medicare on the grounds of cost, and so they have no incentive to price them to meet any cost-effectiveness standard" (Brock, 2010, p. 38). This issue is further compounded by CMS' inability to negotiate prices with pharmaceutical firms, even though it is the largest purchaser of cancer drugs.

Eliminating Waste in Cancer Care

Driven by the IOM's estimate that more than $750 billion in health care spending is wasteful, many clinicians are taking the lead in efforts to eliminate waste and promote high-quality, affordable care. Clinician leadership in these efforts is essential to their success because clinician decisions determine how a majority of health care dollars are spent (Schnipper, 2012). ASCO's policy statement on the cost of cancer care states that physicians have "a societal responsibility to provide care that minimizes waste and is evidence based" (Meropol et al., 2009, p. 3871). The physician charter of the American Board of Internal Medicine (ABIM) Foundation also states that physicians are responsible for "scrupulous avoidance of superfluous tests and procedures" (ABIM, 2013b).

Several clinician-led efforts to improve the quality and affordability of cancer are already under way. Community oncology practices, in collaboration with payers, have been assessing new models of cancer care delivery and payment (Hoverman et al., 2011; IOM, 2013a; Neubauer et al., 2010; Newcomer, 2012; Sprandio, 2010). ASCO has called for physicians to play a leadership role in the development and testing of new payment reform models (see discussion below in the section on "Incentivizing High-Quality Cancer Care") (ASCO, 2013).

The ABIM's Choosing Wisely® initiative is an example of a clinician-led effort targeted at eliminating waste. This program is designed to help clinicians and patients engage in conversations to minimize overuse of tests and procedures and to provide clinicians with the support they need to help patients make informed and effective health care decisions (ABIM, 2013a). It includes an explicit goal of avoiding care that is "unnecessary or whose harm may outweigh the benefits" (Schnipper et al., 2012, p. 1716). ASCO is participating in this initiative and has released a "Top Five" list of common, costly procedures in oncology that are not supported by evidence and that require careful consideration by patients and their clinicians before using (Schnipper et al., 2012) (see Box 8-3). More recently, ASCO identified additional interventions to include on its list, and the American Society for Radiation Oncology released its own "Top Five" list (Choosing Wisely, 2013; Schnipper et al., 2013). Similarly, the Commission on Cancer has also submitted a "Top Five" list to the ABIM. Other professional organizations have developed lists that may be relevant in the cancer care setting as well, including the American Academy of Hospice and Palliative Medicine and the American Geriatrics Society.

The committee recommends that professional societies identify and publicly disseminate evidence-based information about cancer care

---

BOX 8-3
ASCO's "Top Five" List

As a participant in the American Board of Internal Medicine Foundation's Choosing Wisely® initiative, the American Society of Clinical Oncology (ASCO) issued a "Top Five" list of common, costly procedures in oncology that are not supported by evidence in 2012 (shown below). The development of this list was led by ASCO's Cost of Cancer Care Task Force, a multidisciplinary group of oncologists, and selections were based on a comprehensive review of published studies and current guidelines from ASCO and other organizations. The final list also reflects input from more than 200 oncologists and patient advocates.

- For patients with advanced solid-tumor cancers who are unlikely to benefit, do not provide unnecessary anticancer therapy, such as chemotherapy, but instead focus on symptom relief and palliative care.
- Do not use positron emission tomography (PET), computed tomography (CT), and radionuclide bone scans in the staging of early prostate cancer at low risk for metastasis.
- Do not use PET, CT, and radionuclide bone scans in the staging of early breast cancer at low risk for metastasis.
- For individuals who have completed curative breast cancer treatment and have no physical symptoms of cancer recurrence, routine blood tests for biomarkers and advanced imaging tests should not be used to screen for cancer recurrences.
- Avoid administering colony stimulating factors to patients undergoing chemotherapy who have less than a 20 percent risk for febrile neutropenia.

SOURCE: ASCO, 2012.

practices that are unnecessary or where the harm may outweigh the benefits. The Choosing Wisely® initiative is an important step toward eliminating waste in health care and in focusing the nation's attention on solving this problem. However, the current effort is being led by individual professional societies in silos, even though their areas of practice may overlap. In order for this campaign to have a larger impact, it will be important for professional societies to coordinate with each other to identify wasteful practices that cross disciplines and professions. A more systematic, integrated approach to evaluate cancer care practices that are contributing to waste will help establish a consistent message, improve the acceptability of the identified list of wasteful care practices in the cancer community, and, hopefully, result in broader uptake among clinicians. This approach will also be more efficient and reduce duplication of efforts.

It will be important for professional societies to disseminate these findings to their members and the public, and payers should also leverage this work to ensure that their payment policies are consistent with the goal of eliminating waste. **Thus, the committee recommends that CMS and other payers develop payment policies that reflect the evidence-based findings of the professional societies.**

Incentivizing High-Quality Cancer Care

Previous IOM reports have called for payers to reorient their reimbursement policies to reward clinicians for providing high-quality care rather than volume. *Best Care at Lower Cost* recommended that payers structure payments to reward continuous learning and improvement, patient-centered care, and team-based care through outcome- and value-oriented reimbursement models (IOM, 2012a). *Crossing the Quality Chasm* called on federal agencies to work with payers, health care organizations, and clinicians to develop a "research agenda to identify, pilot test, and evaluate various options for better aligning current payment methods with quality improvement goals" (IOM, 2001, p. 182).

Many other organizations have also reached similar conclusions regarding the need for new payment models. For example, the National Commission on Physician Payment Reform recommended that fee-for-service payment be largely eliminated because of its "inherent inefficiencies and problematic financial incentives" (*Report of the National Commission on Physician Payment Reform*, 2013, p. 14). The Commission recommended testing new models of care that reward clinicians for providing high-quality and efficient care over a 5-year period and implementing them on a more widespread scale by the end of the decade. The Partnership for Sustainable Health Care, a collaboration of five organizations representing diverse stakeholders in health care,[7] called for transformation of the current payment paradigm by transitioning away from fee-for-service reimbursement (Partnership for Sustainable Health Care, 2013). It also recommended the dissemination and implementation of alternative payment and delivery models that improve quality and efficiency over the next 5 years. In addition, the Brookings Institution recently recommended that Medicare reimburse the majority of medical services through accountable care organizations (ACOs), medical homes, and bundled payments (Brookings Institution, 2013).

Building on these previous reports, **the committee recommends that CMS and other payers design and evaluate new payment models that incentivize the cancer care team to provide care that is based on the best available evidence and aligns with their patients' needs, values, and preferences.** This recommendation has the potential to facilitate many of the components of the committee's conceptual framework, including incentivizing

- effective patient-clinician communication and shared decision-making that supports patients and caregivers in making informed medical decisions consistent with their needs, values, and preferences, as well as advance care planning, the provision of palliative care and psychosocial support across the cancer continuum, and the timely referral to hospice care at the end of life (Chapter 3);
- team-based cancer care that prioritizes patient-centered care and coordination with a patient's primary care/geriatrics care team and other care teams, especially for patients with comorbidities (Chapter 4);
- evidence-based cancer care that is concordant with clinical practice guidelines and consistent with patients' needs, values, and preferences (Chapter 5);
- clinician participation in the learning health care system and the national quality reporting program (Chapters 6 and 7); and
- reduced use of interventions that do not improve patient outcomes and contribute to unsustainable health care costs (see discussion above in the section on Eliminating Waste in Cancer Care).

It is important that payers be thoughtful in implementing these new reimbursement models because changing financial incentives will lead

---

[7] The Partnership includes America's Health Insurance Plans, Ascension Health, Families USA, the National Coalition on Health Care, and the Pacific Business Group on Health.

to changes in oncology practice (Colla et al., 2012; Jacobson et al., 2006, 2010). The committee hopes that these changes will be beneficial, with the potential to achieve the aims of the committee's conceptual framework. However, they could also be harmful, resulting in unintended adverse consequences, perverse incentives, and lack of improvements to patient care (Biller-Andorno and Lee, 2013; Flodgren et al., 2011; RAND, 2011). Poorly implemented payment models could reduce patients' access to care if clinicians avoid high-risk or high-cost patients, or could lead to the underuse of evidence-based care in an effort to save resources (RAND, 2011).

It is important that payers' implementation of new reimbursement models is embedded within the committee's conceptual framework for improving the quality of cancer care because changing economic incentives is necessary, but insufficient, to improve the quality of cancer care (Biller-Andorno and Lee, 2013). The committee's recommendation to create a more robust quality metrics reporting system (see Chapter 7) and the inclusion of performance metrics in many of the models discussed below will be critical to ensuring that payment reforms maintain or improve the quality of cancer care and do not result in unintended negative consequences. **The committee also recommends that clinicians work with their professional societies to identify and disseminate cancer care practices that are unnecessary or where the harm may outweigh the benefits (see discussion above on eliminating waste)** (ABIM, 2013b).

In addition, many of the committee's recommendations aim to make it easier for clinicians to deliver high-quality cancer care: for example, through improved tools to guide shared decision making and capture it in care plans. A learning health care information technology system for cancer would include clinical decision support that facilitates the delivery of evidence-based cancer care (see Chapter 6). It would also improve care coordination in conjunction with care plans. Moreover, the components of the committee's conceptual framework are interdependent. Thus, removing perverse payment incentives will also have the added benefit of facilitating implementation of the other requirements for a high-quality cancer care delivery system. Ultimately, professional societies will also play an important role in changing the culture by setting expectations for medical professionalism in delivering high-quality cancer care.

The ACA has established the CMS Innovation Center for pilot testing delivery system and payment models that have the potential to reduce health care expenditures and maintain or improve the quality of care (see Box 8-4). The CMS Innovation Center has the authority to expand these innovative models nationally if they demonstrate improvements in quality, reduce costs, or both. Although the models currently being tested are generally not disease specific, the lessons learned from these demonstra-

---

BOX 8-4
The CMS Innovation Center

The Affordable Care Act established the Center for Medicare & Medicaid Innovation (recently renamed the CMS Innovation Center) for testing new delivery system and payment models to improve the quality of care and reduce health care costs. The Secretary of Health and Human Services has the authority to expand the scope and duration of successful models nationwide through a rulemaking process (CMS, 2013a). Each model the CMS Innovation Center tests is evaluated based on the quality of care that clinicians provided when practicing under the parameters of the model (based on patient outcomes and patient-centeredness criteria), as well as changes in costs measured by the Rapid Cycle Evaluation Group (Shrank, 2013).

The CMS Innovation Center is currently testing seven categories of innovation models (CMS, 2013e):

1. Accountable care organizations (ACOs)
2. Bundled payments for care improvement
3. Primary care transformation
4. Initiatives focused on Medicaid and the Children's Health Insurance Program population
5. Initiatives focused on dually eligible Medicare-Medicaid enrollees
6. Initiatives to speed adoption of best practices
7. Initiatives to accelerate the development and testing of new payment and service delivery models

More information on the CMS Innovation Center's work on ACOs and bundled payments, which are most relevant to cancer care, is available in the following section of the chapter.

---

tion projects could be leveraged to advance innovations in cancer care delivery and payment. In addition, the second round of Health Care Innovation Awards specifically solicits proposals for new payment and delivery models for cancer care (CMS, 2013j).

A number of health care payers and oncology practices have also been experimenting with different payment models to improve the quality and reduce the cost of cancer care (Hoverman et al., 2011; Neubauer et al., 2010; Newcomer, 2012; Sprandio, 2010). Table 8-1 summarizes examples of innovative payment models that are currently being explored to realign financial incentives in health care (RAND, 2011). The sections below discuss the most promising examples for cancer care in more detail, including bundled payments, ACOs, oncology patient-centered medical homes (PCMHs), care pathways, coverage with evidence development, and value-based purchasing (VBP) and competitive bidding.

TABLE 8-1 Examples of Payment Reform Models Relevant to Cancer Care

Payment Reform Models	Brief Description
Global payment	A single per-member, per-month payment is made for all services delivered to a patient, with payment adjustments based on measured performance and patient risk.
Accountable care organization (ACO) shared savings program	Groups of clinicians and provider groups that voluntarily assume responsibility for the care of a population of patients (known as ACOs) share payer savings if they meet quality and cost performance benchmarks.
Medical home	A physician practice or other provider group is eligible to receive additional payments if medical home criteria are met. Payment may include calculations based on quality and cost performance using a pay-for-performance-like mechanism.
Bundled payment	A single "bundled" payment, which may be shared by multiple clinicians or provider groups in multiple care settings, is made for services delivered during an episode of care related to a patients' medical condition or procedure.
Hospital-physician gainsharing	Hospitals are permitted to provide payments to physicians that represent a share of savings resulting from collaborative efforts between the hospital and physicians to improve quality and efficiency.
Payment for coordination	Payments are made to clinicians and provider groups furnishing care coordination services that integrate care among clinicians.
Physician pay-for-performance	Physicians receive differential payments for meeting or missing performance benchmarks.
Payment for shared decision making	Reimbursement is provided for shared decision-making services.

SOURCE: Adapted from RAND. 2011. *Payment reform: Analysis of models and performance measurement implications.* http://www.rand.org/pubs/technical_reports/TR841.html (accessed Novembe 1, 2013). © 2011 The RAND Corporation, Santa Monica, CA. Reprinted with permission.

Because the effectiveness of these payment and delivery system reforms is still being evaluated by a number of payers, the committee does not recommend a specific strategy going forward. **However, the committee recommends that if evaluations of specific payment models demonstrate increased quality and affordability, CMS and other payers should rapidly transition from traditional fee-for-service reimbursements to new payment models.** If one payer demonstrates that new payment models are successful, these models will likely be adopted by other payers.

This recommendation is consistent with the IOM study *Variation in Health Care Spending: Target Decision Making, Not Geography,* which recommended that CMS be given the flexibility to accelerate the transition from traditional Medicare to new payment models that demonstrate increased value (IOM, 2013b). The committee also echoes this study's recognition that it is important that CMS monitor the impact of new payment models on patients' access to care. The transition from pilot programs to broader adoption of new payment models will be challenging and require major investments in infrastructure and organizational changes. During this transition, it is critical that patients do not experience reduced access to cancer care.

Bundled Payments

Bundled payments (also called episode-based payments) reimburse care teams for discrete episodes of care and can involve multiple clinicians and care settings (RAND, 2011). They shift financial risk away from insurers and make clinicians more accountable for efficiently using resources. They can also promote better care coordination if a bundle covers multiple modalities in cancer care (e.g., surgery, chemotherapy, and radiation therapy).

There is some evidence that bundled payments reduce health care costs. In 2004, AHRQ undertook an evaluation of bundled payments and concluded that there is "evidence that bundled payment programs have been effective in cost containment without major effects on quality" (AHRQ, 2012a, p. vi). For example, the Medicare Participating Heart Bypass Center Demonstration, conducted in the 1990s, assessed the impact of bundled payments on hospital and physician payments for coronary artery bypass graft surgery. Researchers found that Medicare expenditures declined by about 10 percent in the demonstration program, compared to what Medicare would have spent in the absence of the program. Five hospitals experienced savings of 5 to 10 percent and two hospitals experienced savings of about 20 percent (CBO, 2012b; HCFA, 1998). In an evaluation of eight policy options to reduce health care spending, Hussey et al. (2009) concluded that bundled payments have the greatest potential.

Many efforts are under way to implement bundled payments. Arkansas is incorporating bundled payments in its Medicaid program (Emanuel, 2012). Also, the CMS Innovation Center is evaluating bundled payments through its Bundled Payments for Care Improvement Initiative (CMS, 2013c), which includes four distinct models of care that link payments for multiple services:

1. Retrospective acute care hospital stay only
2. Retrospective acute care hospital stay plus post-acute care
3. Retrospective post-acute care only
4. Acute care hospital stay only

The CMS Innovation Center selected 48 episodes of care that are eligible for bundled payments, none specific to cancer care.

Bundled payments, however, are well suited for cancer care (Bach et al., 2011; Etheredge, 2009; Newcomer, 2012). Bach and colleagues (2011) proposed creating an episode-based payment pilot in Medicare for treating metastatic non-small-cell lung cancer. There are a number of chemotherapy options with similar patient outcomes that the National Comprehensive Cancer Network (NCCN) recommends for this disease. In this proposed pilot, Medicare would set an episode-based payment at a price in between the highest- and lowest-cost treatment regimens, including the cost of chemotherapy drugs, supportive care drugs, and the cost of administering these drugs. This would provide clinicians with a financial incentive to choose the lower cost, equally effective treatment options for their patients. Over time, the episode-based payment would be recalibrated downward to save costs.

Bach and colleagues' episode-based payment pilot could also be effective in treating other cancers where there are comparable treatment regimens at varying prices. It would not be applicable for cancers where it is unclear which treatments result in similar patient outcomes and comparative effectiveness data are unavailable, such as early-stage prostate cancer, for which there are a number of different treatment options, including radical prostatectomy, radiation therapy, and active surveillance (IOM, 2009c).

UnitedHealthcare has also initiated a bundled payment pilot for cancer care (Newcomer, 2012). In this pilot, UnitedHealthcare pays clinicians a set patient care fee regardless of which chemotherapy is prescribed, thus eliminating clinicians' ability to profit from chemotherapy administration. The initial care fee was established by allowing the participating cancer care teams to select what they thought represented the clinically superior treatment for 19 discrete episodes of care among patients with breast, colon, and lung cancer. The participating cancer care teams agreed to an

85 percent treatment compliance rate. The patient care fee was calculated using the drug margin from the selected regimen plus a case management fee. UnitedHealthcare continues to pay the cost of chemotherapy; however, if a clinician switches from the selected treatment regimen to a more expensive one, UnitedHealthcare will not increase the patient care fee. It will only raise the patient care fee based on improved outcomes. If the total cost of care is reduced, UnitedHealthcare will share the savings with the cancer care team. Participating groups have also agreed to meet yearly to compare results for the 19 episodes of care. If the data (including measures of survival, hospitalizations for complications, and total costs of care) identify a best practice, UnitedHealthcare expects all groups to shift to that treatment.

Accountable Care Organizations

RAND (2011) describes ACOs as groups of clinicians or provider groups that assume responsibility for the care of a group of patients and share savings when they satisfy quality and cost performance benchmarks. There are more than 400 public and private ACOs in the United States, including more than 250 public ACOs that provide care for nearly 4 million Medicare beneficiaries (Muhlestein, 2013). The CMS Innovation Center is evaluating several types of ACO programs, including

- Medicare Shared Savings Program for fee-for-service Medicare beneficiaries
- Advance Payment ACO Model for certain eligible providers already in or interested in the Medicare Shared Savings Program
- Pioneer ACO Model for health care organizations and providers already experienced in coordinating care for patients across care settings

Although ACOs were initially focused on primary care, they are now being considered for specialty care, such as cancer (CMS, 2013b; Mehta et al., 2013; Punke, 2013). Cancer Clinics of Excellence, for example, is collaborating with Accretive Health to develop a clinician-led, shared savings model of care in oncology. This shared savings model prioritizes care coordination and appropriate end-of-life care, eliminating unnecessary interventions, and encouraging adherence to care pathways. It also invests heavily in health information technology (IOM, 2013a). Similarly, Florida's largest health insurer, Florida Blue, is collaborating with Moffitt Cancer Center, Baptist Health South Florida, and Advanced Medical Specialties to form oncology ACOs (BCBS, 2012; Conway, 2012).

Oncology Patient-Centered Medical Homes

PCMHs typically refer to a model of primary care delivery in which participating practices receive additional payments for coordinating their patients' care. The AHRQ definition of a PCMH includes five functions and attributes: patient-centeredness; comprehensive care (prevention wellness, as well as chronic and acute care); coordinated care; access to care; and a systems-based approach to quality and safety (AHRQ, 2011).

The National Committee for Quality Assurance's PCMH program recognizes organizations that achieve its PCMH standards. The standards include (1) enhanced access and continuity of care (including afterhours access); (2) data collection to identify and manage patient populations; (3) management of care using evidence-based clinical practice guidelines; (4) assistance with self-care management; (5) the tracking and coordination of care; and (6) continuous quality improvement using performance and patient experience data (NCQA, 2011).

The CMS Innovation Center is evaluating outcomes for medical homes in primary care. In these pilots, clinicians who coordinate care and provide higher-quality care, including care that adheres to guidelines and avoids complications, such as emergency room visits, receive monthly care management fees to help defray the costs of transforming into a PCMH (CMS, 2013d). A number of specialty medical practices are also exploring the use of the PCMH model to improve their quality and coordination of care (NCQA, 2013a). The National Committee for Quality Assurance has developed a recognition program for specialty practices that are successful at achieving the aims of a PCMH (NCQA, 2013b).

One specialty area where clinicians are applying the PCMH model is in cancer care (Fox, 2013; McAneny, 2013; Sprandio, 2010, 2012). The CMS Innovation Center awarded the Community Oncology Medical Homes (COME HOME) project $19.8 million to evaluate a medical home model for Medicare and Medicaid beneficiaries and commercially insured patients with newly diagnosed or relapsed breast, lung, or colorectal cancer (CMS, 2012b). COME HOME includes seven community oncology practices in the United States. These practices will provide comprehensive cancer care in the outpatient setting, including patient education, team-based care, medication management, 24/7 practice access, and inpatient care coordination. COME HOME utilizes Triage Pathways, which provide scripted responses to patients who call with problems about their cancer care. These scripts aim to rapidly send a patient to the right site of service and reduce costly complications and emergency room visits (McAneny, 2013). In addition, the COME HOME project requires clinicians' adherence to care pathways and measures their pathway concordance on a nearly real-time basis.

Similarly, Consultants in Medical Oncology and Hematology (CMOH) became the first oncology practice designated as a level III PCMH by the National Committee for Quality Assurance (Sprandio, 2010, 2012). CMOH reengineered its processes of care and focused on improving coordination and collaboration for all cancer care; streamlining and standardizing the process of patient evaluation; and prioritizing patient engagement and physician accountability (Sprandio, 2010). Like COME HOME, CMOH uses a phone triage system with nurses and symptom management algorithms to address clinical issues. CMOH data suggest that its focus on the medical home model has reduced cancer care costs by reducing emergency room visits by two-thirds, hospital admissions per patient treated with chemotherapy per year by half, and the length of stay for admitted patients by one-fifth (Sprandio, 2012). More research is needed to assess whether the outcomes of the CMOH model are generalizable to other oncology practices.

Care Pathways

The oncology community has also experimented with changes in practice that standardize treatment using evidence-based care pathways. These care pathways "provide an evidence-based algorithm to guide care management for a defined group of patients during a set period of time" (ASCO, 2013). Pathways take into account the evidence base as well as the total cost of care. For example, U.S. Oncology has developed Level I Pathways for 14 common cancers (U.S. Oncology, 2013). Its evaluation of the program found that treating patients according to the Level I Pathways was associated with lower costs and comparable outcomes for patients with non-small-cell lung cancer and colon cancer (Hoverman et al., 2011; Neubauer et al., 2010). NCCN is collaborating with McKesson Specialty Health (the U.S. Oncology Network is a part of McKesson) to develop "Value Pathways," with the goal of creating a single source of information on best practices in cancer care. The pathways and supporting software will initially cover 19 tumor types. These products will provide clinical decision support that is integrated with clinician workflow and compatible with a number of electronic health record systems (Goldberg, 2012; Goldsmith, 2013). Kaiser Permanente has also developed care pathways within its decision support software, including care paths for cancer survivors. This program has reduced the variation in clinical practice, with 90 percent of clinicians adhering to protocols on the first round of cancer treatment (IOM, 2013a).

Coverage with Evidence Development

Many expensive tests and treatments are introduced into clinical practice without evidence of clinical superiority over existing interventions. Once payers agree to cover new interventions, the incentive for manufacturers to conduct additional research on the effectiveness of their product is greatly reduced (Emanuel et al., 2013). Coverage with evidence development (CED) is a policy tool in which payers agree to conditionally cover new medical technologies provided that manufacturers conduct additional research to support more informed coverage decisions (CMTP, 2013a).

CED enables Medicare and other payers to develop more evidence-based coverage policies and fosters the collection of clinical evidence for groups who are often underrepresented in clinical trials, including older beneficiaries and minorities (MedPAC, 2010). The Center for Medical Technology Policy has asserted that the pressures of growing health care costs make CED an "attractive policy mechanism for obtaining the evidence needed for making informed coverage decisions and better understanding of the subgroups and circumstances in which a technology works" (CMTP, 2013b, p. 7).

Legal concerns, however, have hampered CMS' use of CED (MedPAC, 2010). In addition, when CMS launched CED studies in the past, problems with study design, insufficient funding, and inadequate data collection systems impeded the collection of data to inform coverage policies (Tunis et al., 2011). CED has therefore largely been applied on a case-by-case basis (CMTP, 2013b).

CED has previously been used in cancer for fluorodeoxyglucose-positron emission tomography (PET) imaging and identification of bone metastases using PET (sodium-fluoride 18) (CMS, 2013f,g,h). The treatment of localized prostate cancer is an additional area where CED has been suggested (ASTRO, 2013; Emanuel and Pearson, 2012). CED could also be used to incentivize the device industries to participate in evidence generation comparable to the research invested by the pharmaceutical industry in new drugs (Emanuel and Pearson, 2012; IOM, 2013a).

With the goal of improving CED, CMS solicited public comment on the current CED policy and issued a draft guidance policy in 2012 that clarified CMS' authority to use CED (CMS, 2012a; Neumann and Chambers, 2013). The draft guidance also stated that one of AHRQ's roles is to support research that reflects priorities in Medicare, including CED (CMS, 2012a; Daniel et al., 2013).

Value-Based Purchasing and Competitive Bidding Programs

VBP links payments to improved performance by clinicians and holds clinicians accountable for both the cost and the quality of care they provide; "it attempts to reduce inappropriate care and to identify and reward the best-performing [clinicians]" (HealthCare.gov, 2013b). Two VBP programs are relevant to cancer care: hospital VBP and the physician value-based payment modifier. Section 10326 of the ACA requires the Secretary of HHS to initiate VBP for cancer hospitals exempt from the prospective payment system (Albright et al., 2011). In addition, Section 3007 of the ACA mandates CMS to apply a value modifier under the Medicare Physician Fee Schedule (CMS, 2013i). This will adjust physician payments under Medicare Part B based on performance of quality and cost metrics. The first performance assessment period begins in 2013, and the program will begin influencing payment in 2015. The program will be expanded to all physicians by 2017 (VanLare and Conway, 2012; VanLare et al., 2012).

Competitive bidding may also be relevant to cancer care. The ACA requires Medicare to expand competitive bidding for durable medical equipment nationwide (Emanuel et al., 2012). A demonstration project, begun in 2011, found that competitive bidding lowered the prices of oxygen equipment by 41 percent, wheelchairs by 36 percent, hospital beds by 44 percent, and diabetic testing equipment by 72 percent, with no adverse effects on beneficiaries (Emanuel, 2013). A number of health policy leaders have called for this program to be expanded and to include medical devices, laboratory tests, radiologic diagnostic services, and all other commodities (Emanuel et al., 2012).

Designing Insurance Benefits That Promote Affordable Cancer Care

Well-designed insurance benefits could encourage patients to be involved in making cancer care affordable. Some patients may be discouraged from using potentially beneficial treatments because they are responsible for significant levels of cost sharing for their cancer care. For example, the 10 Part D prescription drug plans with the highest enrollment in 2012 had coinsurance rates of 23 to 50 percent (Purvis and Rucker, 2012). For oral cancer drugs approved from 2000 to 2011, the median Part D coinsurance rate was 33 percent, and all of these drugs were included in the plans' highest cost-sharing tiers (Cohen et al., 2013). For physician-administered cancer drugs, there is currently no upper limit for the amount of Medicare Part B cost sharing (MedPAC, 2012), with beneficiaries (or their supplemental insurance plans) responsible for the 20 percent coinsurance. These high coinsurance rates, coupled with the high cost of cancer treatments, can mean that many patients pay several hundreds of dollars per treatment cycle, adding up to thousands of dollars annually (Cohen et al., 2013).

The Medicare Payment Advisory Commission (MedPAC) estimated that 6 percent of Medicare beneficiaries had Part A and B cost-sharing liabilities of more than $5,000 in 2009 (MedPAC, 2012). A study found that of the 10 percent of patients who did not fill their oral cancer treatment prescription, cost sharing was a significant factor in that decision (Streeter et al., 2011). A pilot study of insured cancer patients found that 42 percent of participants reported a significant or catastrophic subjective financial burden from the cost of mediciation, with 20 percent of participants taking less than the prescribed amount of medication, and 24 percent avoiding filling their prescriptions altogether (Zafar et al., 2013).

In contrast, well-insured patients may not be sensitive to the cost of cancer care because they do not bear the full cost of treatment. Thus, they may utilize more care or more expensive care even if it is unlikely to improve their health outcomes. A study commissioned by MedPAC found that individuals with supplemental insurance spent 33 percent more on Medicare compared to individuals without supplemental coverage, after controlling for demographics, income, education, and health status (Hogan, 2009). Almost 90 percent of Medicare beneficiaries have supplemental insurance coverage, either through medigap, employer-sponsored retiree plans, or Medicaid (MedPAC, 2012).

In order to incentivize patients to be more cost conscious in making care decisions, some employers and insurers have created consumer-directed health plans and increased cost-sharing requirements, which place patients at greater risk for the cost of their care. One of the concerns about consumer-directed health plans, however, is that patients have trouble distinguishing between interventions that are likely to be beneficial from those that are wasteful (Bundorf, 2012). Consistent evidence demonstrates that when patients bear more financial risk for their health care, utilization of both necessary and unnecessary health care services declines (IOM, 2009b; Reed et al., 2009; Remler and Greene, 2009; Siu et al., 1986).

Value-based insurance design (VBID) may facilitate patients' ability to be more cost conscious without disincentivizing highly beneficial care. The National Coalition on Health Care suggested that VBID will be a "health system game-changer" (NCHC, 2012). It is intended to encourage patients to choose beneficial treatments and forgo treatments with little or no benefit (Frank et al., 2012). In this design, high-quality cancer interventions would be available at low or no out-of-pocket costs to patients, and interventions that are of questionable benefit to patients would require more cost sharing (IOM, 2009b). For example, palliative care could require little or no cost sharing because, as discussed in Chapter 3, it has been shown to increase survival time for patients, improve symptom management and quality of life, and reduce the cost of cancer care (Morrison et al., 2008; Temel et al., 2010). An important challenge for implementing VBID in cancer is determining which interventions are of the highest quality. This will require both an improved evidence base (see Chapter 5), a learning health care system (see Chapter 6), and expert judgment.

VBID gained national prominence when Pitney Bowes announced $1 million in savings from its VBID program. It lowered patients' cost sharing for asthma and diabetes medications, leading to increased medication compliance and reduced complications for these conditions (Fuhrmans, 2004). Similarly, several evaluations of VBID programs that eliminated generic medicine copays and/or reduced copays for brand-name drugs found that VBID improved patients' medication adherence (Farley et al., 2012; Frank et al., 2012; Maciejewski et al., 2010).

Thus far, VBID has been primarily applied to drug copays, but it may be relevant in other aspects of care. MedPAC recommended that Medicare be given secretarial authority to alter or eliminate patients' cost-sharing requirements for high-quality services and increase cost sharing for ineffective, high-cost services (MedPAC, 2012). In addition, the ACA's call for coverage of preventive services is also a form of VBID (NCHC, 2012). The potential for VBID to improve the quality and affordability of cancer care has not yet been evaluated.

SUMMARY AND RECOMMENDATIONS

The committee's conceptual framework for a cancer care delivery system is one in which all people with cancer have access to high-quality, affordable cancer care. Several IOM reports have called on the U.S. government to ensure that all people have health insurance coverage. Expanding health insurance coverage is a primary goal of the ACA, which is expected to result in 25 million individuals gaining insurance coverage. However, much of the ACA has not yet been implemented and its full impact on access to cancer care is unknown. Many individuals will likely remain uninsured or underinsured. There are also major disparities in cancer outcomes among individuals who are of lower socioeconomic status, are racial or ethnic minorities, or lack insurance coverage. Many of these disparities are exacerbated by these individuals' lack of access to cancer care.

Recommendation 9: Accessible, Affordable Cancer Care

Goal: Reduce disparities in access to cancer care for vulnerable and underserved populations.

To accomplish this, the U.S. Department of Health and Human Services should

- Develop a national strategy that leverages existing efforts by public and private organizations.
- Support the development of innovative programs.
- Identify and disseminate effective community interventions.
- Provide ongoing support to successful existing community interventions.

The affordability of cancer care is equally important as accessibility in a high-quality cancer delivery care system. The committee's conceptual framework (see Figure S-2) illustrates the concept of using quality measurement and new payment models to reward the cancer care team for providing patient-centered, high-quality care and eliminating wasteful interventions. The current fee-for-service reimbursement system encourages a high volume of care, but it fails to reward the provision of high-quality care. This system is leading to higher cancer care costs, which are negatively impacting patients and their families. One survey found that more than one-third of personal bankruptcies in the United States are due to medical problems and that three out of four families studied had insurance at the onset of illness. From a system perspective, health care costs, including the costs of cancer care, are on an unsustainable trajectory and could pose serious fiscal consequences for the United States.

Payers are experimenting with numerous models that could be employed to reward clinicians for providing high-quality cancer care, such as rewarding care that is concordant with clinical practice guidelines; coordinated (based on meaningful patient-clinician communication and shared decision making); and includes palliative care and psychosocial support throughout treatment, advance care planning, and timely hospice services (e.g., bundled payments, ACOs, oncology PCMHs, care pathways, CED, and value-based purchasing and competitive bidding programs). Clinicians are also undertaking efforts to discourage wasteful interventions, such as the Choosing Wisely Campaign.

Recommendation 10: Accessible, Affordable Cancer Care

Goal: Improve the affordability of cancer care by leveraging existing efforts to reform payment and eliminate waste.

To accomplish this:

- **Professional societies should identify and publicly disseminate evidence-based information about cancer care practices that are unnecessary or where the harm may outweigh the benefits.**
- **The Centers for Medicare & Medicaid Services and other payers should develop payment policies that reflect the evidence-based findings of the professional societies.**
- **The Centers for Medicare & Medicaid Services and other payers should design and evaluate new payment models that incentivize the cancer care team to provide care that is based on the best available evidence and aligns with their patients' needs, values, and preferences.**
- **If evaluations of specific payment models demonstrate increased quality and affordability, the Centers for Medicare & Medicaid Services and other payers should rapidly transition from traditional fee-for-service reimbursements to new payment models.**

REFERENCES

Abernethy, A. P., R. R. Coeytaux, K. Carson, D. McCrory, S. Y. Barbour, M. Gradison, R. J. Irvine, and J. L. Wheeler. 2010. *Report on the evidence regarding off-label indications for targeted therapies used in cancer treatment: Technology assessment report.* Rockville, MD: Agency for Healthcare Research and Quality.

ABIM (American Board of Internal Medicine). 2013a. *Choosing wisely.* http://www.abim foundation.org/Initiatives/Choosing-Wisely.aspx (accessed March 28, 2013).

———. 2013b. *Physician charter.* http://www.abimfoundation.org/Professionalism/Physician-Charter.aspx (accessed July 31, 2013).

ACS (American Cancer Society). 2013a. *Find Support Programs and Services in Your Area.* http://www.cancer.org/treatment/supportprogramsservices/index (accessed June 12, 2013).

———. 2013b. *Health Insurance and Financial Assistance for the Cancer Patient.* http://www.cancer.org/treatment/findingandpayingfortreatment/managinginsuranceissues/health insuranceandfinancialassistanceforthecancerpatient/health-insurance-and-financial-assistance-toc (accessed June 12, 2013).

———. 2013c. *National Cancer Information Center.* http://www.cancer.org/aboutus/how wehelpyou/helpingyougetwell/cancer-information-services (accessed June 12, 2013).

AHRQ (Agency for Healthcare Research and Quality). 2010. *Program announcement number: PA-10-168.* http://grants.nih.gov/grants/guide/pa-files/PAR-10-168.html (accessed March 28, 2013).

———. 2011. *Patient centered medical home resource center.* http://pcmh.ahrq.gov/portal/server.pt/community/pcmh__home/1483/what_is_pcmh (accessed March 24, 2013).

———. 2012a. *Bundled payment: Effects on health care spending and quality. Closing the quality Gap: Revisiting the state of the science.* Rockville, MD: AHRQ.

———. 2012b. *2011 National healthcare quality and disparities reports.* http://www.ahrq.gov/research/findings/nhqrdr/nhqrdr11/qrdr11.html (accessed May 15, 2013).

———. 2012c. Disparities report highlights health care challenges for racial and ethnic minorities. http://www.ahrq.gov/news/newsroom/press-releases/2012/qrdr11pr.html (accessed May 15, 2013).

———. 2013. *National healthcare disparities report 2012.* Rockville, MD: U.S. Department of Health and Human Services.

Akscin, J., T. R. Barr, and E. L. Towle. 2007. Key practice indicators in office-based oncology practices: 2007 Report on 2006 Data. *Journal of Oncology Practice* 3(4):200-203.

Albright, H. W., M. Moreno, T. W. Feeley, R. Walters, M. Samuels, A. Pereira, and T. W. Burke. 2011. The implications of the 2010 Patient Protection and Affordable Care Act and the Health Care and Education Reconciliation Act on cancer care delivery. *Cancer* 117(8):1564-1574.

ASCO (American Society of Clinical Oncology). 2012. *Choosing Wisely®: ASCO identifies five key opportunities in oncology toimprove value of patient care.* http://www.asco.org/ASCOv2/Practice+%26+Guidelines/Quality+Care/Access+to+Cancer+Care/Cost+of+Cancer+Care (accessed December 17, 2012).

———. 2013. *ASCO in action brief: Payment reform models explained.* http://ascoaction.asco.org/Home/tabid/41/articleType/ArticleView/articleId/450/ASCO-in-Action-Brief-Payment-Reform-Models-Explained.aspx#.UUYEMmxqNpc.email (accessed March 24, 2013).

ASTRO (American Society for Radiation Oncology). 2013. *ASTRO board of directors approves statement on use of proton beam therapy for prostate cancer.* https://www.astro.org/uploadedFiles/Main_Site/News_and_Media/News_Releases/2013/ASTRO%20Statement%20Proton%20Therapy%20FINAL%20031313.pdf (accessed March 28, 2013).

Bach, P. B. 2007. Costs of cancer care: A view from the centers for Medicare and Medicaid services. *Journal of Clinocal Oncology* 25(2):187-190.

———. 2009. Limits on Medicare's ability to control rising spending on cancer drugs. *New England Journal of Medicine* 360(6):626-633.

Bach, P. B., and M. B. McClellan. 2005. A prescription for a modern Medicare program. *New England Journal of Medicine* 353(26):2733-2735.

Bach, P. B., J. N. Mirkin, and J. J. Luke. 2011. Episode-based payment for cancer care: A proposed pilot for Medicare. *Health Affairs (Millwood)* 30(3):500-509.

Barbash, G. I., and S. A. Glied. 2010. New technology and health care costs: The case of robot-assisted surgery. *New England Journal of Medicine* 363(8):701-704.

BCBS (Blue Cross and Blue Shield). 2012. *Florida Blue and Moffitt Cancer Center create cancer-specific accountable care arrangement.* http://www.bcbs.com/healthcare-news/plans/fl-blue-and-moffitt-cancer-center-create-cancer-specific-aco.html (accessed March 28, 2013).

Bekelman, J. E., G. Suneja, T. Guzzo, C. E. Pollack, K. Armstrong, and A. J. Epstein. 2013. Effect of practice integration between urologists and radiation oncologists on prostate cancer treatment patterns. *Journal of Urology* 10.1016/j.juro.2013.01.103 (epub ahead of print).

Bernard, D. S., S. L. Farr, and Z. Fang. 2011. National estimates of out-of-pocket health care expenditure burdens among nonelderly adults with cancer: 2001 to 2008. *Journal of Clinical Oncology* 29(20):2821-2826.

Biller-Andorno, N., and T. H. Lee. 2013. Ethical physician incentives: From carrots and sticks to shared purpose. *New England Journal of Medicine* 368(11):980-982.

Bolenz, C., S. J. Freedland, B. K. Hollenbeck, Y. Lotan, W. T. Lowrance, J. B. Nelson, J. C. Hu. 2012. Cost of radical prostatectomy for prostate cancer: A systematic review. *European Urology* [epub ahead of print].

Bowman, J., A. Rousseau, D. Silk, and C. Harrison. 2006. Access to cancer drugs in Medi-
    care Part D: Formulary placement and beneficiary cost sharing in 2006. *Health Affairs
    (Millwood)* 25(5):1240-1248.
Brock, D. W. 2010. Ethical and value issues in insurance coverage for cancer treatment.
    Oncologist 15(Suppl 1):36-42.
Brookings Institution. 2013. *Bending the curve: Person-centered health care reform: A framework
    for improving care and slowing health care cost growth.* http://www.brookings.edu/~/
    media/research/files/reports/2013/04/person%20centered%20health%20care%20
    reform/person_centered_health_care_reform.pdf (accessed May 13, 2013).
Bundorf, M. K. 2012. *Consumer-directed health plans: Do they deliver?* Princeton, NJ: Robert
    Wood Johnson Foundation.
CBO (Congressional Budget Office). 2012a. *Estimates for the insurance coverage provisions of the
    Affordable Care Act updated for the recent Supreme Court decision.* http://www.cbo.gov/
    sites/default/files/cbofiles/attachments/43472-07-24-2012-CoverageEstimates.pdf (ac-
    cessed March 22, 2013).
————. 2012b. *Lessons from Medicare's demonstration projects on value-based payment.* http://
    www.cbo.gov/sites/default/files/cbofiles/attachments/WP2012-02_Nelson_
    Medicare_VBP_Demonstrations.pdf (accessed March 24, 2012).
————. 2013. *CBO's estimate of the net budgetary impact of the Affordable Care Act's health
    insurance coverage provisions has not changed much over time.* http://www.cbo.gov/
    publication/44176 (accessed May 15, 2013).
C-Change. 2008. *Increasing access to cancer care: An action guide for comprehensive cancer control
    coalitions.* http://c-changetogether.org/Websites/cchange/images/Publications%20and
    %20Reports/Reports/Access%20to%20Care%20Guidance%20Document%20_final_.pdf
    (accessed March 22, 2013).
————. 2013. *Implementing a National Cancer Health Disparities Strategic Initiative.* http://
    c-changetogether.org/disparities (accessed June 12, 2013).
CDC (Centers for Disease Control and Prevention). 2011a. *Healthy communities: Preventing
    chronic disease by activating grassroots change. At a glance 2011.* http://www.cdc.gov/
    chronicdisease/resources/publications/AAG/healthy_communities.htm#success (ac-
    cessed May 13, 2013).
————. 2011b. *What CDC is doing about health disparities in cancer.* http://www.cdc.gov/
    cancer/healthdisparities/what_cdc_is_doing/index.htm (accessed May 13, 2013).
————. 2012. *Racial and ethnic approaches to community health (REACH).* http://www.cdc.
    gov/reach (accessed May 13, 2013).
CEA (Council of Economic Advisors). 2009. *The economic case for health care reform.* http://
    www.whitehouse.gov/assets/documents/CEA_Health_Care_Report.pdf (accessed
    March 14, 2013).
Chen, A. B., A. Cronin, J. C. Weeks, E. A. Chrischilles, J. Malin, J. A. Hayman, and D.
    Schrag. 2013. Palliative radiation therapy practice in patients with metastatic non–
    small-cell lung cancer: A Cancer Care Outcomes Research and Surveillance Consortium
    (CanCORS) study. *Journal of Clinical Oncology* 31(5):558-564.
Choosing Wisely. 2013. ASTRO releases list of five radiation oncology treatments to ques-
    tion as part of national Choosing Wisely® campaign. http://www.choosingwisely.
    org/astro-releases-list-of-five-radiation-oncology-treatments-to-question-as-part-of-
    national-choosing-wisely-campaign (accessed November 1, 2013).
CMS (Centers for Medicare & Medicaid Services). 2012a. *Draft Guidance for the public, indus-
    try, and CMS staff. Coverage with evidence development in the context of coverage decisions.*
    http://www.cms.gov/medicare-coverage-database/details/medicare-coverage-
    document-details.aspx?MCDId=23 (accessed March 28, 2013).

———. 2012b. *Health care innovation award project profiles.* http://innovation.cms.gov/Files/x/HCIA-Project-Profiles.pdf (accessed March 28, 2013).

———. 2013a. *About the CMS Innovation Center.* http://innovation.cms.gov/about/index.html (accessed March 20, 2013).

———. 2013b. *Accountable care organizations (ACOs): General information.* http://innovation.cms.gov/initiatives/aco/index.html (accessed March 28, 2013).

———. 2013c. *Bundled payments for care improvement initiative: General information.* http://innovation.cms.gov/initiatives/bundled-payments/index.html (accessed March 24, 2013).

———. 2013d. *FQHC Advanced primary care practice demonstration.* http://innovation.cms.gov/initiatives/FQHCs/ (accessed March 24, 2013).

———. 2013e. *Innovations models.* http://innovation.cms.gov/initiatives/index.html (accessed March 20, 2013).

———. 2013f. *(NaF-18) Positron emission tomography to identify bone metastasis of cancer.* http://www.cms.gov/Medicare/Coverage/Coverage-with-Evidence-Development/-NaF-18-Positron-Emission-Tomography-to-Identify-Bone-Metastasis-of-Cancer-.html (accessed March 28, 2013).

———. 2013g. *Positron emission tomography (FDG) for brain, cervical, ovarian, pancreatic, small cell lung, and testicular cancers.* http://www.cms.gov/Medicare/Coverage/Coverage-with-Evidence-Development/Positron-Emission-Tomography-FDG-for-Brain-Cervical-Ovarian-Pancreatic-Small-Cell-Lung-and-Testicular-Cancers.html (accessed March 28, 2013).

———. 2013h. *Positron emission tomography (FDG) for solid tumors.* http://www.cms.gov/Medicare/Coverage/Coverage-with-Evidence-Development/Positron-Emission-Tomography-FDG-for-Solid-Tumors.html (accessed March 28, 2013).

———. 2013i. *Value-based payment modifier.* http://www.cms.gov/Medicare/Medicare-Fee-for-Service-Payment/PhysicianFeedbackProgram/ValueBasedPaymentModifier.html (accessed March 28, 2013).

———. 2013j. *Health Care Innovation Awards round two.* http://innovation.cms.gov/Files/x/HCIA-Two-FOA.pdf (accessed August 8, 2013).

CMTP (Center for Medical Technology Policy). 2013a. *Coverage with evidence development.* http://www.cmtpnet.org/coverage-with-evidence-development (accessed March 28, 2013).

———. 2013b. *Coverage with evidence development: Key issues.* http://www.cmtpnet.org/wp-content/uploads/downloads/2012/03/CED-Key-Issues.pdf (accessed March 28, 2013).

Cohen, J., A. Malins, and Z. Shahpurwala. 2013. Compared to U.S. practice, evidence-based reviews in Europe appear to lead to lower prices for some drugs. *Health Affairs (Millwood)* 32(4):762-770.

Colla, C. H., N. E. Morden, J. S. Skinner, J. R. Hoverman, and E. Meara. 2012. Impact of payment reform on chemotherapy at the end of life. *Journal of Oncology Practice* 8(3 Suppl):e6s-e13s.

Conti, R. M., A. C. Bernstein, V. M. Villaflor, R. L. Schilsky, M. B. Rosenthal, and P. B. Bach. 2013. Prevalence of off-label use and spending in 2010 among patent-protected chemotherapies in a population-based cohort of medical oncologists. *Journal of Clinical Oncology* 31(9):1134-1139.

Conway, L. 2012. *Oncology-specific ACO launches in Florida.* http://www.advisory.com/Research/Oncology-Roundtable/Oncology-Rounds/2012/05/Oncology-specific-ACO-launches-in-Florida (accessed March 28, 2013).

CPCRN (Cancer Prevention and Control Research Network). 2013. *Cancer Prevention and Control Research Network.* http://cpcrn.org/ (accessed May 13, 2013).

Daniel, G. W., E. K. Rubens, M. McClellan. 2013. Coverage with evidence development for Medicare beneficiaries: Challenges and next steps. *JAMA Internal Medicine* doi:10.1001/jamainternmed.2013.6793 (epub ahead of print).

Emanuel, E. 2012. The Arkansas innovation. *New York Times*, September 5. http://opinionator.blogs.nytimes.com/2012/09/05/the-arkansas-innovation (accessed March 24, 2013).

———. 2013. Health care's good news. *New York Times*, February 15, A27.

Emanuel, E., and S. D. Pearson. 2012. It costs more, but is it worth more? *New York Times*, January 2.

Emanuel, E., N. Tanden, S. Altman, S. Armstrong, D. Berwick, F. de Brantes, M. Calsyn, M. Chernew, J. Colmers, D. Cutler, T. Daschle, P. Egerman, B. Kocher, A. Milstein, E. Oshima Lee, J. D. Podesta, U. Reinhardt, M. Rosenthal, J. Sharfstein, S. Shortell, A. Stern, P. R. Orszag, and T. Spiro. 2012. A systemic approach to containing health care spending. *New England Journal of Medicine* 367(10):949-954.

Emanuel, E., A. P. Abernethy, J. E. Bekelman, O. Brawley, R. L. Erwin, P. A. Ganz, J. S. Goodwin, R. J. Green, J. Gruman, J. R. Hoverman, J. Mendelsohn, L. N. Newcomer, J. M. Peppercorn, S. D. Ramsey, L. E. Schnipper, F. M. Schnell, D. Schrag, Y.-C. T. Shih, J. D. Sprandio, T. J. Smith, A. P. Staddon, and J. S. Temel. 2013. A plan to fix cancer care. *New York Times*, SR14.

Etheredge, L. M. 2009. Medicare's future: Cancer care. *Health Affairs (Millwood)* 28(1):148-159.

Farley, J. F., D. Wansink, J. H. Lindquist, J. C. Parker, and M. L. Maciejewski. 2012. Medication adherence changes following value-based insurance design. *American Journal of Managed Care* 18(5):265-274.

Feeley, T. W., H. S. Fly, H. Albright, R. Walters, and T. W. Burke. 2010. A method for defining value in healthcare using cancer care as a model. *Journal of Healthcare Management* 55(6):399-411; discussion 411-392.

Flodgren, G., M. P. Eccles, S. Shepperd, A. Scott, E. Parmelli, and F. R. Beyer. 2011. An overview of reviews evaluating the effectiveness of financial incentives in changing healthcare professional behaviours and patient outcomes. *Cochrane Database of Systematic Reviews*(7):CD009255.

Fox, J. 2013. Lessons from an oncology medical home collaborative. *American Journal of Managed Care* 19(SP1).

Frank, M. B., A. M. Fendrick, Y. He, A. Zbrozek, N. Holtz, S. Leung, and M. E. Chernew. 2012. The effect of a large regional health plan's value-based insurance design program on statin use. *Medical Care* 50(11):934-939.

Fuhrmans. 2004. A radical prescription. *Wall Street Journal*, May 10, R3.

Goldberg, P. 2012. NCCN, McKesson form partnership to build clinical support software. *The Cancer Letter* 38(44):1, 7.

Goldsmith, P. J. 2013. NCCN value pathways: The drive for quality cancer care. *Journal of the National Comprehensive Cancer Network* 11(7):119-120.

Goodwin, J. S., A. Singh, N. Reddy, T. S. Riall, and Y. F. Kuo. 2011. Overuse of screening colonoscopy in the Medicare population. *Archives of Internal Medicine* 171(15):1335-1343.

Goss, E., A. M. Lopez, C. L. Brown, D. S. Wollins, O. W. Brawley, and D. Raghavan. 2009. American Society of Clinical Oncology policy statement: Disparities in cancer care. *Journal of Clinical Oncology* 27(17):2881-2885.

HCFA (Health Care Financing Administration). 1998. *Medicare participating heart bypass center demonstration. Extramural research report.* http://www.cms.gov/Research-Statistics-Data-and-Systems/Statistics-Trends-and-Reports/Reports/downloads/oregon2_1998_3.pdf (accessed March 24, 2013).

HealthCare.gov. 2013a. *Essential health benefits: HHS informational bulletin.* http://www.healthcare.gov/news/factsheets/2011/12/essential-health-benefits12162011a.html (accessed March 28, 2013).

————. 2013b. *Glossary*. http://www.healthcare.gov/glossary/v/vbp.html (accessed March 28, 2013).
HHS (U.S. Department of Health and Human Services). 2010. *HealthyPeople.gov: Disparities*. http://www.healthypeople.gov/2020/about/DisparitiesAbout.aspx (accessed April 21, 2013).
————. 2011. *HHS action plan to reduce racial and ethnic Disparities: A nation free of disparities in health and health care*. Washington, DC: U.S. Department of Health and Human Services.
————. 2013a. *About Healthy People*. http://www.healthypeople.gov/2020/about/default. aspx (accessed April 21, 2013).
————. 2013b. *Million Hearts: The initiative*. http://millionhearts.hhs.gov/aboutmh/overview. html (accessed April 21, 2013).
Himmelstein, D. U., D. Thorne, E. Warren, and S. Woolhandler. 2009. Medical bankruptcy in the United States, 2007: Results of a national study. *American Journal of Medicine* 122(8):741-746.
Hogan, C. 2009. *Exploring the effects of secondary coverage on Medicare spending for the elderly*. Vienna, VA: Direct Research, LLC.
Hoverman, J. R., T. H. Cartwright, D. A. Patt, J. L. Espirito, M. P. Clayton, J. S. Garey, T. J. Kopp, M. Kolodziej, M. A. Neubauer, K. Fitch, B. Pyenson, and R. A. Beveridge. 2011. Pathways, outcomes, and costs in colon cancer: Retrospective evaluations in 2 distinct databases. *American Journal of Managed Care* 17(Suppl 5):SP45-52.
Hussey, P. S., C. Eibner, M. S. Ridgely, and E. A. McGlynn. 2009. Controlling U.S. health care spending: Separating promising from unpromising approaches. *New England Journal of Medicine* 361(22):2109-2111.
IOM (Institute of Medicine). 1993. *Access to health care in America*. Washington, DC: National Academy Press.
————. 1999. *The unequal burden of cancer: An assessment of NIH research and programs for ethnic minorities and the medically underserved*. Washington, DC: National Academy Press.
————. 2001. *Crossing the quality chasm: A new health system for the 21st century*. Washington, DC: National Academy Press.
————. 2003. *Unequal treatment: Confronting racial and ethnic disparities in health care*. Washington, DC: The National Academies Press.
————. 2004. *Insuring America's health: Principles and recommendations*. Washington, DC: The National Academies Press.
————. 2006. *Medicare's quality improvement organization program*. Washington, DC: The National Academies Press.
————. 2009a. *America's uninsured crisis: Consequences for health and health care*. Washington, DC: The National Academies Press.
————. 2009b. *Assessing and improving value in cancer care*. Washington, DC: The National Academies Press.
————. 2009c. *Initial national priorities for comparative effectiveness research*. Washington, DC: The National Academies Press.
————. 2009d. *Value in health care: Accounting for cost, quality, safety, outcomes, and innovation. Workshop summary*. Washington, DC: The National Academies Press.
————. 2011. *Patient-centered cancer treatment planning: Improving the quality of oncology care: Workshop summary*. Washington, DC: National Academies Press.
————. 2012a. *Best care at lower cost: The path to continuously learning health care in America*. Washington, DC: The National Academies Press.
————. 2012b. *How far have we come in reducing health disparities?: Progress since 2000: Workshop summary*. Washington, DC: The National Academies Press.
————. 2012c. *Living well with chronic illness: A call for public health action*. Washington, DC: The National Academies Press.

———. 2013a. *Delivering affordable cancer care in the 21st century: Workshop summary*. Washington, DC: The National Academies Press.

———. 2013b. *Variation in health care spending: Target decision making, not geography*. Washington, DC: The National Academies Press.

IOM and NRC (National Research Council). 1999. *Ensuring quality cancer care*. Washington, DC: National Academy Press.

Jacobson, M., A. J. O'Malley, C. C. Earle, J. Pakes, P. Gaccione, and J. P. Newhouse. 2006. Does reimbursement influence chemotherapy treatment for cancer patients? *Health Affairs (Millwood)* 25(2):437-443.

Jacobson, M., C. C. Earle, M. Price, and J. P. Newhouse. 2010. How Medicare's payment cuts for cancer chemotherapy drugs changed patterns of treatment. *Health Affairs (Millwood)* 29(7):1391-1399.

Jarosek, S., S. Elliott, and B. A. Virnig. 2012. *Proton beam radiotherapy in the U.S. Medicare population: Growth in use between 2006 and 2009*. Rockville, MD: Agency for Healthcare Research and Quality.

Katz, S. J., and M. Morrow. 2013a. Contralateral phophylactic mastectomy for breast cancer: Addressing peace of mind. *Journal of the American Medical Association* (epub ahead of print).

———. 2013b. Addressing overtreatment in breast cancer. *Cancer* (epub ahead of print).

Kenney, G. M., S. Zuckerman, L. Dubay, M. Huntress, V. Lynch, J. Haley, and N. Anderson. 2012. Opting in to the Medicaid expansion under the ACA: Who are the uninsured adults who could gain health insurance coverage? http://www.urban.org/publications/412630.html (accessed July 26, 2013).

KFF (Kaiser Family Foundation). 2013. *Status of state action on the Medicaid expansion decision, as of June 20, 2013*. http://kff.org/medicaid/state-indicator/state-activity-around-expanding-medicaid-under-the-affordable-care-act/# (accessed June 26, 2013).

Koh, H. K., and K. G. Sebelius. 2010. Promoting prevention through the Affordable Care Act. *New England Journal of Medicine* 363(14):1296-1299.

Lee, T. H. 2010. Turning doctors into leaders. *Harvard Business Review* 88(4):50-58.

Maciejewski, M. L., J. F. Farley, J. Parker, and D. Wansink. 2010. Copayment reductions generate greater medication adherence in targeted patients. *Health Affairs (Millwood)* 29(11):2002-2008.

Malin, J. L., J. C. Weeks, A. L. Potosky, M. C. Hornbrook, and N. L. Keating. 2013. Medical oncologists' perceptions of financial incentives in cancer care. *Journal of Clinical Oncology* 31(5):530-535.

McAneny, B. L. 2013. The future of oncology? COME HOME, the oncology medical home. *American Journal of Managed Care* 19(SP1).

McCaskill-Stevens, W., and S. Clauser. 2012. National Cancer Institute Community Oncology Research Program (NCORP). Paper read at National Cancer Advisory Board, November 29, 2012, Bethesda, MD.

MedPAC (Medicare Payment Advisory Commission). 2003. *Report to the Congress: Variation and innovation in Medicare*. http://www.medpac.gov/documents/June03_Entire_Report.pdf (accessed March 18, 2013).

———. 2010. *Report to the Congress: Aligning incentives in Medicare*. http://www.medpac.gov/documents/jun10_entirereport.pdf (accessed March 28, 2013).

———. 2011. *A data book: Health care spending and the Medicare Program*. http://www.medpac.gov/documents/Jun11DataBookEntireReport.pdf (accessed March 18, 2013).

———. 2012. *Report to the Congress: Medicare and the Health Care Delivery System (June 2012)*. http://www.medpac.gov/document_TOC.cfm?id=672 (accessed March 20, 2013).

Mehta, A. J., and R. M. Macklis. 2013. Overview of accountable care organizations for oncology specialists. *Journal of Oncology Practice* 9(4):216-221.

Meropol, N. J., D. Schrag, T. J. Smith, T. M. Mulvey, R. M. Langdon, Jr., D. Blum, P. A. Ubel, and L. E. Schnipper. 2009. American Society of Clinical Oncology guidance statement: The cost of cancer care. *Journal of Clinical Oncology* 27(23):3868-3874.

Morrison, R. S., J. D. Penrod, J. B. Cassel, M. Caust-Ellenbogen, A. Litke, L. Spragens, and D. E. Meier. 2008. Cost savings associated with U.S. hospital palliative care consultation programs. *Archives of Internal Medicine* 168(16):1783-1790.

Moy, B., B. N. Polite, M. T. Halpern, S. K. Stranne, E. P. Winer, D. S. Wollins, and L. A. Newman. 2011. American Society of Clinical Oncology policy statement: Opportunities in the Patient Protection and Affordable Care Act to reduce cancer care disparities. *Journal of Clinical Oncology* 29(28):3816-3824.

Muhlestein, D. 2013. *Continued growth of public and private accountable care organizations.* http://healthaffairs.org/blog/2013/02/19/continued-growth-of-public-and-private-accountable-care-organizations (accessed May 13, 2013).

Nardin, R., L. Zallman, D. McCormick, S. Woolhandler, and D. Himmelstein. 2013. The uninsured after implementation of the Affordable Care Act: A demographic and geographic analysis. http://healthaffairs.org/blog/2013/06/06/the-uninsured-after-implementation-of-the-affordable-care-act-a-demographic-and-geographic-analysis (accessed July 26, 2013).

NCHC (National Coalition on Health Care). 2012. *Curbing costs, improving care: The path to an affordable health care future.* http://www.nchc.org/plan-for-health-and-fiscal-policy (accessed June 18, 2013).

NCI (National Cancer Institute). 2011. Tracking the rise of robotic surgery for prostate cancer. *NCI Cancer Bulletin 8(16).* http://www.cancer.gov/ncicancerbulletin/080911/page4 (accessed March 24, 2013).

———. 2013a. *About CDRP.* http://rrp.cancer.gov/initiatives/cdrp (accessed March 28, 2013).

———. 2013b. *ARRA Research & Training.* http://crchd.cancer.gov/news/ARRA-funding.html (accessed March 28, 2013).

———. 2013c. *The CCOP Network.* http://ccop.cancer.gov (accessed March 28, 2013).

———. 2013d. *Centers for Population Health and Health Disparities. About the initiative (ES-02-009).* http://cancercontrol.cancer.gov/populationhealthcenters/about.html (accessed March 28, 2013).

———. 2013e. *CNP overview.* http://crchd.cancer.gov/cnp/overview.html (accessed March 28, 2013).

———. 2013f. *Comprehensive Partnerships to Reduce Cancer Health Disparities.* http://crchd.cancer.gov/research/cprchd-overview.html (accessed March 28, 2013).

———. 2013g. *Continuing Umbrella of Research Experiences (CURE).* http://crchd.cancer.gov/diversity/cure-overview.html (accessed March 28, 2013).

———. 2013h. *NCI community cancer centers Program.* http://ncccp.cancer.gov (accessed March 28, 2013).

———. 2013i. *Patient Navigation Research Program (PNRP).* http://crchd.cancer.gov/pnp/pnrp-index.html (accessed March 28, 2013).

———. 2013j. *Where can I find cancer statistics by race/ethnicity?* http://surveillance.cancer.gov/statistics/types/race_ethnic.html (accessed July 25, 2013).

NCQA (National Committee for Quality Assurance). 2011. *NCQA patient-centered medical home 2011.* http://www.ncqa.org/Portals/0/PCMH2011%20withCAHPSInsert.pdf (accessed March 28, 2013).

———. 2013a. *Quality profiles: Focus on patient-centered medical homes.* http://www.ncqa.org/PublicationsProducts/OtherProducts/QualityProfiles/FocusonPatientCenteredMedicalHome.aspx (accessed July 29, 2013).

———. 2013b. *Patient-centered specialty practice recognition*. http://www.ncqa.org/Programs/
Recognition/PatientCenteredSpecialtyPracticeRecognition.aspx (accessed July 29, 2013).

Neubauer, M. A., J. R. Hoverman, M. Kolodziej, L. Reisman, S. K. Gruschkus, S. Hoang, A. A.
Alva, M. McArthur, M. Forsyth, T. Rothermel, and R. A. Beveridge. 2010. Cost effectiveness of evidence-based treatment guidelines for the treatment of non-small-cell lung
cancer in the community setting. *Journal of Oncology Practice* 6(1):12-18.

Neumann, P. J., and J. D. Chambers. 2012. Medicare's enduring struggle to define "reasonable and necessary" care. *The New England Journal of Medicine* 367(19):1775-1777.

———. 2013. *Medicare's reset on "coverage with evidence development:"* http://healthaffairs.
org/blog/2013/04/01/medicares-reset-on-coverage-with-evidence-development/?
zbrandid=4337&zidType=CH&zid=16252111&zsubscriberId=1021390268&zbdom=
http://npc.informz.net (accessed May 13, 2013).

Newcomer, L. N. 2012. Changing physician incentives for cancer care to reward better patient
outcomes instead of use of more costly drugs. *Health Affairs (Millwood)* 31(4):780-785.

NIH Record. 2010. *"We have unfinished business." Minority Health Center now an institute*.
http://nihrecord.od.nih.gov/newsletters/2010/10_01_2010/story3.htm (accessed
March 22, 2013).

NPA (National Partnership for Action to End Health Disparities). 2011. *National Stakeholder
Strategy for Achieving Health Equity*. Rockville, MD: U.S. Department of Health & Human Services, Office of Minority Health.

Partnership for Sustainable Health Care. 2013. *Strengthening affordability and quality in America's health care system*. http://rwjf.org/content/dam/farm/reports/reports/2013/
rwjf405432 (accessed April 15, 2013).

Pearson, S. D. 2012. Cost, coverage, and comparative effectiveness research: The critical issues for oncology. *Journal of Clinical Oncology* 30(34):4275-4281.

Perlin, J. B., R. M. Kolodner, and R. H. Roswell. 2004. The Veterans Health Administration:
Quality, value, accountability, and information as transforming strategies for patient-
centered care. *American Journal of Managed Care* 10(part 2):828-836.

Porter, M. E., and E. O. Teisberg. 2006. *Redefining health care: Creating value-based competition
on results*. Boston, MA: Harvard Business School Press.

———. 2007. How physicians can change the future of health care. *Journal of the American
Medical Association* 297(10):1103-1111.

President's Task Force on Environmental Health Risks and Safety Risks to Children. 2012.
Coordinated federal action plan to reduce racial and ethnic asthma disparities. http://www.
epa.gov/childrenstaskforce/federal_asthma_disparities_action_plan.pdf (accessed
April 21, 2013).

Price, C. C., and C. Eibner. 2013. For states that opt out of Medicaid expansion: 3.6 million fewer insured and $8.4 billion less in federal payments. *Health Affairs (Millwood)*
32(6):1030-1036.

Punke, H. 2013. *Specialty ACOs: The next step in accountable care*. http://www.beckers
hospitalreview.com/hospital-physician-relationships/specialty-acos-the-next-step-in-
accountable-care.html (accessed March 28, 2013).

Purvis, L., and N. L. Rucker. 2012. *Open enrollment 2013: Medicare Part D benefits improve
but premiums and cost-sharing rise in many popular plans*. http://www.aarp.org/health/
medicare-insurance/info-11-2012/open-enrollment-2013-medicare-AARP-ppi-health.
html (accessed May 13, 2013).

Ramsey, S., and A. Schickedanz. 2010. How should we define value in cancer care? *Oncologist* 15(Suppl 1):1-4.

Ramsey, S., D. Blough, A. Kirchhoff, K. Kreizenbeck, C. Fedorenko, K. Snell, P. Newcomb,
W. Hollingworth, and K. Overstreet. 2013. Washington State cancer patients found to
be at greater risk for bankruptcy than people without a cancer diagnosis. *Health Affairs
(Millwood)* 32(6):1143-1152.

RAND. 2011. *Payment reform: Analysis of models and performance measurement implications.* Santa Monica, CA: RAND Corporation.

Rawlins, M. 2004. *Scientific and social value judgments.* London, UK: National Institute for Clinical Excellence.

Rawlins, M. D., and A. J. Culyer. 2004. National Institute for Clinical Excellence and its value judgments. *British Medical Journal* 329(7459):224-227.

Reed, M., V. Fung, M. Price, R. Brand, N. Benedetti, S. F. Derose, J. P. Newhouse, and J. Hsu. 2009. High-deductible health insurance plans: Efforts to sharpen a blunt instrument. *Health Affairs (Millwood)* 28(4):1145-1154.

Remler, D. K., and J. Greene. 2009. Cost-sharing: A blunt instrument. *Annual Review of Public Health* 30:293-311.

Report of the National Commission on Physician Payment Reform. 2013. http://physician paymentcommission.org/wp-content/uploads/2013/03/physician_payment_report. pdf (accessed March 28, 2013).

Schnipper, L. E. 2012. The rising cost of cancer care: Physicians take charge. *Journal of Oncology Practice* 8(4):e7e8.

Schnipper, L. E., T. J. Smith, D. Raghavan, D. W. Blayney, P. A. Ganz, T. M. Mulvey, and D. S. Wollins. 2012. American Society of Clinical Oncology identifies five key opportunities to improve care and reduce costs: The top five list for oncology. *Journal of Clinical Oncology* 30(14):1715-1724.

Schnipper, L. E., G. H. Lyman, D. W. Blayney. J. R. Hoverman, D. Raghavan, D. S. Wollins, and R. L. Schilsky. 2013. American Society of Clinical Oncology 2013 top five list in oncology. *Journal of Clinical Oncology* (epub ahead of print).

Schoen, C., S. R. Collins, J. L. Kriss, and M. M. Doty. 2008. How many are underinsured? Trends among U.S. adults, 2003 and 2007. *Health Affairs (Millwood)* 27(4):w298-w309.

Schoen, C., M. M. Doty, R. H. Robertson, and S. R. Collins. 2011. Affordable Care Act reforms could reduce the number of underinsured U.S. adults by 70 percent. *Health Affairs (Millwood)* 30(9):1762-1771.

Shankaran, V., S. Jolly, D. Blough, and S. D. Ramsey. 2012. Risk factors for financial hardship in patients receiving adjuvant chemotherapy for colon cancer: A population-based exploratory analysis. *Journal of Clinical Oncology* 30(14):1608-1614.

Sheets, N. C., G. H. Goldin, A. M. Meyer, Y. Wu, Y. Chang, T. Sturmer, J. A. Holmes, B. B. Reeve, P. A. Godley, W. R. Carpenter, and R. C. Chen. 2012. Intensity-modulated radiation therapy, proton therapy, or conformal radiation therapy and morbidity and disease control in localized prostate cancer. *Journal of the American Medical Association* 307(15):1611-1620.

Shrank, W. 2013. The Center for Medicare and Medicaid Innovation's blueprint for rapid-cycle evaluation of new care and payment models. *Health Affairs (Millwood)* (epub ahead of print).

Siu, A. L., F. A. Sonnenberg, W. G. Manning, G. A. Goldberg, E. S. Bloomfield, J. P. Newhouse, and R. H. Brook. 1986. Inappropriate use of hospitals in a randomized trial of health insurance plans. *New England Journal of Medicine* 315(20):1259-1266.

Smith, G. L., Y. Xu, T. A. Buchholz, B. D. Smith, S. H. Giordano, B. G. Haffty, F. A. Vicini, J. R. White, D. W. Arthur, J. R. Harris, and Y. C. Shih. 2011. Brachytherapy for accelerated partial-breast irradiation: A rapidly emerging technology in breast cancer care. *Journal of Clinical Oncology* 29(2):157-165.

Smith, T. J., and B. E. Hillner. 2011. Bending the cost curve in cancer care. *New England Journal of Medicine* 364(21):2060-2065.

Soares, M. 2005. "Off-label" indications for oncology drug use and drug compendia: History and current status. *Journal of Oncology Practice* 1(3):102-105.

Spinks, T., H. W. Albright, T. W. Feeley, R. Walters, T. W. Burke, T. Aloia, E. Bruera, A. Buzdar, L. Foxhall, D. Hui, B. Summers, A. Rodriguez, R. Dubois, and K. I. Shine. 2012. Ensuring quality cancer care: A follow-up review of the Institute of Medicine's 10 recommendations for improving the quality of cancer care in America. *Cancer* 118(10):2571-2582.

Sprandio, J. D. 2010. Oncology patient-centered medical home and accountable cancer care. *Community Oncology* 7(12):565-572.

———. 2012. Oncology patient-centered medical home *Journal of Oncology Practice* 8(3S): 47s-49s.

Streeter, S. B., L. Schwartzberg, N. Husain, and M. Johnsrud. 2011. Patient and plan characteristics affecting abandonment of oral oncolytic prescriptions. *American Journal of Managed Care* 17(Suppl 5):SP38-S44.

Temel, J. S., J. A. Greer, A. Muzikansky, E. R. Gallagher, S. Admane, V. A. Jackson, C. M. Dahlin, C. D. Blinderman, J. Jacobsen, W. F. Pirl, J. A. Billings, and T. J. Lynch. 2010. Early palliative care for patients with metastatic non-small-cell lung cancer. *New England Journal of Medicine* 363(8):733-742.

Tunis, S. R., R. A. Berenson, S. E. Phurrough, and P. E. Mohr. 2011. *Improving the quality and efficiency of the Medicare program through coverage policy: Timely analysis of immediate health policy issues.* http://www.urban.org/publications/412392.html (accessed May 13, 2013).

U.S. Oncology. 2013. *Level I pathways.* http://www.usoncology.com/cancercareadvocates/AdvancingCancerCare/DeliverHigh-QualityCare/LevelIPathways (accessed June 18, 2013).

VanLare, J. M., and P. H. Conway. 2012. Value-based purchasing: National programs to move from volume to value. *The New England Journal of Medicine* 367(4):292-295.

VanLare, J. M., J. D. Blum, and P. H. Conway. 2012. Linking performance with payment: Implementing the Physician Value-Based Payment Modifier. *Journal of the American Medical Association* 308(20):2089-2090.

Wallerstein, N. B., I. H. Yen, and S. L. Syme. 2011. Integration of social epidemiology and community: Engaged interventions to improve health equity. *American Journal of Public Health* 101(5):822-830.

White House. 2013a. *Executive order—HIV Care Continuum Initiative.* http://www.whitehouse.gov/the-press-office/2013/07/15/executive-order-hiv-care-continuum-initiative (accessed July 30, 2013).

———. 2013b. *Fact sheet: Accelerating improvements in HIV prevention and care in the United States through the HIV Care Continuum Initiative.* http://www.whitehouse.gov/the-press-office/2013/07/15/fact-sheet-accelerating-improvements-hiv-prevention-and-care-united-stat (accessed July 30, 2013).

WHO (World Health Organization). 2013. *Social determinants of health.* http://www.who.int/social_determinants/en (accessed May 13, 2013).

Yeboa, D. R., K. Sunderland, K. Liao, K. Armstrong, and J. Bekelman. 2010. Trends in treatment with intensity modulated (IMRT) vs. 3D conformal (CRT) radiotherapy for non-metastatic prostate cancer. *International Journal of Radiation Oncology, Biology, and Physics* 78(3):s342-s343.

Yu, J. B., P. R. Soulos, J. Herrin, L. D. Cramer, A. L. Potosky, K. B. Roberts, and C. P. Gross. 2013. Proton versus intensity-modulated radiotherapy for prostate cancer: Patterns of care and early toxicity. *Journal of the National Cancer Institute* 105(1):25-32.

Zafar, S. Y., J. M. Peppercorn, D. Schrag, D. H. Taylor, A. M. Goetzinger, X. Zhong, and A. P. Abernethy. 2013. The financial toxicity of cancer treatment: A pilot study assessing out-of-pocket expenses and the insured cancer patient's experience. *Oncologist* 18(4):381-390.

ANNEX 8-1 EXAMPLES OF ONGOING ACTIVITIES DESIGNED TO IMPROVE ACCESS TO CARE FOR VULNERABLE AND UNDERSERVED POPULATIONS

Activity	Description
Department of Health and Human Services (HHS)	
Action Plan to Reduce Racial and Ethnic Health Disparities	The Action Plan outlines goals and actions HHS should take to reduce racial and ethnic health disparities, including promoting integrated approaches, evidence-based programs, and best practices.
National Stakeholder Strategy for Achieving Health Equity	The strategy outlines a comprehensive, community-based approach for achieving health equity. It provides a common set of goals and action steps that local public and private entities and collaborations may adopt to address racial and ethnic disparities within their communities.
Agency for Healthcare Research and Quality (AHRQ)	
National Healthcare Disparities Report	The yearly report tracks national trends in health care disparities. In cancer care, it focuses solely on colorectal and breast cancer in alternating years. The most recent report found that health care quality and access were suboptimal, especially for racial and ethnic minorities and lower income groups. There were disparities with respect to cancer screening, stage of diagnosis, treatment, and death rates among these groups.
Centers for Disease Control and Prevention (CDC)	
Cancer Prevention and Control Research Network (CPCRN)	CPCRN is a network of 10 academic, public health, and community partners that span multiple disciplines and geographic regions, and work together to conduct community-based participatory cancer research. Through implementation and dissemination processes, the network aims to accelerate the adoption of evidence-based cancer prevention and control practices within local communities, focusing on underserved populations disproportionately affected by cancer.
National Comprehensive Cancer Control Program (NCCCP)	NCCCP provides financial and infrastructural support to all 50 states, multiple tribes, and the U.S. Associated Pacific Islands and territories to assist in the development and implementation of comprehensive cancer control plans.

continued

Activity	Description
National Program of Cancer Registries (NPCR)	NPCR compiles data from local cancer registries within each state. CDC uses this data to identify populations with disparities in cancer care. It also assists states in developing and implementing comprehensive cancer control programs designed to alleviate the disparities in these populations.
Racial and Ethnic Approaches to Community Health (REACH)	REACH is a national grant program. It provides financial and infrastructural support to awardees in the identification, development, implementation, evaluation, and dissemination of community-based programs, as well as for culturally tailored interventions that aim to eliminate health disparities among racial and ethnic minority populations. It has prioritized efforts that focus on chronic conditions, including breast and cervical cancer.
National Cancer Institute (NCI)	
Cancer Disparities Research Partnership (CDRP) Program	CDRP was developed by the Radiation Research Program to strengthen the NCI's focus on cancer disparities. The CDRP supports institutions conducting radiation oncology clinical trials focused on medically underserved, low-income, and racial and ethnic minority populations by assisting with the planning, development, and conduct of the trials. The program also assists with the development of partnerships between institutions that are not actively involved in NCI-sponsored research and those that are. These partnerships serve to strengthen cancer disparities research and reduce the cancer disparities burden felt by particular populations.
Center to Reduce Cancer Health Disparities (CRCHD)	The America Recovery and Reinvestment Act of 2009 awarded CRCHD $20 million. It distributed these funds to programs designed to preserve and create jobs, and promote greater scientific impact of research in underserved communities most affected by the recession. In addition, it provided supplemental funds to many of the flagship programs discussed below.
Centers for Population Health and Health Disparities	The Centers fund research assessing the relationship between the environment, behavior, biology, and health outcomes. The Centers uses a community-based participatory research approach to develop a network of research teams to evaluate the multidimensional nature behind health disparities in cancer.

Activity	Description
Community Cancer Centers Program	The NCI has partnered with 21 community hospital-based cancer centers to create this program. Among the partnership's areas of focus are researching ways to reduce health disparities in cancer, increasing participation in clinical trials, improving the quality of cancer care, enhancing cancer survivorship, expanding use of electronic health records, and promoting collection of biospecimens to support genomic research.
Community Networks Program	This program awarded $95 million in 5-year grants to 25 institutions to establish a network of community-based participatory education, training, and research programs among racial and ethnic minorities and other underserved populations.
Comprehensive Partnerships to Reduce Cancer Health Disparities	This program established a network of institutions and NCI Cancer Centers that serve racial, ethnic, and underserved communities. The goal of the program is to train scientists from diverse backgrounds in cancer research and in delivering cancer care to racially and ethnically diverse communities.
Diversity Training Programs	The NCI developed diversity training programs through funding from CRCHD to engage underrepresented investigators in cancer research. The programs provide minorities from high school through the junior investigator level with a continuum of competitive funding opportunities. Programs include, for example, the Continuing Umbrella of Research Experiences and Partnerships to Advance Cancer Health Equity.
Minority-Based Community Clinical Oncology Programs (MB-CCOP)	MB-CCOP is the component of the Community Clinical Oncology Network that is primarily responsible for engaging underserved populations and addressing health disparities in cancer through clinical trials. It has increased access to clinical trials in local communities; recruited many minority participants to clinical trials; and improved researchers' understanding of how new agents, trial designs, and technologies are disseminated and utilized among minority populations.

continued

Activity	Description
National Cancer Institute Community Oncology Research Program (NCORP)	This program includes a research agenda to address cancer disparities. Goals of the research agenda include promoting participation of underserved populations in clinical trials and cancer care delivery research, as well as incorporating specific disparities research questions into clinical trials and cancer care delivery research. It prioritizes research that focuses on the potential drivers of cancer disparities, including health care system factors, health-related quality of life, social determinants, environmental and physical determinants, biological factors, behavioral factors, protective and/or resiliency factors, comorbidities, and biospecimen education and collection.
Patient Navigation Research Program	This program supports the development and evaluation of innovative patient navigation interventions designed to reduce or eliminate health disparities in cancer. Examples of interventions that this program have funded include programs aimed at reducing time between abnormal test results and diagnosis, and improving the quality of cancer care delivery services for cancer patients.
American Cancer Society (ACS)[a]	
Health Insurance Assistance Service	A free resource that connects cancer patients with health insurance specialists who handle inquiries about health insurance coverage and state programs.
National Cancer Information Center	This program provides patients with high-quality information on treatment options, cancer care facilities, community-based programs, clinical trials, and health insurance coverage. Trained oncology nurses answer patients' more complex questions. An interpreter services helps address patients' questions in 160 languages.
Patient Navigator Program	This program hires and trains patient navigators to provide cancer patients and their families with free, one-on-one assistance and support throughout their cancer care, such as helping with the coordination of travel, referring to health care clinicians, providing assistance with psychosocial needs, identifying childcare resources, and recommending sources of financial assistance. Patient navigators are in 122 sites nationwide, with a concentration in public hospitals.

Activity	Description
Transportation Programs	The Road to Recovery Program provides a network of volunteer drivers who provide low-income cancer patients with transportation to and from their treatment. ACS also provides low-income cancer patients with other forms of financial assistance for transportation to and from treatment, including gas cards and tax vouchers.
Hope Lodge and Guest Room Program	Provides cancer patients and their caregivers with a free place to stay or a low cost hotel room when they must travel for treatment. Currently, there are 31 Hope Lodge locations throughout the United States. Accommodations and eligibility requirements vary by location.

American Society of Clinical Oncology (ASCO)[b]

Activity	Description
Disparities Research	ASCO is working with key stakeholders in the cancer community to delineate where future research efforts in cancer disparities should be focused, both in terms of methodology and specific interventions. The resulting work will be developed into a monograph, or series of papers, identifying top research needs, especially in areas of research that have traditionally been underfunded.
Education	ASCO regularly offers educational sessions at its annual meeting designed to help clinicians understand disparities in cancer care. It also offers an expanding array of educational content for providers on ASCO University, as well as resources for patients on Cancer.Net.
Policy and Advocacy	ASCO recently released a policy statement summarizing provisions of the Affordable Care Act that may help alleviate health disparities in cancer care. The statement outlines specific strategies that clinicians can apply to address the barriers to the most vulnerable patient populations accessing high-quality cancer care. In addition, ASCO is developing a policy statement that will make recommendations for ensuring that Medicaid patients have access to high-quality cancer care.
Quality Improvement	ASCO's Quality Oncology Practice Initiative (QOPI) includes a focus on health equity by capturing practice-level information on race/ethnicity, socioeconomic/insurance status, and cultural competency. In addition, ASCO is seeking to assist practices that serve vulnerable and underserved patients with participating in QOPI.

continued

Activity	Description
Workforce Diversity	ASCO has developed and implemented two efforts to diversify the workforce caring for individuals with cancer. The Diversity in Oncology Initiative is an awards program designed to facilitate the recruitment and retention of individuals from populations underrepresented in medicine into careers in oncology. The awards provide individuals the opportunity to participate in an 8- to 10-week clinical or clinical research oncology rotation; pay for individuals to travel to and attend ASCO's Annual Meeting; and repay student loans in exchange for 2 years of service in a medically underserved area. The Diversity Mentoring Program provides physicians who are early in their training and from populations underrepresented in medicine with an oncology mentor. It is designed to encourage these individuals to pursue a career in oncology.
C-Change[c]	
Geographic Intervention Project	C-Change is partnering with local and national organizations to intervene in communities disproportionately affected by four major preventable cancers (breast, cervical, colorectal, and lung). Its first intervention is currently under way in a Mississippi community and will likely involve training lay navigators to guide cancer patients through the cancer care delivery system. The goal of this program is to develop a community-based process of addressing health disparities that is transferable to other communities.
Messaging Project	C-Change worked with a communications firm to develop and test audience-specific messages and associated messaging tools on health disparities in cancer. This project is intended to ensure that C-Change and its membership organizations' communications about health disparities in cancer resonate with the public and policy makers. The overarching goal is to heighten the public's concern about health disparities in cancer care.

[a] Personal communication, Angelina Esparza, American Cancer Society, May 6, 2013.
[b] Personal communication, Dana Wollins, American Society of Clinical Oncology, March 21, 2013.
[c] Personal communication, Tasha Tilghman-Bryant, C-Change, March 21, 2013.
SOURCES: ACS, 2013a,b,c; AHRQ, 2013; C-Change, 2013; CDC, 2011b, 2012; CPCRN, 2013; Goss et al., 2009; HHS, 2011; McCaskill-Stevens and Clauser, 2012; Moy et al., 2011; NCI, 2013a,b,c,d,e,f,g,h,i; NPA, 2011.

Appendix A

Glossary

Access to care—the timely use of personal health services to achieve the best possible health outcomes (IOM, 1993)

Accountable care organization (ACO)—groups of clinicians that voluntarily assume responsibility for the care of a population of patients that share payer savings if they meet quality and cost performance benchmarks (RAND, 2011)

Accreditation—a process whereby a professional association or nongovernmental agency grants recognition to a school or health care institution for demonstrated ability to meet predetermined criteria for established standards (AHRQ, 2012a)

Adjuvant therapy—additional cancer treatment given after primary treatment to lower the risk that the cancer will return. Adjuvant therapy may include chemotherapy, radiation therapy, hormone therapy, targeted therapy, or biological therapy (NCI, 2012)

Advance care planning—making decisions about the care you would want to receive if you happen to become unable to speak for yourself, including consideration of what types of life-sustaining treatments align with your preferences, preparation of an advance directive, and preparation of a durable power of attorney (NHPCO, 2013)

Advance directive—a formal legal document specifically authorized by state laws that allows patients to continue their personal autonomy and that provides instructions for care in case they become incapacitated and cannot make decisions (AHRQ, 2013b)

Advanced cancer—cancer that has spread to other places in the body and usually cannot be cured or controlled with treatment (NCI, 2012)

Ambulatory care—medical care received outside of a hospital setting, such as the use of doctors' offices, home care, outpatient hospital clinics, and daycare facilities (IOM, 2005)

Benefit—a positive or valued outcome of an action or event (IOM, 2011b)

Biomarker—a characteristic that is objectively measured and evaluated as an indicator of normal biologic processes, pathogenic processes, or pharmacologic responses to an intervention (BDWG, 2001)

Bundled payment—a single "bundled" payment, which may be shared by multiple clinicians in multiple care settings, is made for services delivered during an episode of care related to a medical condition or procedure (RAND, 2011)

Cancer—a general term for more than 100 diseases that are characterized by uncontrolled, abnormal growth of cells. Cancer cells can spread locally or through the bloodstream and lymphatic system to other parts of the body (IOM, 2005)

Cancer care continuum—the trajectory from cancer prevention and risk reduction, through screening, diagnosis, treatment, survivorship, and end-of-life care (adapted from NCI, 2013a)

Cancer care team—includes individuals with specialized training in oncology, such as oncologists and oncology nurses, other specialists, and primary care clinicians, as well as family caregivers and direct care workers (see Chapter 4)

Cancer core competencies—the tasks or functions that health care clinicians should be able to perform throughout the cancer care continuum (adapted from Smith and Lichtveld, 2013)

Care coordination—the act of ensuring that care is harmonized across all elements of the broader health care system (adapted from AHRQ, 2013a)

Care plan—information about a patient's diagnosis and prognosis, the planned path of care, and who is responsible for each portion of that care (adapted from IOM, 2011d)

Caregivers—see family caregivers and direct care workers

Chemotherapy—the treatment with drugs that kill cancer cells (NCI, 2012)

Chronic illness—long-term health conditions that threaten well-being and function in an episodic, continuous, or progressive way over many years of life (IOM, 2012)

Clinical decision support—a system that provides clinicians with person-specific information, intelligently filtered or presented at appropriate times, to enhance health and health care (ONC, 2013a)

Clinical practice guidelines (CPGs)—statements that include recommendations intended to optimize patient care that are informed by a systematic review of evidence and an assessment of the benefits and harms of alternative care options (IOM, 2011a)

Clinical trial—a type of research study that tests how well new medical approaches work in people. These studies test new methods of screening, prevention, diagnosis, or treatment of a disease. Also called clinical study (NCI, 2012)

Comorbidity—refers to the co-occurrence of two or more disorders or syndromes (not symptoms) in the same patient (IOM and NRC, 2005)

Comparative effectiveness research (CER)—the generation and synthesis of evidence that compares the benefits and harms of alternative methods to prevent, diagnose, treat, and monitor a clinical condition or to improve the delivery of care. The purpose of CER is to assist consumers, clinicians, purchasers, and policy makers to make informed decisions that will improve health care at both the individual and the population level (IOM, 2009b)

Conflict of interest—a set of circumstances that creates a risk that professional judgment or actions regarding a primary interest will be unduly influenced by a secondary interest (IOM, 2009c)

Cost-effectiveness—a formal method for comparing the benefits of a medical intervention (measured in terms of clinical outcome or utility) with the costs of the medical intervention to determine which alternative provides the maximum aggregate health benefits for a given level of resources, or equivalently, which alternative provides a given level of health benefits at the lowest cost (Sloan, 1996)

Coverage with evidence development (CED)—a policy tool in which payers agree to conditionally cover new medical technologies, provided that manufacturers conduct additional research to support more informed coverage decisions (CMTP, 2013)

Decision aid—a tool that provides patients with evidence-based, objective information on all treatment options for a given condition. Decision aids present the risks and benefits of all options and help patients understand how likely it is that those benefits or harms will affect them. Decision aids can include written materials, Web-based tools, videos, and multimedia programs. Some decision aids are targeted at patients, and others are targeted for clinician use with patients (MedPAC, 2010)

Demonstration project—a project, supported through a grant or a cooperative agreement, generally to establish or demonstrate the feasibility of new methods or new types of services (NCI, 2013c)

Diagnosis—the process of identifying a disease, such as cancer, from its signs and symptoms (NCI, 2012)

Direct care workers—providers of paid hands-on care, supervision, and emotional support for patients. They are typically categorized as nurse aids or nursing assistants, home health aides, and personal and home care aides. They most often provide care in a patient's home, a nursing home, or a hospital (IOM, 2008b)

Electronic health record (EHR)—a real-time, patient-centered record that contains information about a patient's medical history, diagnoses, medications, immunization dates, allergies, radiology images, and lab and test results (ONC, 2013b)

End-of-life care—a term used to describe the support and medical care given during the time surrounding death (NIA and NIH, 2010)

Equity—providing care that does not vary in quality because of personal characteristics such as gender, ethnicity, geographic location, and socio-economic status (IOM, 2001)

Evidence—information on which a decision or guidance is based. Evidence is obtained from a range of sources, including randomized controlled trials, observational studies, and the expert opinions of clinical professionals and/or patients (IOM, 2011b)

Family caregivers—relatives, friends, or neighbors who provide assistance related to an underlying physical or mental disability but are unpaid for those services (IOM, 2008b)

Harm—a hurtful or adverse outcome of an action or event, whether temporary or permanent (IOM, 2011b)

Health care proxy—a document that allows the patient to designate a surrogate, a person who will make treatment decisions for the patient if the patient becomes too incapacitated to make such decisions (AHRQ, 2013b)

Health information technology (IT)—a technical system of computers and software that operates in the context of a larger sociotechnical system; that is, a collection of hardware and software working in concert within an organization that includes people, processes, and technology (IOM, 2011c)

Health literacy—the degree to which individuals have the capacity to obtain, process, and understand basic health information and services needed to make appropriate health care decisions (IOM, 2004)

Hospice care—the most intensive form of palliative care; a service delivery system that provides palliative care for patients who have a limited life expectancy and require comprehensive biomedical, psychosocial, and spiritual support as they enter the terminal stage of an illness or condition. It also supports family members coping with the complex consequences of illness, disability, and aging as death nears. Hospice care further addresses the bereavement needs of the family following the death of the patient (NQF, 2006)

Incidence—the number of new cases of a disease diagnosed over a certain period of time (adapted from NCI, 2013b)

Late effects—side effects of cancer treatment that appear months or years after treatment has ended. Late effects include physical and mental problems and second cancers (NCI, 2012)

Learning health care information technology (IT) system—a health care system that uses advances in information technology to continuously and automatically collect and compile the evidence needed to deliver the best, most up-to-date personalized care for each patient from clinical practice, disease registries, clinical trials, and other information sources. That evidence is made available as rapidly as possible to users of a [learning health care IT system], which include patients, physicians, academic institutions, hospitals, insurers, and public health agencies. A [learning health care IT system] ensures that this data-rich system learns routinely and iteratively by analyzing captured data, generating evidence, and implementing new insights into subsequent care (IOM, 2010 [adapted from Etheredge, 2007])

Metastasis—the spread of cancer from one part of the body to another (NCI, 2012)

Morbidity—a disease or the incidence of disease within a population. Morbidity also refers to adverse effects caused by a treatment (NCI, 2012)

Mortality—the state of being mortal (destined to die). Mortality also refers to the death rate, or the number of deaths in a certain group of people in a certain period of time. Mortality may be reported for people who have a certain disease, live in one area of the country, or who are of a certain gender, age, or ethnic group (NCI, 2012)

Needs—a patient's physical or emotional requirements (adapted from IOM, 2001, 2003)

Observational study—research in which investigators observe the course of events (IOM, 2011b)

Oncology—the study of cancer (IOM and NRC, 2005)

Out-of-pocket cost—expenses for medical care that are not reimbursed by insurance. Out-of-pocket costs include deductibles, coinsurance, and copayments for covered services plus all costs for services that are not covered (HealthCare.gov, 2013b)

Palliative care—patient- and family-centered care that optimizes quality of life by anticipating, preventing, and treating suffering. Palliative care throughout the continuum of illness involves addressing physical, intellectual, emotional, social, and spiritual needs and facilitating patient autonomy, access to information, and choice (NQF, 2006)

Patent—an exclusive right to the benefits of an invention or improvement granted by the U.S. Patent Office, for a specific period of time, on the basis that it is novel (not previously known or described in a publication), "nonobvious" (a form which anyone in the field of expertise could identify), and useful (The Free Dictionary, 2013)

Patient-centered care—providing care that is respectful of and responsive to individual patient, needs, values, and preferences and ensuring that patient values guide all clinical decisions (IOM, 2001)

Patient-centered communication—processes and outcomes of the patient-clinician interaction that elicit, understand, and validate the patient's perspective (e.g., concerns, feelings, expectations); understand the patient within his or her own psychological and social context; reach a shared understanding of the patient's problem and its treatment; help a patient share power by offering him or her meaningful involvement in choices relating to his or her health; build a stronger patient-clinician relationship characterized by mutual trust, respect, and commitment; and enhance the patient's well-being to reduce suffering after the patient leaves the consultation (adapted from Epstein and Street, 2007)

Patient-clinician interactions—the communication, shared decision making, and provision of care that occurs between patients and their care teams (see Chapter 3)

Patient navigation—individualized assistance offered to patients, families, and caregivers to help overcome health care system barriers and facilitate timely access to high-quality medical and psychosocial care from pre-diagnosis through all phases of the cancer experience (C-Change, 2005)

Patient-reported outcome—health data provided by patients, including feedback on their feelings or what they are able to do as they are dealing with chronic diseases or conditions, delivered through a system of reporting (PROMIS, 2012)

Patient safety—freedom from accidental or preventable injuries produced by medical care. Thus, practices or interventions that improve patient safety are those that reduce the occurrence of preventable adverse events (AHRQ, 2012b)

Payment models—methods for reimbursing clinicians. Examples include capitation, fee-for-service, and pay-for-performance (see Chapter 8)

Performance improvement initiatives—systematic, data-guided activities designed to bring about immediate, positive change in the delivery of health care in a particular setting (Baily, 2008)

Preferences—a patient's concerns, expectations, and choices regarding health care, based on a full and accurate understanding of care options (adapted from IOM, 2001, 2003)

Prevalence—the number of existing cases of a disease at one point in time (adapted from NCI, 2013b)

Prognosis—the likely outcome or course of a disease; the chance of recovery or recurrence (NCI, 2012)

Psychosocial health services—psychological and social services and interventions that enable patients, their families, and health care providers to optimize biomedical health care and to manage the psychological/behavioral and social aspects of illness and its consequences so as to promote better health (IOM, 2008a)

Quality measure or metric—quantitative indicators that reflect the degree to which care is consistent with the best available, evidence-based clinical standards (IOM, 2005)

Quality of care—the degree to which health services for individuals and populations increase the likelihood of desired health outcomes and are consistent with current professional knowledge (IOM, 1990)

Quality of life—the overall enjoyment of life. Many clinical trials assess the effects of cancer and its treatment on the quality of life. These studies measure aspects of an individual's sense of well-being and ability to carry out various activities (IOM and NRC, 2005)

Radiation therapy—the use of high-energy radiation from X-rays, gamma rays, neutrons, and other sources to kill cancer cells and shrink tumors.

Radiation may come from a machine outside of the body (external-beam radiation therapy), or it may come from radioactive material placed in the body near cancer cells (internal radiation therapy, implant radiation, or brachytherapy). Systemic radiotherapy uses a radioactive substance, such as a radiolabeled monoclonal antibody, that circulates throughout the body, also called radiation therapy (NCI, 2012)

Randomized clinical trial—a study in which the participants are assigned by chance to separate groups that compare different treatments; neither the researchers nor the participants can choose the group to which they are assigned. Using chance to assign people to groups means that the groups will be similar and the treatments they receive will be compared objectively. At the time of the trial, it is not known which treatment is best. It is the patient's choice to be in a randomized trial (NCI, 2012)

Recurrence—cancer that has recurred (come back), usually after a period of time during which the cancer could not be detected. The cancer may come back to the same place as the original (primary) tumor or to another place in the body (NCI, 2012)

Remission—a decrease in or disappearance of signs and symptoms of cancer. In partial remission, some, but not all, signs and symptoms of cancer have disappeared. In complete remission, all signs and symptoms of cancer have disappeared, although cancer may still be in the body (NCI, 2012)

Shared decision making—the process of negotiation by which physicians and patients arrive at a specific course of action, based on a common understanding of the goals of treatment, the risks and benefits of the chosen treatment versus reasonable alternatives, and the patient's needs, values, and preferences (adapted from IOM, 2011d)

Staging—performing exams and tests to learn the extent of the cancer within the body, especially whether the disease has spread from the original site to other parts of the body. It is important to know the stage of the disease in order to plan the best treatment (NCI, 2012)

Survivor—an individual is considered a cancer survivor from the time of cancer diagnosis through the balance of his or her life, according to the National Coalition for Cancer Survivorship and the NCI Office of Cancer Survivorship. Family members, friends, and caregivers are also impacted by the survivorship experience and are therefore included in this definition (IOM and NRC, 2005)

Survivorship care—a distinct phase of care for cancer survivors that includes four components: (1) prevention and detection of new cancers and recurrent cancer; (2) surveillance for cancer spread, recurrence, or second cancers; (3) intervention for consequences of cancer and its treatment; and (4) coordination between specialists and primary care providers to ensure that all of the survivor's health needs are met (IOM and NRC, 2005)

Survivorship research—encompasses the physical, psychosocial, and economic sequelae of cancer diagnosis and its treatment among both pediatric and adult survivors of cancer. It also includes within its domain issues related to health care delivery, access, and follow-up care as they relate to survivors. Survivorship research focuses on the health and life of a person with a history of cancer beyond the acute diagnosis and treatment phase. It seeks both to prevent and to control adverse cancer diagnosis and treatment-related outcomes, such as late effects of treatment, second cancers, and poor quality of life; to provide a knowledge base regarding optimal follow-up care and surveillance of cancers; and to optimize health after cancer treatment (IOM and NRC, 2005)

Systematic review—a scientific investigation that focuses on a specific question and uses explicit, planned scientific methods to identify, select, assess, and summarize the findings of similar but separate studies. It may or may not include a quantitative synthesis of the results from separate studies (meta-analysis) (IOM, 2011b)

Team-based care—the provision of health services to individuals, families, and/or their communities by at least two health care clinicians who work collaboratively with patients and their caregivers—to the extent preferred by each patient—in order to accomplish shared goals within and across settings to achieve coordinated, high-quality care (Mitchell et al., 2012)

Total cost—the direct medical costs resulting from the provision of cancer care (see Chapter 3)

Toxicity—a measure of the degree to which something is toxic or poisonous (IOM and NRC, 2005)

Value-based insurance design (VBID)—a benefit design that is intended to encourage patients to choose beneficial treatments and forgo treatments with little or no benefit. High-quality cancer interventions would be available at little or no out-of-pocket costs to patients, and interventions that are of questionable benefit to patients would require more cost sharing (IOM, 2009a)

Value-based purchasing (VBP)—links provider payments to improved performance by health care providers. This form of payment holds health care clinicians accountable for both the cost and the quality of care they provide. VBP attempts to reduce inappropriate care and to identify and reward the best-performing providers (HealthCare.gov, 2013a)

Values—a patient's concerns, expectations, and choices regarding health care, based on a full and accurate understanding of care options (adapted from IOM, 2001, 2003)

Vulnerable and underserved—people who may have difficulty accessing high-quality cancer care, including but not limited to racial and ethnic minorities, older adults, individuals living in rural and urban underserved areas, uninsured and underinsured individuals, and populations of lower socioeconomic status (see Chapter 8)

REFERENCES

AHRQ (Agency for Healthcare Research and Quality). 2012a. *National quality measures clearinghouse: Glossary.* http://www.qualitymeasures.ahrq.gov/about/glossary.aspx (accessed May 1, 2012).
———. 2012b. *Patient safety network: Glossary.* http://www.psnet.ahrq.gov/glossary.aspx (accessed March 21, 2012).
———. 2013a. *Coordinated care.* http://pcmh.ahrq.gov/portal/server.pt/community/pcmh__home/1483/pcmh_tools___resources_coordinated_care_v2 (accessed April 22, 2013).
———. 2013b. *Advance care planning, preferences for care at the end of life.* http://www.ahrq.gov/research/findings/factsheets/aging/endliferia/index.html (accessed April 1, 2013).
Baily, M. A. 2008. Harming through protection? *New England Journal of Medicine* 358(8):768-769.
BDWG (Biomarkers Definitions Working Group). 2001. Biomarkers and surrogate endpoints: Preferred definitions and conceptual framework. *Clinical Pharmacology and Therapeutics* 69(3):89-95.
C-Change. 2005. *Cancer patient navigation.* http://www.cancerpatientnavigation.org (accessed May 2, 2012).
CMTP (Center for Medical Technology Policy). 2013. *Coverage with evidence development.* http://www.cmtpnet.org/coverage-with-evidence-development (accessed March 28, 2013).
Epstein, A., and R. Street. 2007. *Patient-centered communication in cancer care: Promoting healing and reducing suffering.* Bethesda, MD: National Cancer Institute.
The Free Dictionary. 2013. *Patent.* http://legal-dictionary.thefreedictionary.com/patent (accessed April 22, 2013).
HealthCare.gov. 2013a. *Glossary.* http://www.healthcare.gov/glossary/v/vbp.html (accessed March 28, 2013).
———. 2013b. *Out-of-pocket costs.* http://www.healthcare.gov/glossary/O/oop-costs.html (accessed April 22, 2013).

IOM (Institute of Medicine). 1990. *Medicare: A strategy for quality assurance.* Vol. 1. Washington, DC: National Academy Press.

———. 1993. *Access to health care in america.* Washington, DC: National Academy Press.

———. 2001. *Crossing the quality chasm: A new health system for the 21st century.* Washington, DC: National Academy Press.

____. 2003. *Unequal treatment: Confronting racial and ethnic disparities in health care.* Washington, DC: The National Academies Press.

———. 2004. *Health literacy: A prescription to end confusion.* Washington, DC: The National Academies Press.

———. 2005. *Assessing the quality of cancer care: An approach to measurement in Georgia.* Washington, DC: The National Academies Press.

———. 2008a. *Cancer care for the whole patient: Meeting psychosocial health needs.* Washington, DC: The National Academies Press.

———. 2008b. *Retooling for an aging america: Building the health care workforce.* Washington, DC: The National Academies Press.

———. 2009a. *Assessing and improving value in cancer care.* Washington, DC: The National Academies Press.

———. 2009b. *Initial national priorities for comparative effectiveness research.* Washington, DC: The National Academies Press.

———. 2009c. *Conflict of interest in medical research, education, and practice.* Washington, DC: The National Academies Press.

———. 2010. *A foundation for evidence-driven practice: A rapid learning system for cancer care: Workshop summary.* Washington, DC: The National Academies Press.

———. 2011a. *Clinical practice guidelines we can trust.* Washington, DC: The National Academies Press.

———. 2011b. *Finding what works in health care: Standards for systematic reviews.* Washington, DC: The National Academies Press.

———. 2011c. *Health IT and patient safety: Building safer systems for better care.* Washington, DC: The National Academies Press.

———. 2011d. *Patient-centered cancer treatment planning: Improving the quality of oncology care: Workshop summary.* Washington, DC: National Academies Press.

———. 2012. *Living well with chronic illness: A call for public health action.* Washington, DC: The National Academies Press.

IOM and NRC (National Research Council). 2005. *From cancer patient to cancer survivor: Lost in transition.* Washington, DC: The National Academies Press.

MedPAC (Medicare Payment Advisory Commission). 2010. *Report to the Congress: Aligning incentives in Medicare.* http://www.medpac.gov/documents/jun10_entirereport.pdf (accessed March 28, 2013).

Mitchell, P., M. Wynia, R. Golden, R. McNellis, S. Okun, C. E. Webb, V. Rohrbach, and I. Von Korhorn. 2012. *Core principles and values of effective team-based health care.* Washington, DC: Institute of Medicine.

NCI (National Cancer Institute). 2012. *National cancer institute: Dictionary of cancer terms.* http://www.cancer.gov/dictionary (accessed May 2, 2012).

———. 2013a. *Cancer control continuum.* http://cancercontrol.cancer.gov/od/continuum.html (accessed April 22, 2013).

———. 2013b. *Cancer health disparities.* http://www.cancer.gov/cancertopics/factsheet/disparities/cancer-health-disparities (accessed April 22, 2013).

———. 2013c. *Extramural glossary.* deais.nci.nih.gov/glossary (accessed April 22, 2013).

NHPCO (National Hospice and Palliative Care Organization). 2013. *Advance care planning.* http://www.nhpco.org/advance-care-planning (accessed April 1, 2013).

NIA (National Institute on Aging) and NIH (National Institutes of Health). 2010. *End of life: Helping with comfort and care.* http://www.nia.nih.gov/health/publication/end-life-helping-comfort-and-care (accessed May 2, 2012).

NQF (National Quality Forum). 2006. *A national framework and preferred practices for palliative and hospice care quality.* http://www.qualityforum.org/Publications/2006/12/A_National_Framework_and_Preferred_Practices_for_Palliative_and_Hospice_Care_Quality.aspx (accessed May 22, 2013).

ONC (Office of the National Coordinator for Health Information Technology). 2013a. Clinical decision support. http://www.healthit.gov/policy-researchers-implementers/clinical-decision-support-cds (accessed February 14, 2013).

———. 2013b. Learn HER basics.

PROMIS (Patient-Reported Outcomes Measurement Information System). 2012. *What patient reported outcomes are.* http://www.nihpromis.org/Patients/PROs (accessed September 18, 2012).

RAND. 2011. *Payment reform: Analysis of models and performance measurement implications.* Santa Monica, CA: RAND Corporation.

Sloan, F. A. 1996. *Valuing health care: Costs, benefits, and effectiveness of pharmaceuticals and other medical technologies.* Edited by F. A. Sloan. New York: Cambridge University Press.

Smith, A. P., and M. Y. Lichtveld. 2013. *A competency-based approach to expanding the cancer care workforce.* http://c-changetogether.org/Websites/cchange/Images/MedSurg%20Journals/2007/MSJApril07_C-Change.pdf (accessed April 22, 2013).

Appendix B

Committee Member and Staff Biographies

COMMITTEE MEMBER BIOGRAPHIES

Patricia A. Ganz, M.D. (*Chair*), a medical oncologist, received her B.A. magna cum laude from Harvard University and her M.D. from the University of California, Los Angeles (UCLA). She completed her training in internal medicine and hematology/oncology at UCLA Medical Center and has been a member of the UCLA School of Medicine faculty since 1978 and the UCLA School of Public Health since 1992. In 1993, she became the director of the Division of Cancer Prevention & Control Research at the Jonsson Comprehensive Cancer Center. She was awarded an American Cancer Society Clinical Research Professorship in 1999 and was elected to the Institute of Medicine (IOM) in 2007. In 2010, she received the American Cancer Society Medal of Honor. She served on the National Cancer Institute (NCI) Board of Scientific Advisors from 2002-2007 and on the American Society of Clinical Oncology (ASCO) Board of Directors from 2003-2006. She was a founding member of the National Coalition for Cancer Survivorship (NCCS) in 1986, and has directed the UCLA-LIVE**STRONG** Survivorship Center of Excellence at the Jonsson Comprehensive Cancer Center since 2006. Dr. Ganz's current research is focused on two major areas: understanding the biological mechanisms of late effects of cancer treatment (e.g., fatigue, cognitive disturbance), and developing interventions to mitigate these effects. Since serving on the IOM committee study on adult cancer survivors (From Cancer Patient to Cancer Survivor: Lost in Transition, 2006), she has led a national effort to improve the post-treatment quality and coordination of care for cancer patients and survivors. In addition, she served on the IOM committee study focused on the psychosocial needs of cancer survivors (Cancer Care for the Whole Patient: Meeting Psychosocial Health Needs, 2008). Dr. Ganz has been a member of the IOM National Cancer Policy Forum (NCPF) since 2005, and currently serves as its vice chair. She has conducted much of her recent policy work through her participation in NCPF workshops on, for example, the Rapid Learning Health System, Cancer Genetics, Obesity in Cancer Survivors, Cancer in the Elderly, and others.

Harvey Jay Cohen, M.D., currently serves in several professional roles at Duke University Medical Center in Durham, North Carolina, including Walter Kempner professor; director, Center for the Study of Aging and Human Development; chair emeritus, Department of Medicine; and principal investigator of the Duke Claude Pepper Older Americans Independence Center, and of the Partnership for Anemia: Clinical and Translational Trials in the Elderly. He received his medical degree, cum laude, from Downstate Medical College of the State University of New York. He served his internship in medicine at Duke University Medical Center, where he was later a resident and fellow in hematology-oncology. He was also a staff associate for the National Institutes of Health (NIH), National Institute of Arthritis and Metabolic Diseases. Dr. Cohen chairs the Cancer in the Elderly Committee for Alliance for Clinical Trials in Oncology, and co-chaired the Task Force on Cancer and Aging for the American Association for Cancer Research. He is a past president of the American Geriatrics Society, the Gerontologic Society of America, and the International Society of Geriatric Oncology. He is also a member of the International Association of Gerontology Governing Board and the Board of the American Federation for Aging Research. Dr. Cohen is on the editorial board of *Journal of Gerontology: Medical Sciences* and of *Clinical Geriatrics*. He is also on the international editorial board of *Geriatrics & Gerontology International*. He has published extensively, with more than 300 peer-reviewed papers as well as book chapters on topics in geriatrics and hematology/oncology, including special emphasis on aspects of cancer and immunologic disorders in the elderly and geriatric assessment. His current interests are geriatric assessment, biologic basis of functional decline, and cancer and hematologic problems in the elderly. He is author of the book *Taking Care After 50*, and co-editor of *The Link Between Religion and Health: Psychoneuroimmunology and the Faith Factor; Geriatric Medicine*, 4th Edition; and *Practical Geriatric Oncology*. Dr. Cohen is listed in Who's Who in America, Who's Who Among American Teachers, Who's Who in Frontiers of Science and Technology, Who's Who in Science, International Who's Who in Medicine, and American Men and Women of Science and Biography International. He has received the Joseph T. Freeman Award and the Kent Award from the Gerontological Society of America, the Jahnigen Memorial Award from the American Geriatrics Society, the B.J. Kennedy Award from the American Society of Clinical Oncology, the Paul Calabresi Award from the International Society of Geriatric Oncology, and the Clinically Based Research Mentoring Award from Duke University. Dr. Cohen has been named one of the "Best Doctors" in the United States continuously since 1992 and has been awarded grants from the John A. Hartford Foundation for the Center of Excellence, the Academic Geriatrics Recruitment Initiative, the National Institute on Aging, and the Donald W. Reynolds Foundation.

Timothy J. Eberlein, M.D., is the Bixby Professor of Surgery and Professor of Pathology and Immunology at the Washington University School of Medicine in St. Louis. He is also the chairman of the Department of Surgery and the surgeon-in-chief at Barnes-Jewish Hospital. Dr. Eberlein serves as the Olin distinguished professor and director of the Siteman Cancer Center at Barnes-Jewish Hospital and Washington University Medical Center. Siteman Cancer Center is now an NCI Comprehensive Cancer Center and a member of the National Comprehensive Cancer Network (NCCN). It is one of the largest clinical cancer centers in the United States and its integrated research programs involve all school of medicine departments, as well as the schools of engineering, social work, and arts and sciences. Prior to moving to St. Louis, Dr. Eberlein served as the Richard E. Wilson professor of surgery at Harvard Medical School in Boston, chief of the Division of Surgical Oncology and vice chairman for research in the Department of Surgery at Brigham and Women's Hospital. Dr. Eberlein has been very active in the work of the NCI, having served on the Board of Scientific Counselors and having been a chairperson for a NIH Study Section. He is a past board member of the American Association of Cancer Institutes and is currently vice chair of the board of directors of the NCCN. In 2004, Dr. Eberlein was elected a member of the IOM. He received the John Wayne Clinical Research Award from the Society of Surgical Oncology in 1999 and the Sheen Award in 2006 for outstanding contributions to the medical profession. He has served as president of the Society of Surgical Chairs, the Society of Surgical Oncology, and the American Surgical Association. Recently he was named president of the Southern Surgical Association. Dr. Eberlein serves on a number of editorial boards of peer-reviewed journals and is currently the editor in chief of the *Journal of the American College of Surgeons* and associate editor of *Annals of Surgical Oncology*.

Thomas W. Feeley, M.D., is a senior faculty member at The University of Texas MD Anderson Cancer Center and is the Helen Shafer Fly Distinguished Professor of Anesthesiology. Dr. Feeley is the head of the Institute for Cancer Care Innovation and the Division of Anesthesiology and Critical Care. He came to MD Anderson in 1997, following 19 years on the anesthesiology faculty at Stanford University, to create a new division devoted to anesthesiology, critical care, and pain management for cancer patients. Since 2008, he has led the development of the MD Anderson Cancer Center's Institute for Cancer Care Innovation. The institute is designed to study the value of MD Anderson's cancer care delivery system using the framework created by the 10 recommendations of 1999 IOM report *Ensuring Quality Cancer Care* and Harvard Business School Professor Michael Porter's principles of value-based health care. In June 2009, he presented a proposal to the NCPF to reexamine the volume outcome recommendation of the 1999 report; however, the forum had a number of projects under way at the time. With his colleagues, he went on to perform an analysis of the current state of quality of cancer care in the United States as a follow-up to the 1999 IOM report and *Cancer* published the findings in a November 2011 paper titled "Ensuring Quality Cancer Care: A Follow-Up Review of the Institute of Medicine's 10 Recommendations for Improving the Quality of Cancer Care in America." He also presented MD Anderson's work on value in cancer care using Porter's value-based health care model at the IOM regional meeting in Houston in April 2010. He published a summary from that presentation in the *Journal of Healthcare Management* and that paper, titled "A Method for Defining Value in Healthcare Using Cancer Care as a Model," earned the 2012 Edgar C. Hayhow Article of the Year Award from the American College of Healthcare Executives. Dr. Feeley's team at MD Anderson has also published work on cancer quality metrics, the effect of the Affordable Care Act on cancer care delivery, and the use of medical records by cancer patients, and it has contributed to a major article in the *Harvard Business Review* on the measurement of cancer care delivery costs. Dr. Feeley's Division of Anesthesiology and Critical Care is one of the world's largest programs of its kind delivering anesthesia, critical care, and pain management services to cancer patients in conjunction with a major basic and clinical research program. Dr. Feeley also provides anesthesia care to cancer patients undergoing surgery at MD Anderson.

Betty R. Ferrell, RN, Ph.D., M.A., FAAN, FPCN, has been in oncology nursing for 35 years and has focused her clinical expertise and research on pain management, quality of life, and palliative care. Dr. Ferrell is a professor and research scientist at the City of Hope Medical Center in Los Angeles. She is a fellow of the American Academy of Nursing, and she has contributed to more than 350 publications in peer-reviewed journals and texts. She is principal investigator of a project funded by the NCI on "Palliative Care for Quality of Life and Symptom Concerns in Lung Cancer" and of the "End-of-Life Nursing Education Consortium" project. She directs several other projects related to palliative care in cancer centers and quality-of-life issues. Dr. Ferrell is a member of the NCI's Board of Scientific Advisors and was chairperson of the National Consensus Project for Quality Palliative Care. She served on the National Quality Forum (NQF) Committee for Preferred Practices in palliative care. She is also the chairperson of the Southern California Cancer Pain Initiative. She has authored nine books, including *Cancer Pain Management* (1995), *Pain in the Elderly* (1996), and the *Oxford Textbook of Palliative Nursing* (3rd edition, Oxford University Press, 2010). She co-authored the text *The Nature of Suffering and the Goals of Nursing* (Oxford University Press, 2008) and *Making Health Care Whole: Integrating Spirituality into Patient Care* (Templeton Press, 2010). Dr. Ferrell completed a master's degree in theology, ethics, and culture from Claremont Graduate University in 2007.

James A. Hayman, M.D., M.B.A., received his M.D. and M.B.A. degrees simultaneously from the University of Chicago in 1991. Following a 1-year internship at Evanston Hospital in Evanston, Illinois, he moved to Boston, Massachusetts, and completed his radiation oncology residency at the Joint Center for Radiation Therapy, Harvard Medical School. Since joining the faculty in the Department of Radiation Oncology at the University of Michigan in 1996, he has achieved the rank of professor and is also associate chair for clinical activities at the university hospital. His clinical and research interests include the management of thoracic and breast cancers, as well as skin, ocular, and central nervous system malignancies. He is among the few radiation oncologists in the United States who has been active in the field of health services research and who is board certified in hospice and palliative medicine. He has served on numerous local and national committees related to quality of care. Dr. Hayman is the chair of the American Society for Radiation Oncology's Clinical Affairs and Quality Committee and is a long-serving member of ASCO's Quality of Care Committee. He has also been involved with projects related to quality of care coordinated by NQF, the American Medical Association (AMA) Physician Consortium for Performance Improvement, the Cancer Quality Alliance, and the NCCN. He is helping to lead a new statewide collaborative quality initiative supported by Blue Cross Blue Shield of Michigan, the Michigan Radiation Oncology Quality Consortium.

Katie B. Horton, J.D., M.P.H., is a research professor at the George Washington University (GWU) School of Public Health and Health Services, Department of Health Policy. Professor Horton has more than 20 years of public policy experience. Currently, she conducts research in a variety of issue areas related to the implementation of the new health reform law, including the public health and prevention provisions, delivery system reforms, quality improvement initiatives, and the health insurance exchange system. Much of Professor Horton's research involves issues specific to individuals with chronic illness. Prior to joining GWU, Professor Horton was president of Health Policy R&D, a health policy firm in Washington, DC, and she served as senior professional health staff specializing in Medicare financing issues for the U.S. Senate Committee on Finance. She was an advisor to Senator Daniel Patrick Moynihan (D-NY) and other Democratic senators and their staffs on federal health insurance issues and drafted a variety of legislative proposals involving improvements to Medicare and patient protections in the private health insurance market. Prior to her work with the Senate Committee on Finance, Ms. Horton served as the legislative director for Congressman Pete Stark (D-CA), during which she was responsible for the representative's legislative agenda regarding Medicare, Medicaid, welfare reform, and social security issues. As a nurse, Ms. Horton also served as director of clinical services for Operation Smile, an organization providing health services to indigent children in developing countries.

Arti Hurria, M.D., is a geriatrician and oncologist, focusing on care of the older patient with cancer. She completed a geriatric fellowship in the Harvard Geriatric Fellowship Program, followed by a hematology-oncology fellowship at Memorial Sloan-Kettering Cancer Center (MSKCC). She subsequently joined the faculty at MSKCC, where she served as co–principal investigator on the institutional NIH P20 grant "Development of an Aging and Cancer Center at MSKCC." In the fall of 2006, Dr. Hurria joined the City of Hope as director of the Cancer and Aging Research Program. Dr. Hurria is a recipient of the Paul Beeson Career Development Award in Aging Research (K23 AG026749-01) and American Society of Clinical Oncology–Association of Specialty Professors' Junior Development Award in Geriatric Oncology. She is chair of the NCCN Senior Adult Oncology Panel, editor in chief of the *Journal of Geriatric Oncology*, vice co-chair of the Alliance Cancer in the Elderly Committee, and president of the International Society of Geriatric Oncology. Dr. Hurria serves as principal investigator on a U13 grant in collaboration with the National Institute on Aging and the NCI to identify and develop research methodology that will lead to evidence-based recommendations for improved clinical care for older adults with cancer. She also serves as principal investigator on an R01-funded grant evaluating clinical and biological predictors of chemotherapy toxicity in older adults with breast cancer. These grants are executed in collaboration with members from the Cancer and Aging Research Group, which Dr. Hurria founded and leads.

Mary S. McCabe, RN, M.A., is director of the Cancer Survivorship Program at MSKCC. Since 2003, she has been responsible for developing and implementing a center-wide program for cancer survivors focused on research, clinical care, professional training, and education. She is also a faculty member in the Division of Medical Ethics at the Cornell Weill Medical College, and chair of the MSKCC Ethics Committee. A graduate of Trinity College, Emory University, and Catholic University, she was previously the nursing director at the Lombardi Cancer Center, Georgetown University, in Washington, DC. She held several positions at the NCI before joining MSKCC, including assistant director of the Division of Cancer Treatment and Diagnosis, director of the Office of Clinical Research, and faculty in the Department of Bioethics at NIH. Ms. McCabe serves on many committees, including the Committee on Improving the Quality of Cancer Care at the IOM, the Survivorship Steering Committee of the American Cancer Society, the National Comprehensive Cancer Network Survivorship Panel, the Scientific Advisory Board of the LIVE**STRONG** Foundation, and the NCI Clinical Trials and Translational Research Advisory Committee. Ms. McCabe is chair of the ASCO Survivorship Committee. She is a member of the Oncology Nursing Society, ASCO, and the American Society for Bioethics and Humanities. Ms. McCabe has published many peer-reviewed articles, serves on the editorial boards for *Seminars in Oncology Nursing*, *Oncology*, and *Oncology for Nurses*, and writes a column on cancer survivorship for the *ASCO Post*. She has received numerous awards, including the American Cancer Society Merit Award, Oncology Nursing Society Leadership Award, NIH Outstanding Performance Award, NIH Director's Award, and Emory University's Outstanding Alumnae Award.

Mary D. Naylor, Ph.D., RN, FAAN, is the Marian S. Ware Professor in Gerontology and director of the New Courtland Center for Transitions and Health at the University of Pennsylvania, School of Nursing. Since 1989, Dr. Naylor has led an interdisciplinary program of research designed to improve the quality of care, decrease unnecessary hospitalizations, and reduce health care costs for vulnerable community-based older adults and their family caregivers. In the 1990s, Dr. Naylor co-led the establishment of a program of all-inclusive care at Penn's School of Nursing called Living Independently for Elders. Dr. Naylor is the national program director for the Interdisciplinary Nursing Quality Research Initiative (INQRI), sponsored by the Robert Wood Johnson Foundation. The primary goal of INQRI is to generate, disseminate, and translate research that demonstrates nursing's contribution to the quality of patient care. In recognition of her research and leadership, Dr. Naylor has received numerous awards. She was elected to the IOM in 2005. She is also a member of the RAND Health Board, the NQF board of directors, and the founding board chair of the Long-Term Quality Alliance. She was appointed to the Medicare Payment Advisory Commission in 2010.

Larissa Nekhlyudov, M.D., M.P.H., is currently associate professor and director of cancer research at Harvard Medical School's Department of Population Medicine. She is also a practicing general internist at Harvard Vanguard Medical Associates in Boston, Massachusetts. Dr. Nekhlyudov has published numerous original manuscripts in leading cancer and general medicine journals on topics related to cancer treatment and outcomes, specifically focusing on quality of life, surveillance for recurrences, adherence, communication, and coordination of care. She has also co-authored book chapters focusing on cancer screening, detection, and survivorship. Dr. Nekhlyudov is particularly interested in improving the care of cancer survivors and the interplay between primary and oncology care, and has extensive clinical and research expertise in this area. She served as guest editor of a supplement to the *Journal of General Internal Medicine* on cancer survivorship care for the general internist and has both led and participated in numerous educational programs in cancer survivorship. Dr. Nekhlyudov currently serves as the director of the NCI-funded Community Practice Research Core at the Dana-Farber/Harvard Cancer Center. She is an active member of the Society of General Internal Medicine and the American Society of Clinical Oncology. She serves on the Advisory Board at the Massachusetts Cancer Registry. Dr. Nekhlyudov received her M.D. at the Mount Sinai School of Medicine, and then pursued her residency training at the Yale-New Haven Hospital and the Yale Primary Care Residency programs. She was chief resident at the Hospital of Saint Raphael, affiliated with the Yale School of Medicine. Following her training, Dr. Nekhlyudov was a fellow in the Harvard Medical School Fellowship Program in general medicine and received an M.P.H. at the Harvard School of Public Health.

Michael N. Neuss, M.D., is the chief medical officer of the Vanderbilt-Ingram Cancer Center and professor of clinical medicine in the Vanderbilt University Medical Center. After receiving training at Duke University, leading to board certification in internal medicine and medical oncology, he was in private practice in Cincinnati from 1986 through 2011. As the first medical oncologist at Oncology Hematology Care, he has been the vice president of the Oncology Hematology Care Group from 1986 to 2011, a time during which the group expanded from 2 to 48 doctors. Since arriving at Vanderbilt in July 2011, he has served as chair of the American Society of Clinical Oncology Clinical Practice Committee, is current chair of the Quality Oncology Practice Initiative Steering Group, and is on the

AMA Innovators' Committee, which is examining care delivery and payment reform models.

Noma L. Roberson, Ph.D., is a retired cancer research scientist with expertise in cancer control, epidemiology, and health services research. Currently, she is president and owner of Roberson Consulting International, a health research consulting firm. She is also the owner of Noma's Fine Apparel, an upscale women's dress shop located in Amherst, New York. Dr. Roberson received her graduate degree in experiential pathology and epidemiology from the State University of New York at Buffalo School of Medicine and Biomedical Sciences. She is author of three books and numerous articles. During her 29-year tenure at Roswell Park Cancer Institute in Buffalo, New York, Dr. Roberson served as the director of community intervention and research. In addition to her research, Dr. Roberson is credited for the development of several training curricula and health promotional materials for the early detection of breast and lung cancer. Dr. Roberson is also credited for the design and operation of a 34-foot mobile van that provided health education and screening services throughout western New York. With more than 40 years of experience as a health care professional, Dr. Roberson's research has carried her across the United States as well as to several international locations, including Budapest, Hungary; Rio de Janeiro, Brazil; New Delhi, India; Toronto, Canada; and Jamaica, West Indies. Dr. Roberson currently serves on the NIH/NCI Scientific Review Board/Special Emphasis Panel, the National Surgical Adjuvant Breast and Bowel Project Diversity Strategic Planning Group and Behavioral and Health Outcomes Committee, the American Cancer Society Eastern Division Board of Advisors, the National Federation for Just Communities board of directors, and the Faith-Based Health Initiative of Buffalo Committee. Throughout her career, she has served on numerous boards and committees and is the recipient of more than 40 awards and certificates for her contributions to research and the community. As the wife of businessman and contractor Willie Roberson, Dr. Roberson served as the president of the National PHC Contractors Auxiliary, where she oversaw 6 U.S. zones and 13 national committees.

Ya-Chen Tina Shih, Ph.D., is associate professor of health economics in the Section of Hospital Medicine, Department of Medicine, at the University of Chicago's Pritzker School of Medicine. Dr. Shih is also the director of the Economics of Cancer Program, affiliated faculty at the Center for Health and the Social Sciences at the University of Chicago, and member of the University of Chicago Comprehensive Cancer Center. Prior to joining the University of Chicago in March 2011, she was associate professor at the Section of Health Services Research, Department of Biostatistics, at the University of Texas MD Anderson Cancer Center. Prior to that, she was assistant professor at the Division of Pharmaceutical Policy and Evaluative Sciences, School of Pharmacy, University of North Carolina, Chapel Hill. Born in Taipei, Taiwan, Dr. Shih came to the United States in 1990 for graduate study. She received her Ph.D. in economics from Stanford University, with a concentration on labor/health economics and econometrics. She has served as principal investigator on research grants related to various economic aspects of cancer funded by the NCI, National Human Genome Research Institute, Agency for Healthcare and Quality, American Cancer Society, Lance Armstrong Foundation, and Robert Wood Johnson Foundation. Dr. Shih has more than 15 years of experience with economic evaluation, health services, and comparative effectiveness research, using both modeling approaches and econometric techniques applied to observational and trial data. Major themes in her work include studying the diffusion of new medical technologies among various patients/provider subgroups and/or geographic areas; examining the impact of new technologies on the outcomes and costs of cancer care; and exploring the effect, especially the unintended consequences, of technology diffusion, health policies, and regulations on cancer patients. Her other research interests are assessing the cost-effectiveness of medical and behavioral interventions. Dr. Shih is co-editor of *Value in Health*, and is on the editorial board of *PharmacoEconomics*. She has been a member of the NCPF at the IOM since 2011 and serves on the American Cancer Society Guidelines Development Panel.

George W. Sledge, Jr., M.D., is the oncology chief at Stanford University School of Medicine, where he is currently a professor of medicine. He specializes in the study and treatment of breast cancer and directed the first nationwide study on the use of paclitaxel to treat advanced breast cancer. His recent research focuses on novel biologic treatments for breast cancer. He has published more than 250 articles in medical journals about breast cancer and has chaired several national clinical trials involving new breast cancer treatments. He conducts both laboratory and clinical work. Dr. Sledge serves as editor in chief of *Clinical Breast Cancer* and was past president of the American Society of Clinical Oncology. He served as chairman of the Breast Cancer Committee of the Eastern Cooperative Oncology Group from 2002 to 2009, where he played an important role in the development of several nationwide clinical trials. He has also been chair of ASCO's Education Committee, a member of the Department of Defense's Breast Cancer Research Program's Integration Panel, and a member of the Food and Drug Administration's Oncology Drug Advisory Committee. He is currently a member of the External Advisory Committee for The Cancer Genome Atlas Project. Dr. Sledge was the recipient of the 2006 Komen Foundation Brinker Award for Scientific Distinction, the 2007 Breast Cancer Research Foundation's Jill Rose Award, and the 2010 William L. McGuire Award from the San Antonio Breast Cancer Symposium.

Thomas J. Smith, M.D., is a medical oncologist and palliative care specialist with a lifelong interest in better symptom management, open and accurate communication, and improving access to high-quality affordable care. He is now the director of palliative medicine for Johns Hopkins Medicine, charged with integrating palliative care into all the Johns Hopkins venues. Johns Hopkins has opened a hospital-wide PC consult service that will see more than 1,000 patients each year, an inpatient unit as of March 1, and has a growing research agenda. Dr. Smith has a long track record of starting innovative programs while their impact on care and costs are being evaluated concurrently; examples of those programs include the Rural Cancer Outreach Program, the Thomas Palliative Care Program, the Virginia Initiative on Palliative Care, and the Rural Palliative Care Program. The palliative medicine group at Johns Hopkins was the first to show improved care with substantial cost savings from coordinated rural-urban care, inpatient palliative care, and rural palliative care. He has been influential within the oncology community, working to improve care at a cost society can afford, maintaining his credentials as a treating oncologist while integrating palliative care. Dr. Smith received the national Humanism in Medicine Award in 2000, and in 2000 and 2006 he was voted the Distinguished Clinician on the Virginia Commonwealth University's School of Medicine faculty. He has been recognized in "Best Doctors in America" for many years. In June 2008, he received the ASCO "Statesman" award for continued service to oncology, and is now a fellow with the American Society of Clinical Oncology and the American Academy of Hospice and Palliative Medicine. In 2012, Dr. Smith and Bruce Hillner received the ABIM "Professionalism" Prize for their *New England Journal of Medicine* article "Bending the Cost Curve in Cancer Care" and leading the "Choosing Wisely" initiatives. He serves as an attending physician on the Longcope Service of the Osler Medical Housestaff training program as well as in palliative care.

Neil S. Wenger, M.D., M.P.H., is a professor in the Division of General Internal Medicine and Health Services Research at UCLA, and a practicing general internist with an interest in patients with complex illness. He also directs the UCLA Health System Ethics Center. At RAND, he is a senior scientist and directs the Assessing Care of Vulnerable Elders project. Dr. Wenger's research focuses on measuring and improving the quality of care for vulnerable older persons. He has led assessments of care for various groups of older individuals and has recently participated in a team that implements practice redesign efforts aimed at improving primary care for older patients, with an emphasis on falls, incontinence, and dementia care. He is particularly interested in measuring and improving care toward the end of life. Dr. Wenger's educational efforts focus on training physician fellows in health services and primary care research, training resident physicians in primary care general internal medicine, and teaching clinical ethics. He directs the National Research Service Award Primary Care Research Fellowship, funded by the U.S. Health Resources and Services Administration, in the Division of General Internal Medicine at UCLA. Dr. Wenger received his M.D. from the UCLA School of Medicine and his M.P.H. from the UCLA School of Public Health.

IOM STAFF BIOGRAPHIES

Laura Levit, J.D., is a program officer at the IOM, where she has worked with the Board on Health Care Services and the NCPF. She started at the IOM as a Christine Mirzayan Science and Technology Graduate Fellow in the winter of 2007 and that year received the IOM Rookie Award. Her previous work at the IOM has focused on topics that include the Health Insurance Portability and Accountability Act (HIPAA) Privacy Rule, comparative effectiveness research, the oncology workforce, and regulatory hurdles to personalized medicine. She graduated from the University of Virginia School of Law and is a member of the Virginia Bar Association. In law school, Ms. Levit worked for several different nonprofit organizations that focused on health and mental health care policy, including the Treatment Advocacy Center, the National Research Center for Women & Families, the Bazelon Center, and the World Federation for Mental Health. She completed her undergraduate studies at the College of William and Mary, receiving a B.S. with honors in psychology. Ms. Levit was the 2009 recipient of the National Academies' Group Distinguished Service Award, and the 2012 recipient of the IOM staff team achievement award.

Erin Balogh, M.P.H., is an associate program officer for the IOM Board on Health Care Services and the NCPF. She has directed NCPF workshops on patient-centered cancer treatment planning, affordable cancer care, precompetitive collaboration, combination cancer therapies, and reducing tobacco-related cancer incidence and mortality. She has staffed IOM consensus studies focusing on the quality of cancer care, omics-based test development, the national cancer clinical trials system, and the evaluation of biomarkers and surrogate endpoints. She completed her M.P.H. in health management and policy at the University of Michigan School of Public Health, and graduated summa cum laude from Arizona State University with bachelor's degrees in microbiology and psychology. Ms. Balogh interned with AcademyHealth in Washington, DC, and worked as a research site coordinator for the Urban Institute in Topeka, Kansas. Previously, Ms. Balogh was a management intern with the Arizona State University Office of University Initiatives, a strategic planning group for the university.

Pamela Lighter, M.P.H., is a research assistant on the Board on Health Care Services. She is currently working with the NCPF and Committee on Improving Quality of Cancer Care. She has previously worked with the Committee on Living Well with Chronic Disease; the Roundtable on Environmental Health Sciences, Research, and Medicine; and the Roundtable on the Promotion of Health Equity and the Elimination of Health Disparities. She received her M.P.H. and a certificate on health disparities and health inequality from Johns Hopkins University Bloomberg School of Public Health in August 2013 and received bachelor's degrees in mathematics and general biology from the University of Maryland, College Park, in August 2008.

Michael Park served as senior program assistant for the NCPF and Board on Health Care Services at the IOM from September 3, 2007, to September 2, 2013. He received his B.A. in Germanic language and literature from the University of Maryland, College Park, in 2006 after studying 2 years abroad (on scholarship) in Germany and Italy. Having completed his final year of high school in Zaragoza, Spain, he is fluent in Spanish, Italian, and German. In 2013, Mr. Park graduated from Duke University, The Fuqua School of Business, with a Master of Management in Clinical Informatics degree. He is enthusiastic about developing apps, tools, and processes to facilitate personalized medicine, clinical decision support, and real-time insight discovery.

Sharyl Nass, Ph.D., is director of the NCPF. As a study director and senior program officer at the IOM, she has worked with the Board on Health Sciences Policy, the Board on Health Care Services, and the National Cancer Policy Board and Forum. Her previous work at the IOM focused on topics that include developing cancer biomarkers and omics-based tests to guide patient care, improving cancer clinical trials, formulating strategies for large-scale biomedical science, developing technologies for the early detection of breast cancer, improving breast imaging quality standards, assessing the impact of the HIPAA Privacy Rule on health research, and facilitating contraceptive research and development. She has also served as an adjunct faculty member at the University of Maryland School of

Nursing, lecturing on cancer biology, detection, and treatment. With a Ph.D. in cell and tumor biology from Georgetown University and post-doctoral training at the Johns Hopkins University School of Medicine, she has published research on the cell and molecular biology of breast cancer. She also holds a B.S. in genetics and an M.S. in endocrinology/reproductive physiology, both from the University of Wisconsin, Madison. In addition, she studied developmental genetics and molecular biology at the Max Planck Institute in Germany under a fellowship from the Heinrich Hertz-Stiftung Foundation. Dr. Nass was the 2007 recipient of the IOM's Cecil Award for Excellence in Health Policy Research, the 2010 recipient of a National Academy of Sciences Distinguished Service Award, and the 2012 recipient of the IOM staff team achievement award.

Roger Herdman, M.D., is director of the IOM Board on Health Care Services. He received his undergraduate and medical school degrees from Yale University. Following an internship at the University of Minnesota and a stint in the U.S. Navy, he returned to Minnesota, where he completed a residency in pediatrics and a fellowship in immunology and nephrology, and also served on the faculty. He was a professor of pediatrics at Albany Medical College until 1979. In 1969, Dr. Herdman was appointed director of the New York State Kidney Disease Institute in Albany, New York, and shortly thereafter was appointed deputy commissioner of the New York State Department of Health (1969-1977). In 1977, he was named New York state's director of public health. From 1979 until joining the U.S. Congress Office of Technology Assessment (OTA), he served as a vice president of MSKCC in New York City. In 1983, Dr. Herdman was named assistant director of OTA, where he subsequently served as director from 1993 to 1996. He later joined the IOM as a senior scholar and directed studies on graduate medical education, organ transplantation, silicone breast implants, and the Department of Veterans Affairs national formulary. Dr. Herdman was appointed director of the IOM/National Research Council National Cancer Policy Board from 2000 through 2005. From 2005 until 2009, Dr. Herdman directed the IOM National Cancer Policy Forum. In 2007, he was also appointed director of the IOM Board on Health Care Services. During his work at the IOM, Dr. Herdman has worked closely with the U.S. Congress on a wide variety of health care policy issues.